T0329591

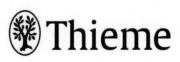

Distal Radius Fractures and Carpal Instabilities

FESSH IFSSH 2019 Instructional Book

Editor-in-Chief:
Francisco del Piñal, MD, PhD
Former Secretary General and Former President of EWAS
Hand and Microvascular Surgeon
Madrid and Santander, Spain

Co-Editors:
Max Haerle, MD, PhD
Professor
Former General Secretary of FESSH
Former President of EWAS
Director of Hand and Plastic Surgery Department
Orthopädische Klinik Markgröningen
Markgröningen, Germany

Hermann Krimmer, MD, PhD
Professor
Chief of Hand Center
St. Elisabeth Hospital
Ravensburg, Germany

645 illustrations

Thieme
Stuttgart • New York • Delhi • Rio de Janeiro

Library of Congress Cataloging-in-Publication Data is available from the publisher.

© 2019. Thieme. All rights reserved.

Thieme Publishers Stuttgart
Rüdigerstrasse 14, 70469 Stuttgart, Germany
+49 [0]711 8931 421, customerservice@thieme.de

Thieme Publishers New York
333 Seventh Avenue, New York, NY 10001, USA
+1-800-782-3488, customerservice@thieme.com

Thieme Publishers Delhi
A-12, Second Floor, Sector-2, Noida-201301
Uttar Pradesh, India
+91 120 45 566 00, customerservice@thieme.in

Thieme Publishers Rio de Janeiro,
Thieme Publicações Ltda.
Edifício Rodolpho de Paoli, 25º andar
Av. Nilo Peçanha, 50 – Sala 2508
Rio de Janeiro 20020-906 Brasil
+55 21 3172 2297 / +55 21 3172 1896

Cover design: Thieme Publishing Group
Typesetting by DiTech Process Solutions Pvt. Ltd., India

Printed in Germany by Aprinta GmbH, Wemding   5 4 3 2 1

ISBN 978-3-13-242379-4

Also available as an e-book:
eISBN 978-3-13-242380-0

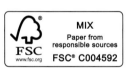

Contents

31 Chronic Distal Radioulnar Joint Instability... 271

Michael C. K. Mak, Pak-Cheong Ho

Preface

It is a great privilege that the International Federation of Societies for Surgery of the Hand (IFSSH) and the Federation of European Societies for Surgery of the Hand (FESSH) have considered me as editor-in-chief of this book on the burning issue of distal radius fractures and ligamentous injuries.

Management of distal radius fractures and wrist ligamentous injuries has seen dramatic changes in the last few decades. For those of us who have lived this on the front line, it has been a very exciting experience. Beginning from casts, external fixateurs, intramedullary devices, volar or dorsal plates, and finally to arthroscopy, all have contributed to making it possible to provide our patients with outstanding results. One thing we have learned is that no one method can be used for all injuries, as the personality of each fracture or ligamentous injury demand a different approach. For this reason, every available treatment has its own space in our armamentarium.

Fully conscious of this, we have compiled here an up-to-date selection of the techniques available to tackle all injury types. The topics have been carefully selected to cover the subjects of greatest interest or higher impact. In this endeavor, we have had the fortune to count on world-renowned surgeons, who have championed the changes we are now using in our everyday practice. Some chapters provide new answers or refinements to recurrent problems.

This book will hopefully improve the care of our patients and, furthermore, inspire the creativity of future generations of surgeons.

Finally, I would like to thank my co-editors and all the authors who have devoted their precious time to sharing their knowledge with us.

Paco Piñal
Madrid, 2019

Contributors

Yukio Abe, MD, PhD
Director
Department of Orthopaedic Surgery
Saiseikai Shimonoseki General Hospital
Shimonoseki, Japan

Joshua M. Abzug, MD
Associate Professor
Departments of Orthopedics and Pediatrics
University of Maryland School of Medicine
Director of Pediatric Orthopedics
University of Maryland Medical Center
Deputy Surgeon-in-Chief
University of Maryland Children's Hospital
Baltimore, Maryland, USA

Dirck Ananos, MD
Fellow
Kaplan Hand Institute
Barcelona, Spain

Rohit Arora, MD
Department of Trauma Surgery
Medical University Innsbruck
Innsbruck, Austria

Andrea Atzei, MD
Fenice Hand Surgery and Rehabilitation Team
Treviso, Italy

Gregory Bain, MD
APWA President
Professor of Upper Limb and Research
Department of Orthopaedic Surgery
Flinders University
Adelaide, South Australia, Australia

Marion Burnier, MD
Wrist Surgery Unit
Department of Orthopaedics
Claude-Bernard Lyon 1 University
Herriot Hospital
Lyon, France

Alexandria L. Case, MD
Clinical Research Coordinator
Department of Orthopedics
University of Maryland School of Medicine
Baltimore, Maryland, USA

Scott G. Edwards, MD
Chief of Hand and Upper Extremity Surgery
Banner University Medical Center
The CORE Institute Specialty Hospital
Phoenix, Arizona, USA

Mitchell G. Eichhorn, MD
Hand Surgery Fellow
University of Arizona Banner Hand Surgery Fellowship
Phoenix, Arizona, USA

Markus Gabl, MD
Department of Trauma Surgery
Medical University Innsbruck
Innsbruck, Austria

Thais Galissard, MD
Wrist Surgery Unit
Department of Orthopaedics
Claude-Bernard Lyon 1 University
Herriot Hospital
Lyon, France

Marc Garcia-Elias, MD, PhD
Consultant and Co-Founder
Kaplan Hand Institute
Barcelona, Spain
Honorary Consultant
Pulvertaft Hand Center
Derby, UK

Rohit Garg, MBBS
Hand and Upper Extremity Orthopaedic Surgeon
Massachusetts General Hospital
Boston, Massachusetts, USA

Patrick Groarke, MD
Brisbane Hand and Upper Limb Research Institute
Brisbane Private Hospital
Brisbane, Queensland, Australia
Orthopaedic Department
Princess Alexandra Hospital
Woolloongabba, Queensland, Australia

Max Haerle, MD, PhD
Professor
Former General Secretary of FESSH
Former President of EWAS
Director of Hand and Plastic Surgery Department
Orthopädische Klinik Markgröningen
Markgröningen, Germany

Mark Henry, MD
Practicing Hand Surgeon
Hand and Wrist Center of Houston
Houston, Texas, USA

Guillaume Herzberg, MD, PhD
Professor of Orthopaedic Surgery
Lyon Claude Bernard University
Herriot Hospital
Lyon, France

Pak-Cheong Ho, MD, MBBS, FRCS, FHKCOS, FHKAM(Ortho)
EWAS Former President
APWA Founder and Former President
Department of Orthopaedics and Traumatology
Prince of Wales Hospital
Chinese University of Hong Kong
Hong Kong, SAR China

Haroon M. Hussain, MD
Greater Washington Orthopaedic Group PA
Rockville, Maryland, USA

Rames Mattar Junior, MD
Associate Professor
Department of Orthopedic
Hand and Microsurgery Unit
University Of São Paulo
São Paulo, Brazil

Jesse Jupiter, MD
Hansjorg Wyss AO Professor
Department of Orthopedic Surgery
Massachusetts General Hospital
Harvard Medical School
Boston, Massachusetts, USA

Kenji Kawamura, MD, PhD
Tamai Susumu Memorial Hand and Extremity
    Trauma Center
Nara Medical University
Kashihara, Japan

Jong-Pil Kim, MD, PhD
Professor
Department of Orthopedic Surgery
Dankook University College of Medicine
Cheonan, South Korea

Christopher Klifto, MD
Assistant Professor
Department of Orthopaedic Surgery
Hand Division
Duke University Medical Center
Durham, North Carolina, USA

Hermann Krimmer, MD, PhD
Professor
Chief of Hand Center
St. Elisabeth Hospital
Ravensburg, Germany

Riccardo Luchetti, MD
Rimini Hand Surgery and Rehabilitation Center
Rimini, Italy

Simon MacLean, MBChB, FRCS(Tr&Orth), PGDipCE
Consultant Orthopaedic and Upper Limb Surgeon
Tauranga Hospital, BOPDHB
Tauranga, New Zealand

Michael C. K. Mak, MD
Division of Hand and Microsurgery
Department of Orthopaedics and Traumatology
Prince of Wales Hospital
Chinese University of Hong Kong
Hong Kong, SAR China

Stephanie Malliaris, MD
Assistant Professor
Plastic and Reconstructive Surgery
University of Colorado School of Medicine
Attending Surgeon
Denver Health Medical Center
Denver, Colorado, USA

Christophe Mathoulin, MD, FMH
Vice-President
Institut de la Main
Founder and Honorary Chairman
European (International) Wrist Arthroscopy Society
    (EWAS - IWAS)
Founder and Chairman
International Wrist Center–Wrist Clinic
Clinique Bizet
Paris, France

Tiago Guedes da Motta Mattar, MD
Department of Orthopedic
Hand and Microsurgery Unit
University of São Paulo
São Paulo, Brazil

Robert J. Medoff, MD
Assistant Professor
Department of Surgery
University of Hawaii
Honolulu, Hawaii, USA

Ladislav Nagy, MD
Professor
Hand Surgery Division
University Clinic Balgrist
Zürich, Switzerland

Shohei Omokawa, MD, PhD
Department of Hand Surgery
Nara Medical University
Kashihara, Japan

Tadanobu Onishi, MD
Department of Orthopedic Surgery
Nara Medical University
Kashihara, Japan

Jorge L. Orbay, MD
Hand & Upper Extremity Surgeon
The Miami Hand & Upper Extremity Institute
Miami, Florida, USA

Lee Osterman, MD
Professor, Hand and Orthopedic Surgery
Thomas Jefferson University
President
Philadelphia Hand to Shoulder Center
Philadelphia, Pennsylvania, USA

Min Jong Park, MD
Department of Orthopaedic Surgery
Samsung Medical Center
Sungkyunkwan University School of Medicine
Seoul, South Korea

Emygdio Jose Leomil de Paula, MD, PhD
Department of Orthopedic
Hand and Microsurgery Unit
University Of São Paulo
São Paulo, Brazil

Gabriel Pertierra, BA
The Miami Hand & Upper Extremity Institute
Miami, Florida, USA

Christoph Pezzei, MD
Department of Traumatology
AUVA Trauma Hospital Lorenz Böhler–European Hand
    Trauma Center
Vienna, Austria

Francisco del Piñal, MD, PhD
Former Secretary General and Former President of EWAS
Hand and Microvascular Surgeon
Madrid and Santander, Spain

Benjamin F. Plucknette, DO, DPT
Orthopaedic, Hand, and Microvascular Surgeon
Department of Orthopaedic Surgery
San Antonio Military Medical Center
JBSA-Fort Sam Houston, Texas, USA

Karl-Josef Prommersberger, MD
Professor
Clinic for Hand Surgery
Rhön Klinikum AG
Salzburger Leite
Bad Neustadt an der Saale, Germany

Stefan Quadlbauer, MD
AUVA Trauma Hospital Lorenz Böhler–European Hand
    Trauma Center
Ludwig Boltzmann Institute for Experimental and Clinical
    Traumatology
AUVA Research Center
Austrian Cluster for Tissue Regeneration
Vienna, Austria

Peter C. Rhee, DO, MS
Orthopedic Surgery
Mayo Clinic
Rochester, Minnesota, USA

Mark Ross, MD
Brisbane Hand and Upper Limb Research Institute
Brisbane Private Hospital
Brisbane, Queensland, Australia
Orthopaedic Department
Princess Alexandra Hospital
Woolloongabba, Queensland, Australia
School of Medicine
The University of Queensland
St Lucia, Queensland, Australia

Tamara D. Rozental, MD
Chief, Hand and Upper Extremity Surgery
Associate Professor
Department of Orthopaedic Surgery
Beth Israel Deaconess Medical Center
Harvard Medical School
Boston, Massachusetts, USA

David Ruch, MD
Professor and Chief of Division of Hand and
 Microvascular Surgery
Adjunct Professor of Plastic and Reconstructive Surgery
Duke University Medical Center
Durham, North Carolina, USA

Gustavo Mantovani Ruggiero, MD
São Paulo Hand Center
Hospital Beneficência Portuguesa de São Paulo
São Paulo, Brazil
Hand Surgery Department
Plastic Surgery School
Ospedale San Giuseppe
Università Degli Studi Di Milano
Milan, Italy

James M. Saucedo, MD
The Hand Center of San Antonio
Adjunct Assistant Professor
Department of Orthopaedics
University of Texas Health San Antonio
San Antonio, Texas, USA

Frédéric Schuind, MD, PhD
Full Professor
Université libre de Bruxelles
Head, Department of Orthopaedics and Traumatology
Erasme University Hospital
Brussels, Belgium

Jae Woo Shim, MD
Department of Orthopaedic Surgery
Samsung Medical Center
Sungkyunkwan University School of Medicine
Seoul, South Korea

Takamasa Shimizu, MD, PhD
Department of Orthopedic Surgery
Nara Medical University
Kashihara, Japan

Alexander Y. Shin, MD
Orthopedic Surgery
Mayo Clinic
Rochester, Minnesota, USA

Gustavo Bersani Silva, MD
Department of Orthopedic
Hand and Microsurgery Unit
University Of São Paulo
São Paulo, Brazil

Luciano Ruiz Torres, MD
Department of Orthopedic
Hand and Microsurgery Unit
University of São Paulo
São Paulo, Brazil

Oliver Townsend, BSc, MBBS, MRCS
Core Surgical Fellow
Southampton General Hospital
University Hospital Southampton
Southampton, UK

David Warwick, MD, FRCSOrth, Eur Dip Hand Surg
Professor and Consultant Hand Surgeon
University Hospital Southampton
Southampton, UK

Tracy Webber, MD, BIDMC
Harvard Orthopaedic Hand Fellowship
Department of Orthopaedic Surgery
Beth Israel Deaconess Medical Center
Harvard Medical School
Boston, Massachusetts, USA

Scott Wolfe, MD
Professor
Department of Orthopaedic Surgery
Hospital for Special Surgery
Weill Medical College of Cornell University
New York, New York, USA

1 Anatomy of the Fracture

Simon MacLean, Gregory Bain

Abstract

This chapter discusses the importance of the anatomy of distal radius in relation to fracture. First, we describe the microanatomy of the distal radius. Its microanatomy resembles that seen in everyday engineering structures; the subchondral bone plate and arrangement of trabeculae enabling the wrist to handle high multidirectional loads. Stability of the wrist is achieved by multiple ligamentous rings that confer stability within and between the rows and columns of the wrist. Ligamentous insertions play an important role in fracture morphology, both initiation and propagation of the fracture lines.

Hand position at impact determines the position of the carpus on the distal radius. When a line of differential load occurs in the scapholunate interval, scapholunate ligament injury (SLI) may result. SLI is associated with specific fracture types. "Unmasking" with scapholunate diastasis occurs when there is compromise to the secondary stabilizers.

The volar marginal rim fracture represents an important subset of fractures. These are associated with a higher rate of carpal ligamentous injury and fixation failure. Distal radius plate design has evolved to attempt to capture this fragment.

Lastly, we present a biomechanical model for distal radius fracture.

Keywords: distal radius fracture, microstructure, scapholunate injury, volar rim fracture, radiocarpal ligaments

1.1 Introduction

Distal radius fractures (DRFs) are one of the most commonly treated injuries in orthopaedic practice. A bimodal distribution exists; in younger patients, caused by high-energy and in older patients, caused by low-energy falls. Osteoporotic DRFs reflect a change in the microarchitecture of the distal radius with aging and are a predictor for subsequent fracture of long bones. Classification systems have attempted to provide clarity to the morphology and treatment of these injuries.

With an improved understanding of the anatomy of distal radius, we are better equipped to treat the patient, respecting not just the fracture components but also the contribution of the surrounding ligaments, carpal bones, and other associated injuries. This chapter will explore the importance of each component and its interaction in the mechanism of fracture. First, we will study the *microanatomy* of the distal radius; and then we will focus on *fracture initiation* and the role of the carpus; and third, the role of the carpal ligaments and *fracture propagation*. We will look at the specific anatomy of the *volar rim fracture*. We will propose a biomechanical model for DRF.

1.2 Microanatomy of the Distal Radius: A Feat of Evolutionary Engineering

Singh reported the trabecular structure of the proximal femur and changed our approach to the understanding and management of these injuries.[1] The microstructure of the distal radius assists in understanding its behavior under load. We performed an analysis of the architecture of cadaveric distal radii on micro-computed tomography (CT)[2,3] and found it resembled many of the engineering concepts in everyday man-made structures. Interestingly, an engineer once advised us that he knew when he had the design correct and when it resembled the structures identified in nature.

1.2.1 The Subchondral Bone Plate: The "Leaf Spring" of the Wrist

The subchondral bone plate is a 2-mm-thick multilaminar plate that absorbs impact and transmits the load to the radial metaphysis. The superficial "primary" bone plate bridges the entire articular margin. Multiple deeper layers resemble a leaf spring used in the suspension of heavy motor vehicles.

Between these laminae, and connecting them, lie intralaminar struts. These are initially perpendicular to the joint line, but more proximally align with the radial shaft. Voids between the struts and laminae absorb impact and enable vessels to perforate. The struts between the laminae are mini "I-beams," which make the structure strong but still enable it to bend. Engineers refer to this multilayered lamina construct as a "honeycomb sandwich panel."

With physiological wrist extension, the volar capsule becomes taut, and the scaphoid and lunate load the distal radius subchondral bone plate.

The multilayered subchondral bone plate resists buckling and transmits the load to the intermediate trabeculae and then the metaphyseal arches (▶Fig. 1.1).

On a magnified view, areas can be seen where these trabeculae coalesce to form a rod and extend as longitudinal ridges down the diaphysis (▶Fig. 1.2). These align in the direction of load through the cortical bone and reinforce the radius, similar to the longerons in a plane's fuselage (▶Fig. 1.3), and prevent torsional failure and buckling.

The load bearing area of the lunate is very volar. The sagittal images demonstrate the thick volar trabecular columns spanning to the volar cortex of the metaphyseal radius (▶Fig. 1.4). This explains the devastating effect of Barton volar lip fracture, as the carpus will simply dislocate volarly.

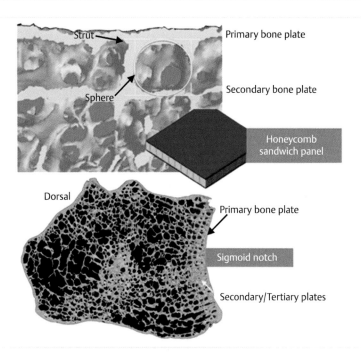

Fig. 1.1 Anatomy of the subchondral bone plate of the distal radius. (Copyright © Gregory Bain, MD)

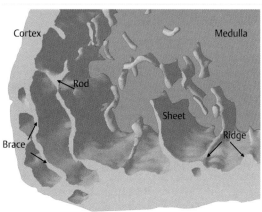

Fig. 1.2 The radial styloid cortex is quite thin but is reinforced by bracing trabeculae. The trabeculae are thin sheets of bone, which are designed to transmit load. There the sheets meet and coalesce into rods, which then become the ridges on the endosteal cortex. (Copyright © Gregory Bain, MD)

Further dorsal on the lunate facet, trabeculae course dorsally forming a curve in the shape of a gothic arch, with an underlying intramedullary "vault." From medial to lateral through the distal radius, these gothic arches are in series—connected by interarch struts. In normal bone under normal loads, the parabolic shape of the arch transfers loads in a longitudinal and lateral direction, to the base of the arch without creating tension (▶ Fig. 1.4).

At the base of each arch, the trabeculae merge with the cortex, which then becomes thickened—therefore buttressing the arch. In contrast, at the articular margin, the cortex is thin. It acts to suspend the subchondral bone plate and serves as a site for ligament attachment, rather than to bear the load.

1.2.2 The Arch Bridge Concept

The microstructure of the distal radius resembles an arch bridge with the following equivalent: deck—SBP, intermediate struts—intermediate trabeculae, arches—arches, and bridge foundation—cortex. The deck is a tightly held lattice with multiple "I-beams" in a multilayer sandwich panel construct. This resists buckling, absorbs impact, and takes the entire load (▶ Fig. 1.5).

The arches and intermediate struts are a semiflexible construct, which distributes compressive forces from the deck to the base (diaphysis).[4] The orientation of the microstructure ensures that forces are distributed in compression rather than tension (where the bone is weakest).

1.2.3 Multiple Rings Concept of the Wrist

Force transfer from the hand to the radius at the time of DRF involves the transmission of force through the three columns of the wrist. The three columns are bound by a series of ligamentous rings. These ligamentous rings provide stability within and between the proximal and distal rows of the wrist (▶ Fig. 1.6).

Within Rows

The distal radioulnar joint is bound by a fibroligamentous ring. Disruption of this at the time of DRF can lead to dislocation of this joint and distal radioulnar instability, if not addressed at the time of surgery.

Within the proximal carpal row, interosseous ligaments on the volar and dorsal aspects of the scapholunate and lunotriquetral joints form a ring. Transmission of force

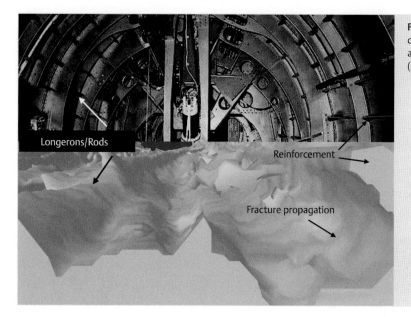

Fig. 1.3 Longitudinal ridges in the diaphysis of the distal radius resembling a plane's fuselage. (Copyright © Gregory Bain, MD)

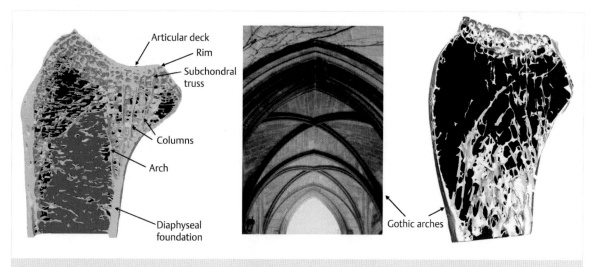

Fig. 1.4 The sagittal microanatomy of the distal radius resembling a gothic arch.(Copyright © Gregory Bain, MD)

from the central column to the scaphoid, lunate, or both can lead to a disruption of these ligaments and a "greater arc" injury or an impaction fracture of the distal radius.

The distal carpal row is tightly bound by interosseous ligaments, allowing for minimal motion within the row. Disruption of this ring rarely occurs at the time of DRF but is seen with high-energy axial fracture-dislocations of the carpus.

Between Rows

A series of ligaments connect the rows of the wrist. Kuhlmann ring refers to the volar radiotriquetral ligament and the dorsal radiocarpal ligament (DRC) complexes.[5] Disruption of this ring in complex high-energy DRFs can lead to ulnar translocation of the carpus. The DRC also acts as a secondary stabilizer to the scapholunate joint.

The scaphotrapeziotrapezoid (STT) ligament stabilizes the scaphoid to the distal carpal row. As a secondary stabilizer of the scapholunate joint, disruption of this complex can lead to scapholunate diastasis and dorsal intercalated segmental instability (DISI) deformity.

1.3 The Role of the Carpal Ligaments

The dorsal and volar ligamentous complexes surrounding the wrist are anatomically and functionally distinct. The stout volar capsular ligaments are a complex series of condensations in the thick volar capsule.[6,7] In contrast, there are only two named dorsal ligaments: the dorsal radiocarpal and dorsal intercarpal

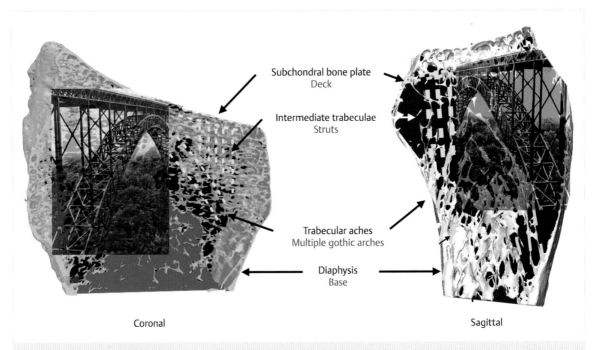

Subchondral bone plate
Deck

Intermediate trabeculae
Struts

Trabecular aches
Multiple gothic arches

Diaphysis
Base

Coronal

Sagittal

Fig. 1.5 The microstructure of the distal radius resembling an arch bridge. (Copyright © Gregory Bain, MD)

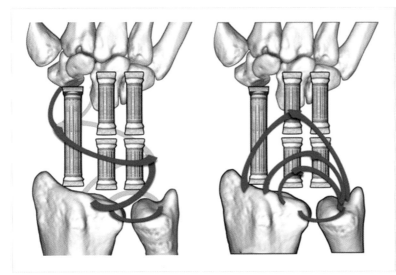

Fig. 1.6 The "multiple rings" of the wrist. (Copyright © Gregory Bain, MD)

(DIC) ligaments. The remainder of the dorsal capsule is extremely elastic.

Both Melone and Medoff described the importance of the ligamentous attachments of the distal radius.[8-11] Melone highlighted the role of the two medial fragments for the articular function: "the medial complex" and its strong ligamentous attachments.[10] Medoff recognized the contributions of ligaments to fracture displacement, and described radiocarpal instability and the contribution of ligament avulsion to the creation of "rim" fragments, leading to catastrophic failure of fixation.[11]

In our study by Mandziak et al,[12] we performed CT mapping of 100 distal radius intra-articular fractures

and identified that fracture lines were significantly more likely to occur *between* the ligament insertions (▶Fig. 1.7).[6,7] In low-energy injuries, the fractures almost never include the ligament attachments but are between the ligaments. High-energy injuries are more random and reflect the forces placed on the wrist.

The ligaments are designed to resist tension, which is maximal at the extremes of motion. Bone is designed to take the compressive load and fail in tension. The ligaments play two key roles in the mechanism of fracture.

Our study, however, suggests that ligament insertion points may be protective for DRFs, as most fracture

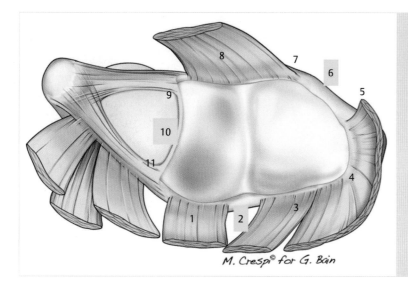

Fig. 1.7 Fractures most commonly involve the interligamentous zones 10, 2, and 6. (Copyright © Gregory Bain, MD)

lines avoided these sites. This would correlate with the role of ligamentotaxis with fracture reduction. In the exception of the isolated "die-punch" fracture, ligamentotaxis reduces distal radius morphology. Even in cases of extreme comminution, an initial almost anatomical reduction may be possible by the creation of radiocarpal ligament tension across the joint. This would not be possible in the setting of radiocarpal ligament avulsion. Failure of the microarchitecture and the intraosseous arches may lead to later collapse—hence the high rate of redisplacement in fractures with comminution in osteoporotic bone.[13] "Bridge plating" is an example of ligamentotaxis in the case of articular comminution. The "bridge" is used to maintain ligamentotaxis and neutralize deforming forces before osseous union occurs.

1.4 Fracture Initiation and Propagation

We hypothesized that the position of the wrist at injury and subsequent position of the carpus *initiates* the fracture, leading to specific DRF patterns. We retrospectively reviewed a series of CT scans of two-part articular fractures of the distal radius. The DRF and specific points on the scaphoid and lunate were precisely mapped. The images were overlaid, and the proximity of the fracture to these points was measured and statistically analyzed (▶ Fig. 1.8).

We used the classification of two-part fractures that Bain et al[14] described (▶ Fig. 1.9). Each of the defined fractures had an association with various parts of the lunate or scaphoid. For example, radial styloid oblique (RSO) fractures were associated with the volar ulnar aspect of the scaphoid. Intermediate column fractures with the radial border of the lunate. Dorsal ulnar corner (DUC)

fractures with the dorsal radial aspect of the lunate. The volar ulnar corner and volar coronal (VC) fractures were associated with the position of the volar lunate and midposition of the lunate and scaphoid, respectively.

There is an association between the position of the carpal bones and the type of articular fracture that occurs in the distal radius. The vast majority of fractures involve the scapholunate interval. We propose that a compressive load transmitted from the carpus initiates the fracture along the radial aspect of the lunate or the ulnar aspect of the scaphoid. Second, the fracture propagates to the periphery of the articular surface between the sites of ligamentous insertion (▶ Fig. 1.10). Wrist position is important; radial deviation causes impaction of the scaphoid, and ulnar deviation—impaction of the lunate. A neutral position will cause corresponding impaction of the scaphoid *and* lunate.

This theory fits with the work of Pechlaner, who used a cadaveric model to produce a DRF and found concomitant lesions in 63% of cases. The majority of these lesions involved either disruption to the articular disc of the triangular fibrocartilaginous complex or the scapholunate ligament complex.[15]

1.5 Scapholunate Dissociation and Two-Part Fractures of the Distal Radius

There is a high incidence of intercarpal soft tissue injuries (34–54%) in association with DRF although the mechanism and relevance are unclear.[16–18] Forward showed that intra-articular fractures were associated with a twofold increase in scapholunate dissociation as seen radiographically at 1 year.[16] Mrkonjic reported long-term follow-up of untreated scapholunate injuries in association with DRF. No significant difference in functional scores was

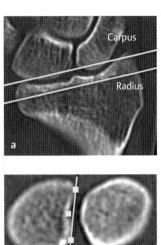

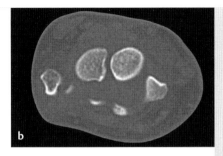

Fig. 1.8 (a–e) Representative axial slices of the articular surface and proximal carpal row. Neighboring points on the scaphoid and lunate and a line of best fit are drawn to mark the orientation of the scapholunate joint to the articular surface. (Copyright © Gregory Bain, MD)

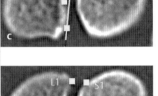

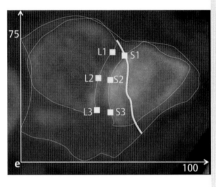

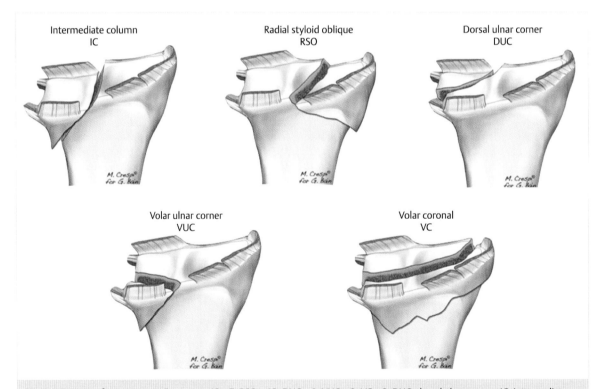

Fig. 1.9 Two-part fracture types. Frequency: IC = 7, RSO = 12, DUC = 9, VUC = 3, VC = 3. DUC, dorsal ulnar corner; IC, intermediate column; RSO, radial styloid oblique; VC, volar coronal; VUC, volar ulnar corner. (Copyright © Gregory Bain, MD)

found; however, numbers in his series were low, no Geissler grade 4 injuries were included, and most injuries were in the nondominant hand.[19]

We performed a CT study, comparing of two-part DRFs with a control group. The significant increase in the scapholunate distance was noted in fracture subtypes RSO, DUC, sagittal ulnar column, and VC. In particular, both the dorsal and volar aspects of the scapholunate gap were significantly widened in the RSO and DUC groups. This may relate to the level or vector of force at the time of

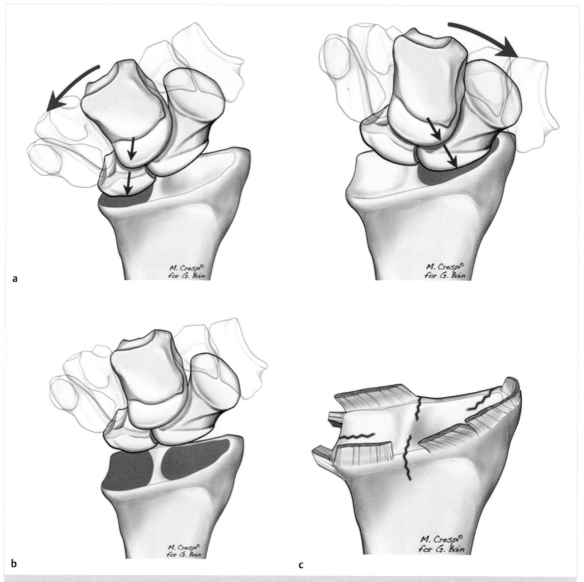

Fig. 1.10 Fracture mechanism of injury. Diagrammatic representation of initiation followed by propagation of articular distal radius fractures. **(a)** Force is transmitted from the hand—capitate—scaphoid or lunate to the distal radius. **(b)** Fracture of the articular surface of the radius is initiated at a point along the line of differential load (scapholunate interval). The lunate facet is compressed with ulnar deviation, while the scaphoid is not as loaded. **(c)** The fracture then propagates to the periphery of the articular surface, preferentially between protected areas of ligamentous insertion. (Copyright © Gregory Bain, MD)

injury (▶Fig. 1.11). The scaphoid, lunate, or both bones as a unit may die-punch the distal radius articular surface, leading to scapholunate rupture and predictable fracture subtypes.

1.6 Volar Marginal Rim Fractures

The volar marginal rim of the distal radius contains the lunate fossa and is the "keystone" for loadbearing through the distal radius. The volar rim also contains important volar radiolunate ligament insertions. These act as check reins, preventing volar subluxation and ulnar translocation of the carpus.

As previously described, the fracture can propagate between avulse radiocarpal ligaments. The volar marginal rim fracture represents the failure of the volar radiocarpal ligaments in tension and disruption of these important stabilizers to the rim of the distal radius (▶Fig. 1.12). The radioscaphocapitate (RSC) ligament acts as a secondary stabilizer to the scapholunate joint. Disruption of this ligament may unmask scapholunate injury as diastasis seen on preoperative imaging or under fluoroscopy.

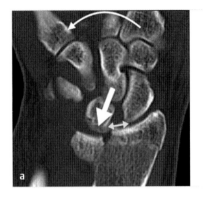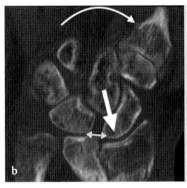

Fig. 1.11 Scapholunate dissociation with different fracture subtypes: sagittal ulnar column **(a)** and radial styloid oblique **(b)**. Note the position of the wrist (radial or ulnar deviation). The capitate hinges on either the lunate or scaphoid and drives into the scapholunate gap, causing scapholunate ligamentous injury and diastasis. The scaphoid, lunate, or the scapholunate unit impact the distal radius, initiating the fracture. (Copyright © Gregory Bain, MD)

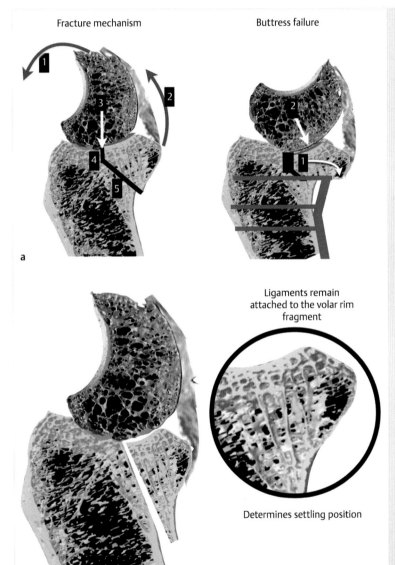

Fig. 1.12 (a) The mechanism of injury is often a fall on an outstretched hand, with hyperextension (1), which produces a tension band effect of the volar carpal ligaments (2), producing a localized impaction of the carpus on the radius (3). This causes initiation of a fracture (4) and subsequent fracture propagation (5). The volar plating is designed to provide a buttress of the volar fragments. If these fragments are small or osteoporotic, they can "flow" over the top of the buttress wall (1) and produce a volar collapse of the carpus (2). **(b)** If the fracture is not reduced and buttressed, the ligaments remain attached to the volar rim fragment, which determines the settling position of the carpus. (Copyright © Gregory Bain, MD)

We performed a retrospective radiological review of 25 volar marginal rim fractures and then compared to a control group of 25 consecutive intra-articular fractures not involving the volar rim.

Volar rim fractures have significantly higher incidence of scapholunate instability (48 vs. 20%), DISI deformity (44 vs. 20%), ulnar styloid fracture (88 vs. 68%), and ulnar translocation of the carpus (20 vs. 8%).

Following fixation, the volar rim fractures had a significantly higher incidence of scapholunate diastasis (48 vs. 20%) and failure of fixation (24 vs. 0%) (▶Fig. 1.13).

Distal radius plate design has evolved to attempt to capture the volar marginal rim fragment. Despite the placement of these plates distal to the watershed line, failure of the carpus can still occur (▶Fig. 1.14). This can be due to very distal comminuted avulsion fragments not being identified at the time of surgery or separation of the ligamentous attachment from the fragment. In these instances, we recommend fragment-specific hook or pin plates (▶Fig. 1.15) and ligament repair or reinforcement through transosseous repair or suture anchor fixation.

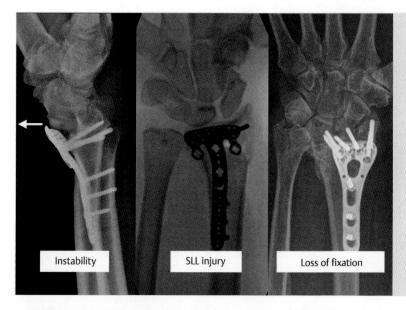

Instability

SLL injury

Loss of fixation

Fig. 1.13 Volar rim fractures have a higher incidence of volar instability (*white arrow*, showing volar subluxation of the carpus), scapholunate instability, and loss of fixation.

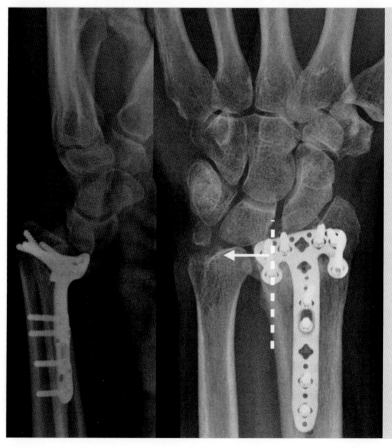

Fig. 1.14 Specific volar rim plating. Despite initial capture and support of the lunate fossa fragment, the carpus has subluxated volarly and ulnocarpal translocation has occurred.

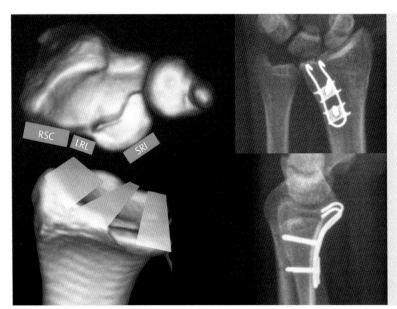

Fig. 1.15 Fragment-specific fixation of the volar rim. Note the ligamentous origins on the distal radius in relation to the fracture. (Copyright © Gregory Bain, MD)

1.7 A Biomechanical Model for Distal Radius Fracture

We propose a uniting theory incorporating the findings of our studies with the published literature. The fracture event occurs as two distinct stages: fracture initiation followed by propagation.

When the patient falls on the outstretched hand, the wrist is taken past the normal physiological arc of motion. In a dorsally displaced fracture, the volar ligaments and flexor tendons become taut, acting as a tension band, which accentuates the compressive force on the distal radius articular surface.

Force is transmitted from the hand through the midcarpal joint predominantly by the capitate to the proximal carpal row over the scapholunate interval. With the wrist in extension and ulnar deviation, the force is transmitted to the lunate and then the lunate facet. With the wrist in extension and radial deviation, the force is transmitted to the scaphoid and then to the scaphoid facet (▶ Fig. 1.10).

When there is disparity between load transmitted across the radiocarpal joint by the scaphoid and the lunate, a line of differential load exists along the scapholunate interval (SLI). Similar to the industrial die-punch analogy where sheet metal fails at the margin of the die, the distal radius subchondral bone plate fails in compression along this line of differential load. In this manner, articular fractures are initiated along the margin of the distal radius corresponding to the scapholunate interval. The scapholunate ligament complex can undergo stretch or complete rupture, depending on the magnitude and direction of force propagation. Intact secondary stabilizers, including the RSC, DRC, DIC, and STT ligaments, will prevent scapholunate diastasis. If there is compromise to

these insertion points on the distal radius, such as in the context of a volar marginal fracture, static instability and diastasis will result. The specific point along the SLI ligament depends on a number of variables, including wrist position at the time of injury and both the magnitude and direction of the external force.

The energy of the fracture then dissipates throughout the subchondral bone plate, propagating along the path of least resistance to the periphery of the articular surface, fracturing between protected areas of ligamentous insertion. Predictable articular osteoligamentous fragments are created (▶ Fig. 1.8).

In extreme wrist extension, the predominant force on the wrist is tensile over the volar carpal ligament complex. In this case, an avulsion fracture of the volar carpal ligaments will occur, leading to a volar marginal rim fracture. If the wrist is in radial deviation at the time of impact, the ulnar-sided short radiolunate is under most tension and likely to avulse. If the wrist is in ulnar deviation, the long radiolunate or RSC will avulse. After impact, the wrist settles; the lunate flexes and the carpus subluxates volarly (▶ Fig. 1.12).

Fracture reduction methods rely on ligamentotaxis, creating a tensile force on the ligaments attached to the fracture fragments. This allows the fragments to realign in their anatomical position. It is imperative when performing surgery on distal radius malunion, therefore to respect this principle and avoid soft tissue stripping of these ligamentous insertions.

1.8 Summary

DRFs occur in low energy in compromised osteoporotic bone and high energy in younger patients. The distal radius functions as an "arch bridge"; its microarchitecture is a complex evolutionary design and resembles other common engineering structures used to absorb and transmit load safely.

Distal radius follows a predictable sequence of events from initiation through propagation. The bone fails in tension, compression, or both. The fracture pattern is dependent on the vector of force and position of ligaments. Fracture fixation as described in the following chapters should, therefore, respect the pathomechanics of the fracture and the role of the soft tissue stabilizers.

References

[1] Singh M, Nagrath AR, Maini PS. Changes in trabecular pattern of the upper end of the femur as an index of osteoporosis. J Bone Joint Surg Am 1970;52(3):457–467

[2] Bain GI, MacLean SBM, McNaughton T, Williams R. Microstructure of the Distal Radius and Its Relevance to Distal Radius Fractures. J Wrist Surg 2017;6(4):307–315

[3] Bain GI, MacLean SBM, McNaughton T, Williams R. Erratum: Microstructure of the Distal Radius and Its Relevance to Distal Radius Fractures. J Wrist Surg 2017;6(4):e1–e2

[4] Roth L, Clark A. Understanding Architecture: Its Elements, History, and Meaning. Colorado, USA: Westview Press; 2013

[5] Kuhlmann JN, Luboinski J, Laudet C, et al. Properties of the fibrous structures of the wrist. J Hand Surg [Br] 1990;15(3):335–341

[6] Berger RA. The ligaments of the wrist. A current overview of anatomy with considerations of their potential functions. Hand Clin 1997;13(1):63–82

[7] Berger RA. The anatomy of the ligaments of the wrist and distal radioulnar joints. Clin Orthop Relat Res 2001(383):32–40

[8] Melone CP Jr. Articular fractures of the distal radius. Orthop Clin North Am 1984;15(2):217–236

[9] Melone CP Jr. Open treatment for displaced articular fractures of the distal radius. Clin Orthop Relat Res 1986(202):103–111

[10] Melone CP Jr. Distal radius fractures: patterns of articular fragmentation. Orthop Clin North Am 1993;24(2):239–253

[11] Medoff RJ. Essential radiographic evaluation for distal radius fractures. Hand Clin 2005;21(3):279–288

[12] Mandziak DG, Watts AC, Bain GI. Ligament contribution to patterns of articular fractures of the distal radius. J Hand Surg Am 2011;36(10):1621–1625

[13] Mackenney PJ, McQueen MM, Elton R. Prediction of instability in distal radial fractures. J Bone Joint Surg Am 2006;88(9):1944–1951

[14] Bain GI, Alexander JJ, Eng K, Durrant A, Zumstein MA. Ligament origins are preserved in distal radial intraarticular two-part fractures: a computed tomography-based study. J Wrist Surg 2013;2(3):255–262

[15] Pechlaner S, Kathrein A, Gabl M, et al. [Distal radius fractures and concomitant lesions. Experimental studies concerning the pathomechanism] Handchir Mikrochir Plast Chir 2002;34(3):150–157

[16] Forward DP, Lindau TR, Melsom DS. Intercarpal ligament injuries associated with fractures of the distal part of the radius. J Bone Joint Surg Am 2007;89(11):2334–2340

[17] Lindau T, Arner M, Hagberg L. Intraarticular lesions in distal fractures of the radius in young adults. A descriptive arthroscopic study in 50 patients. J Hand Surg [Br] 1997;22(5):638–643

[18] Geissler WB, Freeland AE, Savoie FH, McIntyre LW, Whipple TL. Intracarpal soft-tissue lesions associated with an intra-articular fracture of the distal end of the radius. J Bone Joint Surg Am 1996;78(3):357–365

[19] Mrkonjic A, Lindau T, Geijer M, Tägil M. Arthroscopically diagnosed scapholunate ligament injuries associated with distal radial fractures: a 13- to 15-year follow-up. J Hand Surg Am 2015;40(6):1077–1082

2 Radiology of the Fractured Radius

Mark Ross, Patrick Groarke

Abstract

This chapter provides guidelines for the radiographic assessment of distal radius fractures. We discuss plain radiographic parameters and their relationship in predicting stability and outcome and determining the adequacy of reduction and fixation strategy where indicated. We will review how to interpret computed tomography in the different planes and the relevance of fragmentation patterns. The value of magnetic resonance imaging and other modalities in assessing the fractured distal radius will be reviewed.

Keywords: radiographs, stability, reduction, parameters, CT, MRI, fragments

2.1 Introduction

Radiographic assessment of the distal radius should be undertaken when the mechanism of injury and presence of deformity or bony tenderness leads to clinical suspicion of a fractured distal radius. Understanding the imaging that needs to be obtained is a key element in the surgeon's ability to decide on appropriate management. The interpretation of the imaging is an even more important element in planning management, and if fixation is indicated, what fixation method should be employed. It is also critical to understand that each option in the imaging process provides very specific information, which may not be available in other images. In this way, prereduction radiographs (XRs) inform certain aspects, postreduction XRs provide different information, and each plane of computed tomography (CT) imaging is best suited for specific anatomic components of the injury pattern.

The functional demands of each patient differ. As a consequence, the age (physiologic as well as chronologic), employment, and lifestyle of each patient must be used to place the radiographic parameters into context. The goal of treatment is to provide a painless extremity with good function. In surgical decision-making, special attention should be given to the patient's bone quality. In addition, elderly patients with low demands may tolerate greater variance in many of the radiographic parameters that will be discussed in this chapter. However, with increasing activity level and functional expectations in an aging population, it is increasingly difficult to predict what may be tolerated by elderly patients.[1]

One of the most challenging considerations is whether the fracture pattern (pre- or postreduction) is stable. That is, is this the position that the fracture will ultimately heal in? The injury (prereduction) XR is very important in determining stability as it provides more information about maximum displacement and the energy of the injury. It is vital that the surgeon considers this series of images when making clinical decisions. Wherever possible, every effort should be made to obtain and assess the injury film. Consideration should also be given to this issue when the fracture has undergone some form of traction or closed reduction *prior* to initial radiographic assessment as the degree of displacement may be underestimated. A careful history of the interventions following injury is, therefore, vital. Following reduction and institution of closed treatment, it may be possible, with careful attention to cast changes, to control dorsal tilt; however, it is frequent to see the recurrence of radial shortening back to the injury position; thus, this must be considered when deciding on management.

Both increasing age of patients and increasing obesity in younger patients[2] have led to an increase in fractures that are comminuted. Comminuted fractures can be difficult to assess on plain XRs, but by applying the same system to evaluate them and with the proper interpretation of the CT, the surgeon can plan the fixation technique where indicated.

2.2 Plain Radiographs

Standard XRs are indicated in all suspected distal radius fractures (DRFs). We recommend XR before and after reduction. As noted above, the assessment of stability is best conducted using the injury (prereduction) XRs. Standard views include posteroanterior (PA) and lateral XR. Oblique views can also be helpful in bringing the volar portion of the radial and ulnar aspect of the radius as well as the dorsal ulnar corner (DUC) into view. These provide a two-dimensional image of a three-dimensional (3D) structure but understanding the normal parameters on each view can allow clarification of articular fragments even where CT images are not available. It is important to be able to determine what constitutes a true PA and lateral because many images can be rotated due to patient's inability to position the arm correctly due to pain, and many parameters are validated in relation to the orthogonal XRs.

2.2.1 Injury (Prereduction) Radiographs

The value of these films should not be understated to those carrying out emergent management such as closed manipulation so as to discourage reduction before imaging. This can happen where a grossly deformed wrist presents. Clearly, if the skin is threatened or there are significant neurological symptoms and XRs cannot be obtained emergently, the restoration of gross alignment takes priority; however, careful documentation of the deformity should be made. Injury films can reveal small, nondisplaced, and intra-articular fragments. These fragments might not be visible after anatomical reductions and cast application, which might mask the severity of the fracture. The original displacement and angulation of the fracture can be an indicator of instability. In a study of 406 DRFs, initial displacement was associated with worse QuickDASH score, worse EQ-5D score, reduced grip strength, and reduced range of motion (ROM).[3]

2.2.2 Postreduction Radiographs

Although potentially obscured by cast material, these images guide where fragments lie in relation to each other and what type of fixation should be considered. In addition, they guide the adequacy of reduction although should not be used for determining the stability of the fracture and propensity for loss of position (▶Fig. 2.1).

2.2.3 Parameters Can Change with Time

Where nonoperative management is undertaken, follow-up XRs at 1- and 2-week intervals would be considered a minimum and we have observed ongoing loss of position out to 6 weeks and beyond in cast treatment.

CT is more accurate in measuring the change in dorsal angulation over time in DRFs when compared to XRs.[4] However, the cost and high dose of radiation are prohibitive in most healthcare systems, and benefits from this increased accuracy have not been clarified.

2.2.4 Radiograph of the Opposite Side

In severely comminuted fractures, or where the fragments have been inadequately reduced, it might be difficult to establish what the patient's normal parameters should be. An XR of the uninjured opposite side can be helpful for comparison. Coronal plane translation, as will be discussed later, can be guided by the uninjured side. Contralateral XRs can also give an indication to the energy load to failure of the distal radius by defining normal ulna variance for that patient, given the significant variance in radial length. Increased ulnar variance (loss of radial length) after fracture is also associated with reduced bone mineral density in the distal radius.[5]

Parameters may vary between populations but the difference is likely to lie within the ranges described below.[6]

2.2.5 Posteroanterior View

The ulnar border of the ulnar styloid should be continuous with the ulnar border of the shaft. Pronation or supination can result in the ulnar styloid being partially overshadowed by the distal ulna shaft. The radial border of the ulna shaft is concave on a true PA view. Moreover, if the shafts of the radius and ulna are seen to converge, this indicates pronation. A full pronation view has the effect of shortening the radius by at least 0.5 mm.

The PA view presents the carpal facet horizon. This is a radiodense line that represents the volar rim of the lunate facet and medial half of the scaphoid facet, in a radius with normal volar tilt. It extends ulnarward to the sigmoid notch. In a wrist with preserved volar tilt, the XR beam is tangential to the volar half of the articular surface (▶Fig. 2.2). The DUC and dorsal rim are distal to this horizon and less well visualized (▶Fig. 2.3). In a dorsally angulated fracture, the radiodense line will represent the dorsal rim and DUC as the XR beam will be tangential to it (▶Fig. 2.4). The main value of the carpal facet horizon is that a step-off in it will indicate an articular step-off, and understanding whether one is viewing the dorsal or volar half of the joint will help to locate that articular involvement.[7]

The other implication of the separate representation of the volar and dorsal aspects of the ulnar corner is where to measure ulnar variance and radial inclination from. It has been suggested that true radial length is represented by the average point between the dorsal and volar ulnar corner on the PA view. This may be termed the central

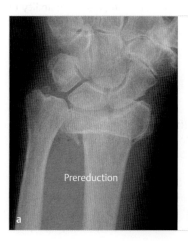
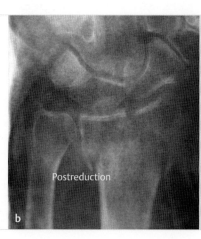

Fig. 2.1 (a) Prereduction film demonstrates significant displacement and implies an unstable fracture. **(b)** Postreduction image demonstrates articular surface involvement more clearly.

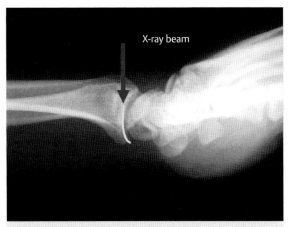

Fig. 2.2 The radiograph (XR) beam is tangential to the volar half of the joint in an intact or undisplaced radius.

reference point (CRP).[7] Many studies published up until this point have failed to clarify their method for determining the measuring point for ulnar variance. Perhaps radial length may be a more reproducible measure of true shortening of the radius than ulnar variance because of this factor.

2.2.6 Lateral View

It should be taken in neutral rotation. On a true lateral XR, the pisiform is located directly over the distal pole of the scaphoid. If the pisiform lies dorsal to the distal pole of the scaphoid, the forearm is rotated into pronation.

Another method of ensuring the wrist is in neutral rotation and is to use the scaphopisocapitate relationship.[8] This is described where the rotation of the wrist is set at a position in which the volar margin of the pisiform bone lies at

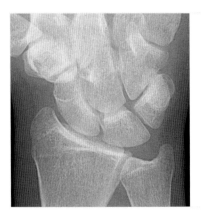
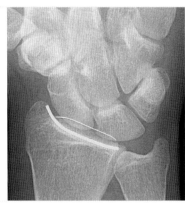

Fig. 2.3 The denser line represents the volar rim when the radius is intact or not dorsally tilted.

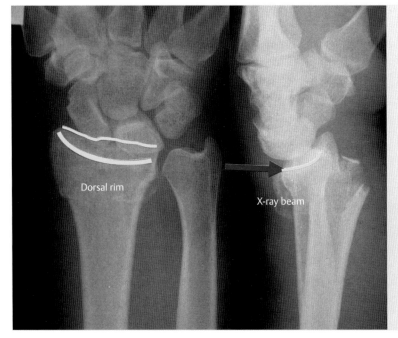

Fig. 2.4 In the dorsally tilted radius, the denser line becomes the dorsal rim as it rotates into a tangential relationship to the radiograph (XR) beam.

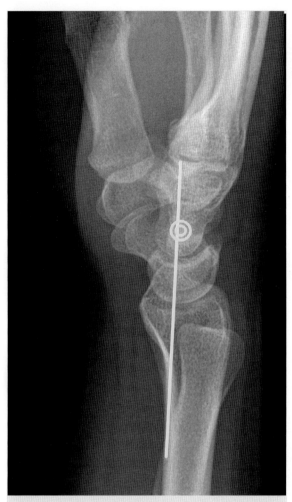

Fig. 2.5 Carpal alignment with the distal radius is assessed using a line up the volar surface of the radial shaft, which should intersect the center of the head of the capitate.[7]

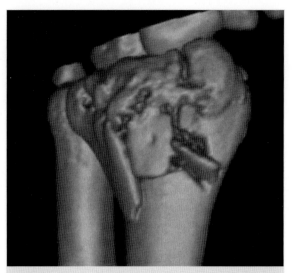

Fig. 2.6 Significant dorsal comminution implies a higher energy injury that would have had more displacement at the time of injury and may be less stable.

the central third of the interval between the volar cortex of the scaphoid tubercle and volar capitate. Wrist position is also important although may be compromised by pain or deformity in the acute setting. Larsen et al defined the true lateral XR as when the long axis of the radius and third metacarpal bone are collinear in neutral rotation.[9]

Carpal alignment is determined on the lateral. A line extending from the volar surface of the radial shaft (not the metaphysis) should bisect the center of rotation of the proximal pole of the capitate[7] (▶ Fig. 2.5).

2.3 Plain Radiographic Parameters

Radiographic parameters are assessed in terms of extra-articular alignment and intra-articular fragmentation/congruence to determine stability and acceptability of reduction.

In general terms, comminution is a key extra-articular factor in assessing fracture stability (▶ Fig. 2.6). It is an indirect measure of the energy of the injury and implies a more unstable fracture pattern. Volar comminution, in particular, is associated with a significantly higher chance of secondary displacement. Malalignment of the volar cortex on the lateral projection after closed reduction is a significant risk factor for loss of position. Comminution remains a subjective assessment, which is difficult to quantify.

The following parameters are listed as the average measure with normal ranges as defined by Geissler et al[10] The wide variability in these parameters necessitates consideration of obtaining XRs of the opposite side where any concerns regarding the adequacy of reduction exist.

It should be noted that there have been some concerns raised regarding the interobserver error for these parameters when assessed visually as opposed to digitally, which has raised caution in relation to formulating treatment plans based on purely visual assessments.[11]

2.3.1 Posteroanterior View

- Radial inclination—the angle between the ulnar aspect of the articular surface of the radius and the radial styloid is 23° (range: 13–30°).
  - The reference point on the ulnar side of the radius should be halfway between the dorsal and volar rims (CRP; ▶ Fig. 2.7).
- Assessment of the degree of shortening of the radius relative to the ulna—there are a number of methods for quantifying shortening of the radius:
  - Radial height (also called radial length)—the difference in length between the distal surface of the ulnar head and the tip of the radial styloid: 12 mm (range: 8–18 mm) (▶ Fig. 2.8).

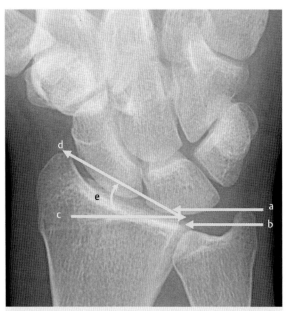

Fig. 2.7 Radial inclination angle is calculated by the angle between the ulnar aspect of the radius and the radial styloid. **(a)** Dorsal rim of radius. **(b)** Volar rim of radius. **(c)** Average of a and b. **(d)** Radial styloid. **(e)** Radial inclination angle.

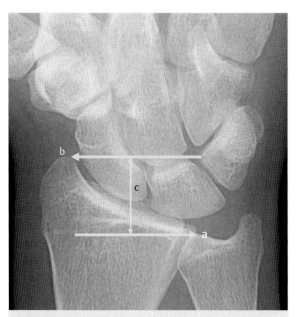

Fig. 2.8 Radial height (length). **(a)** Distal ulnar surface. **(b)** Radial styloid. **(c)** Radial height.

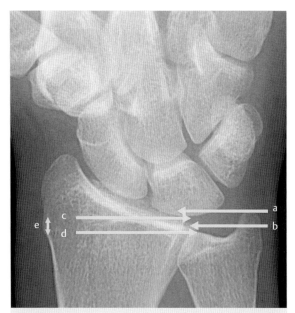

Fig. 2.9 Ulnar variance. **(a)** Dorsal rim of radius. **(b)** Volar rim of radius. **(c)** Average of a and b. **(d)** Distal ulnar surface. **(e)** Ulnar variance.

- Ulnar variance—refers to the relative lengths of the distal articular surfaces of the ulnar part of the radius and the ulna. Where the ulnar is shorter, the value is negative: negative 1 mm (range: positive 2 mm to negative 4 mm). As noted by Medoff, it is important to utilize CRP when calculating this parameter (►Fig. 2.9).

- Coronal plane translation—is measured by drawing a line along the ulnar aspect of the radial shaft proximal to the metaphyseal flare and extended distally through the proximal row of the carpus on the PA XR. This line intersects the lunate. The point of intersection is evaluated by drawing a second line along the widest part of the transverse width of the lunate on the anteroposterior (AP) XR, parallel to the distal radial articulation. The point of intersection of these two lines is measured from the radial side of the lunate to determine the percentage of lunate radial to this point (►Fig. 2.10). Ross et al looked at 100 PA XRs of normal wrists. The mean was 45.48% of the lunate, radial to the bisecting line. This showed high levels of inter- and intraobserver agreement between three fellowship-trained upper limb surgeons.[12]

It has been suggested that radial translation of the distal fragments is a marker for distal radioulnar joint (DRUJ) instability.[13] Residual radial translation contributes to DRUJ instability because malpositioning of the distal fragment results in loss of tension of the distal portion of the interosseous membrane (IOM) and pronator quadratus (PQ). A consequence of this tension loss is that even if the sigmoid notch is well positioned in all other respects (length, coronal tilt, and sagittal tilt), the ulnar head may not be held firmly into the concavity of the sigmoid notch, possibly contributing to the instability of the DRUJ (►Fig. 2.11).

Wolfe et al contributed to this observation by confirming in a cadaver study that residual translation of the distal radius fragment in DRFs can indeed contribute to DRUJ instability by detensioning the IOM.[14]

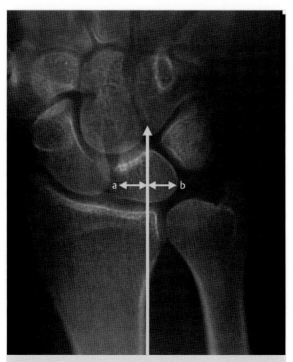

Fig. 2.10 Coronal translation is calculated by determining how much of the lunate lies radial to a line drawn along the ulnar shaft of the radius before the metaphyseal flare. Normally, less than half of the lunate lies radial to this line.

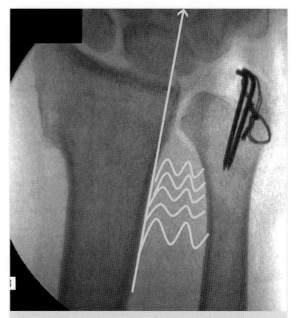

Fig. 2.11 This patient has residual radial translation. The fixation of the ulnar styloid may have been unnecessary if the translation had been corrected, thereby tensioning the distal interosseous membrane (IOM).

Volar locking plate fixation typically addresses the parameters of volar tilt, radial height, and radial inclination. However, it does not routinely force the surgeon to look for and correct radial translation because it is essentially a flat plate on a flat surface. If the radial translation is not looked for and addressed intraoperatively, DRUJ instability may exist postoperatively. Although preoperative radial translation deformity may be more likely to occur when there is greater disruption of the ulnar-sided stabilizing structures, this makes it even more important for the surgeon to be aware of this deformity and to ensure that from a technical perspective, the radial deformity is corrected at the time of surgery.[15]

- Other measurements in the literature include radiolunate relations, but these are less commonly used.[16]

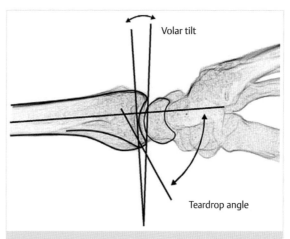

Fig. 2.12 Volar tilt and teardrop angle. (Reproduced with permission of Medoff R.)

2.3.2 Lateral View

- Volar tilt—At the articular surface of the radius, a tangent line is drawn from dorsal to volar, followed by a line perpendicular to the long axis of the radius. The angle between these lines is the volar tilt of 12° (range: 1–21°) (▶Fig. 2.12).
- Teardrop angle[7]—The teardrop is best seen on the inclined lateral view. It represents the U-shaped outline of the volar rim of the lunate facet. A line drawn down the central axis of the teardrop (parallel to the subchondral bone of the volar rim) subtends an angle of

70° to a line extended from the central axis of the radial shaft (▶Fig. 2.12, ▶Fig. 2.13). Loss of the relationship between the lunate and the teardrop can also reveal carpal subluxation. Where there are separate dorsal and volar articular fragments, a diminished teardrop angle may imply dorsal rotation of the volar fragments independent of dorsal fragments, which may exist in spite of apparent maintenance of volar tilt. The teardrop angle can also give a clue to the causative mechanism of volar rim fragments and therefore inform reduction strategies. A volar shear injury will often have a maintained teardrop angle with no rotation of

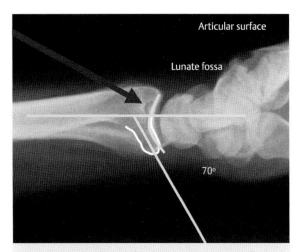

Fig. 2.13 The teardrop angle is best assessed on a radially inclined lateral view.

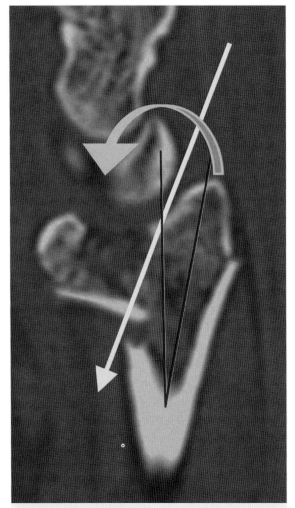

Fig. 2.15 Dorsally tilted fracture with volar rim fragment rotated by volar extrinsic ligament.

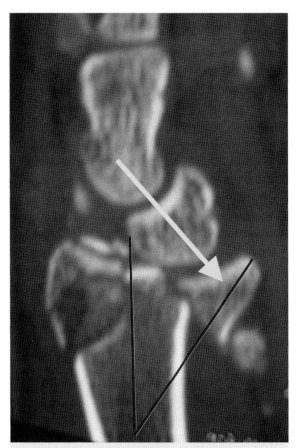

Fig. 2.14 Volar shear injury with maintained teardrop angle. This may be fixed with simple buttress fixation and articular congruence will not be affected.

the volar rim fragment (▶Fig. 2.14). In this case, simple buttressing of the fragment will adequately reduce and stabilize it. Conversely, a diminished teardrop angle implies dorsal rotation of the volar rim fragment. This is usual in a dorsally directed axial load injury with traction on the volar rim fragment from the volar wrist ligaments (▶Fig. 2.15). In this circumstance, a simple buttress-type fixation will not derotate the fragment and an alternate fixation strategy may be required.

• AP distance[7]—This is the distance described by Medoff between the apices of the dorsal and the volar rims of the lunate facet of the radius[7] (▶Fig. 2.16). This is sometimes better appreciated on a 10 to 15° tilt lateral (with the forearm elevated up towards the XR beam). The optimum angle is determined by the radial inclination of the distal radial articular surface. If the AP distance of the radius is significantly greater than the AP dimension of the lunate, it implies an intra-articular fracture with separation between the dorsal and volar rim (▶Fig. 2.17, ▶Fig. 2.18). When there is a fracture in the coronal plane with significant separation, this may be the only plain radiographic parameter that is abnormal. Importantly, this articular incongruity may involve the sigmoid notch.

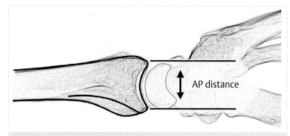

Fig. 2.16 Anteroposterior (AP) distance.

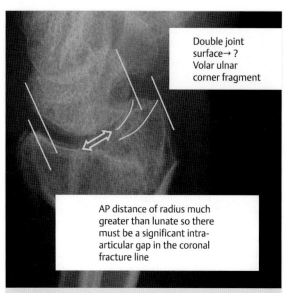

Double joint surface→ ?
Volar ulnar corner fragment

AP distance of radius much greater than lunate so there must be a significant intra-articular gap in the coronal fracture line

Fig. 2.17 Increased Anteroposterior (AP) distance of radius compared to lunate implies a significant intra-articular separation. A double shadow of the volar articular surface raises a suspicion of a volar ulnar (critical corner) fragment. (Reproduced with permission of Medoff R.)

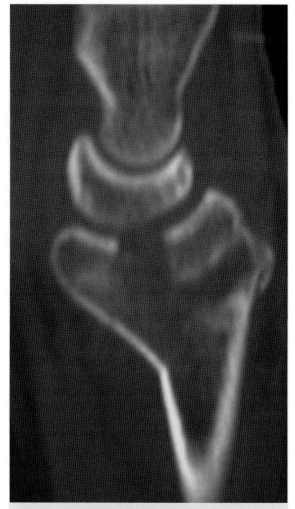

Fig. 2.18 Computed tomography (CT) scan corresponding to ▶Fig. 2.17 confirms the articular separation.

2.4 Effect of Wrist Position on Carpal Indices

Koh et al looked at the position of the wrist and the change in carpal indices on the lateral XR. They took lateral XR of 25 wrists every 5° ranging from 20° wrist flexion to 20° wrist extension. Measurements included: radioscaphoid

(RS) angle, scapholunate (SL) angle, and scaphocapitate angle, among others. Almost all of these measurements were shown to change at each 5° of flexion through extension relative to the neutral position. The exception was the SL angle at 5 and 10° of flexion and 5° extension. This highlights the importance of getting an accurate lateral.[17]

If the position of the wrist is standardized, the carpal alignment indices can be reliably reproduced between observers. Lee at al performed XR and CT on 30 volunteers who did not have fractures. The position of the wrist was standardized for each by placing it into a custom-designed positioning device. Three observers then independently measured the distal radius articular angle, radiolunate angle, RS angle, radiocapitate angle, radius–third metacarpal angle, SL angle, and others. Interobserver reliability was high for XR and CT.[4,18]

2.5 Reproducibility of Indices

It is important to point out that visual estimation of these values can vary between observers when compared to digital measuring techniques as done by a musculoskeletal radiologist.[11,19] Nevertheless, it has not been demonstrated that this difference is significant in terms of clinical decision-making.

2.6 Effect of Lateral Inclination on Volar Tilt

It is important to acknowledge that the scaphoid and lunate fossae are not exactly similar. The scaphoid fossa is deeper than the lunate.[20] Nevertheless, a cadaveric study on 38 distal radii demonstrates that as the wrist is elevated from the standard lateral position, the value for volar tilt does not significantly change. This is particularly relevant when using an image intensifier intraoperatively to assess restoration of volar tilt.[20]

2.7 Intra-articular Components

Specific fracture components have been identified in relation to articular involvement. It should be remembered that while the radiocarpal articulation is the more obvious (scaphoid and lunate facets), the sigmoid notch and DRUJ congruence influence recovery of forearm rotation significantly and this is often a greater determinant of patient satisfaction than radiocarpal ROM. The description of articular components has seen two similar but differing approaches and each offers some benefits:

• The column approach popularized by Rikli and Regazoni[21]: The wrist is divided into three columns, which must each be considered in planning any proposed stabilization. The medial column is the distal ulna, the triangular fibrocartilage, and the DRUJ. The intermediate column is the medial part of the radius, including the lunate fossa and the sigmoid notch. The lateral column includes the lateral radius with the scaphoid fossa and the styloid process.

• The fragment-specific approach popularized by Medoff: It represents an evolution of the work by Melone in defining fragmentation patterns[22,23] (▶ Fig. 2.19). The main categories of intra-articular fragments are:

  - Radial column or scaphoid facet—not just the radial styloid.
  - DUC/sigmoid notch.
  - Dorsal rim.
  - Volar rim (teardrop).
  - Intra-articular—including the "die-punch" fragment.

More recent work by Bain et al[24] has suggested that the consistent articular fracture line locations are a result of "fault lines" where the bone is weaker between ligamentous insertions and stronger at the insertion of the extrinsic ligaments (▶ Fig. 2.20).

The final fragment is the pedestal, which is the metaphysis upon which the radial and intermediate columns sit. In essence, the pedestal is the entire axial circumference of the metaphysis and may be variably involved. It may be more substantially in high-energy injuries and in the presence of osteopenia. It is a challenging problem as radial height can be difficult to restore and maintain, especially in the setting of significant metaphyseal bone comminution.

Different fragments are best appreciated on certain views. The radial column is best visualized on the PA view, although the radial styloid can be identified on a standard lateral projection (▶ Fig. 2.21).[7] The volar rim fragment can be evaluated on a standard lateral or 10°

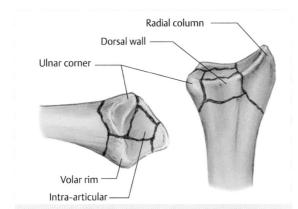

Fig. 2.19 Medoff description of common fragments. (Reproduced with permission of Medoff R.)

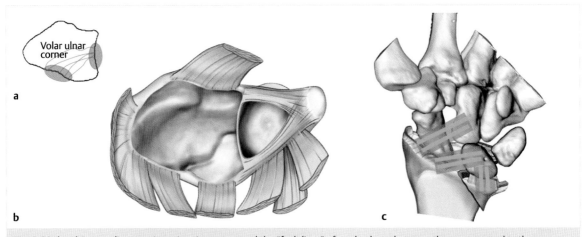

Fig. 2.20 (a–c) Bone at ligament insertions is stronger and the "fault lines" of weaker bone between them correspond to the common fracture lines according to Bain et al. (Reproduced with permission of Bain G.)

tilt lateral by measuring the teardrop angle (normal is 70°; ▶Fig. 2.13). The scaphoid fossa is best seen with a 10° tilt lateral or a 45° pronated lateral view. The DUC fragment is assessed on the PA and oblique views. The lateral view can determine if there is DRUJ instability by checking for dorsal displacement of the ulna relative to the radius, although a true lateral projection is important to make this determination. This can be due to an unstable DUC fragment or a triangular fibrocartilage complex (TFCC) injury associated with unreduced coronal plane translation.[12,15]

Dorsal wall alignment, dorsal angulation, and dorsal wall comminution are seen on the lateral image. The lateral view also shows radiocarpal alignment in the sagittal plane—a line along the volar aspect of the shaft of the radius should bisect the capitate.[7] The free intra-articular or die-punch fragment can be difficult to appreciate

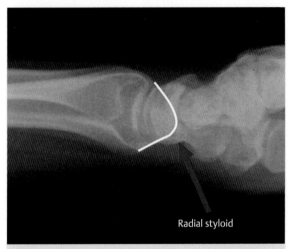

Fig. 2.21 The standard lateral projection demonstrates the outline of the radial styloid portion of the radial column.

on plain XRs but is best seen on the PA, 10° tilt PA, lateral, or 10° tilt lateral. Comminution into the pedestal is shown on the PA with neutral rotation and the lateral and the presence of a radiodense line on the PA may give an indication of significant metaphyseal comminution (▶Fig. 2.22).

A more complete characterization of articular fragments may be undertaken with CT scanning. Determination of fracture components may be more reproducible using CT, for the less experienced assessor.

2.8 Are the Parameters Reproducible?

There are many studies in the literature that evaluate how reproducible the radiological parameters for DRF alignment are. Stirling et al took a random sample from over 3,000 DRFs. Four weeks later, a second random sample was taken. High inter- and intraobserver correlations were found for measurements of radial height, radial inclination, and volar tilt. It was poor for articular step.[25]

Another study, involving five observers, showed intra- and interobserver reliability. Intraobserver reliability was high for dorsal shift and palmar tilt; moderate for radial angle, radial height, ulnar variance, and radial shift; and low for intra-articular gap and step. Interobserver reliability was high for palmar tilt; moderate for dorsal shift, ulnar variance, radial angle, and radial height; and low for radial shift and articular step. Therefore, evaluating articular step is not readily reproducible across different grades of surgeons on XRs.[25,26] Ross et al demonstrated good inter- and intraobserver agreement for the coronal plane translation index, which gives a more reproducible measurement of radial shift.[12]

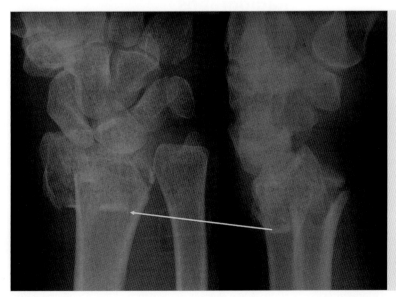

Fig. 2.22 A proximal radiodense line is a clue to metaphyseal comminution.

2.9 Determination of Stability of Fracture Pattern and Adequacy of Reduction

2.9.1 Extra-articular Stability

A fracture of the distal radius is considered to be unstable if it is unable to resist displacement once it has been reduced anatomically.[27]

Lafontaine et al published a series of criteria for determining whether a fracture was unstable based on the prereduction XRs[28]:

- Dorsal tilt > 20°.
- Dorsal comminution.
- Intra-articular fracture.
- Distal ulnar fracture.
- Age greater than 60 years.

In contrast, Nesbitt et al reviewed Lafontaine criteria and concluded that only increased age was associated with a greater risk of displacement.[29]

Cai et al attempted to ascertain indicators of an unstable fracture by assessing the initial parameters in those elderly patients who were treated nonoperatively and noting which patients required corrective osteotomy.[30] They found that radial height of < 4.5 mm and dorsal tilt of > 7.7° were significant.

Batra and Gupta concluded that radial length was the most significant factor affecting fracture stability and outcome, although they did note a relatively weak correlation between anatomic parameters and final functional scores.[31] In contrast, Altissimi et al noted that while some patients with a poor anatomical position could still achieve reasonable function, the superior function was far more likely with a good position at final union.[32]

Mackenney et al concluded that patient age, metaphyseal comminution of the fracture, and ulnar variance were the most consistent predictors of radiographic outcome.[33]

A systematic review published in 2016 by Walenkamp et al revealed a significantly increased risk of secondary displacement in fractures with dorsal comminution in females and patients over 60 years.[34] There was no increased risk with an associated ulna fracture or intra-articular involvement.

Ultimately, consensus on what parameters define an unstable fracture remains elusive. Furthermore, although restoration of these parameters is the goal of surgical fixation, evidence in the literature has differing opinions on how these parameters affect the outcome. Dario et al suggest that ulnar variance and volar tilt are the most important for improving outcome. Small variations of the carpal indices do not influence the final functional outcome in DRFs.[35]

2.9.2 Intra-articular Reduction

In a landmark and much-quoted paper, Knirk and Jupiter retrospectively reviewed 43 intra-articular fractures in 40 young adults (mean age 27.6 years) with a mean follow-up of 6.7 years.[36] Thirty-eight fractures were treated with cast or pins and plaster. Accurate reduction of the articular surface was the most critical factor in achieving a successful result. Radiographic evidence of arthritis developed in all fractures with 2 mm or more articular incongruity, whereas it was seen in only 11% of the fractures that healed with a congruous joint. In 2009, Haus and Jupiter published a critique of the original 1986 paper and concluded that there were possibly methodological shortcomings, which made the original conclusions more difficult to support.[37] Nevertheless, they argued that the reduction of articular incongruence should remain a goal.

Altissimi et al reviewed 59 patients with comminuted intra-articular fractures of the distal radius who were treated nonoperatively.[38] Average follow-up was 3.5 years. Thirty-one percent of the patients with greater than 2 mm of residual articular malalignment were noted to have degenerative arthritis. Catalano et al followed 21 patients less than 45 years of age who had undergone internal fixation of displaced intra-articular fractures.[39] At an average of 7.1 years, osteoarthrosis of the radiocarpal joint was radiographically apparent in 16 wrists (76%). A strong association was found between the development of osteoarthrosis of the radiocarpal joint and residual displacement of articular fragments at the time of bony union.

Fernandez et al observed that intra-articular incongruence of 1 mm or greater resulted in the development of arthrosis.[40] These studies suggest that articular incongruity following a DRF is the most significant factor in the development of post-traumatic radiocarpal arthritis. There remains uncertainty as to whether the critical dimension is 1 or 2 mm. The articular step may be more damaging than articular separation.[36]

2.10 Other Signs on Radiographs

PQ fat pad sign is a shadow deep to PQ that can be a subtle finding to indicate a fracture hematoma. A positive PQ sign was defined as a PQ complex thickness > 8.0 mm (female) or > 9.0 mm (male). A positive PQ fat pad sign shows high specificity but low sensitivity for detection of DRFs. The PQ complex thickness cannot predict the severity of DRFs.

This is more commonly seen in undisplaced extra-articular fractures that very rarely require surgical intervention.[41]

2.11 Frequency of Radiographic Assessment

A final consideration is that too many XRs of DRFs are performed unnecessarily at follow-up after internal fixation. When there is no evidence of bony tenderness and no clinical concern for ROM, then an XR is not indicated. Weil et al found that only 2.6% of XRs resulted in treatment being affected.[19] In our institution, we reviewed over 700 cases of distal radius fixation and identified 7 cases where medium-term management was changed postoperatively on the basis of follow-up XRs within the first 3 months. In all seven cases that underwent a return to the theater for malpositioned hardware or loss of position, a careful inspection of the recorded intraoperative fluoroscopy images from the index procedure identified the problem. We concluded that careful and experienced review of the intraoperative images is more important than the routine performance of postoperative imaging in the first 3 months. Indeed, systematic intraoperative fluoroscopic imaging by an experienced surgeon offers the best opportunity to assess articular reduction and hardware placement. Our current indications for repeat XRs where adequate intraoperative images are available are a significant change in symptomatology or unexpected poor progress, or a significant traumatic event with associated increased pain.

Reducing unnecessary follow-up XRs could reduce workload and cost in the treatment of DRFs.

2.12 Classification of Distal Radius Fractures

In general terms, no single classification system has offered a clear algorithm for decision-making regarding treatment of DRFs. Careful consideration of stability and articular reduction, in the context of expected patient functional demands, utilizing the parameters discussed above is far more helpful in the day-to-day management of these fractures. The Association for Osteosynthesis (AO) concept of the "personality" of the fracture considering both injury factors and patient factors is perfectly applied to DRFs. However, classifications do offer some benefits. Those such as Melone and later fragment-specific classifications do make one consider the various fragmentation patterns when planning internal fixation.[22,23] Mechanistic classifications such as Jupiter and Fernandez shed light on injury patterns, energy involved, and likely modes of secondary displacement.[42] Finally, while having had some concerns raised about inter-/intraobserver error, the AO classification provides a useful tool in the research setting where comparison between groups is needed.

2.13 Computed Tomography

CTs are not indicated for undisplaced stable extra-articular DRFs that will not require fixation. A CT may be warranted for fractures undergoing internal fixation, although the threshold is determined by the degree of comminution, the possibility of articular involvement, and the experience of the surgeon. CT scanning is best performed after a closed reduction. CT defines the number of fragments

involved and the size/comminution of these fragments. This helps set a surgical plan for fixation.[43]

Coronal, sagittal, and axial series should all be viewed carefully as each provides different information on the personality of the fracture. Three-dimensional reconstructions, where provided, are helpful in certain circumstances but are not mandatory.

The die-punch or lunate fossa fragment is characterized by the CT. CT identifies die-punch fragments more frequently than XRs. It can also be used to reliably classify these fragments but the clinical relevance of this has not documented in the literature.[44]

CT is usually associated with higher cost and radiation dose. Radiation dosage can be reduced in focused protocols for DRFs such that the dose is smaller or equivalent to XRs. Such protocols have been shown to be diagnostically comparable and sometimes more favorable than XRs. The cost would still be higher. Both XRs and CT have a role.[45]

In a study that compared plain XRs to CT in 168 patients with acute wrist injuries, plain XRs showed high sensitivity, specificity, and accuracy. Radiography still remains as the first screening tool in acute traumatic wrist injuries and CT is complementary to it.[35] After fixation, CT can be useful for identifying intra-articular hardware.

2.13.1 Sagittal Computed Tomography

Sagittal CT gives the best appreciation of volar and dorsal articular shear fractures (▶ Fig. 2.14, ▶ Fig. 2.15) and carpal subluxation (▶ Fig. 2.23). This is particularly insidious when associated with the volar ulnar corner (critical corner) fragment. Central articular fragments are also shown well (▶ Fig. 2.24).

2.13.2 Coronal Computed Tomography

Coronal CT gives an excellent characterization of the radial column (▶ Fig. 2.25a, b), central articular fragments (▶ Fig. 2.26), and the distal ulna.

2.13.3 Axial Computed Tomography

Axial CT is best for assessing the sigmoid notch and the dorsal ulnar fragment as well as DRUJ congruence and subluxation (▶ Fig. 2.27), and the volar ulnar critical corner fragment (▶ Fig. 2.28).

2.13.4 Computed Tomography and DRUJ Stability

At the initial time of injury, it is often too painful to assess DRUJ instability, although the axial CT may raise the index of suspicion if there is a dorsally displaced dorsal ulnar fragment with associated dorsal displacement of the ulnar head relative to the volar sigmoid notch. CT is a static test and may not elucidate DRUJ instability. A study comparing DRUJ stability parameters on the injured and uninjured side in 46 patients with unilateral DRF showed poor agreement between clinical findings and CT for DRUJ instability.[46,47]

It is important to perform an intraoperative clinical check after the DRF has been internally fixed. There remains debate as to what degree of intraoperative increased dorsal/volar translation is associated with

Fig. 2.23 Sagittal computed tomography (CT) is best for demonstrating marginal shear fractures and carpal subluxation.

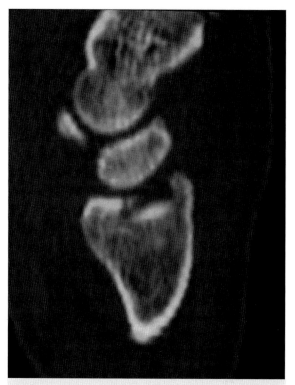

Fig. 2.24 Sagittal computed tomography (CT) demonstrates central articular fragments.

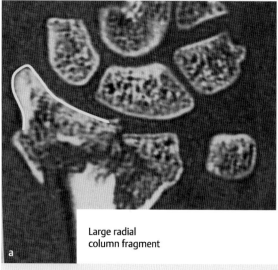

Large radial column fragment

a

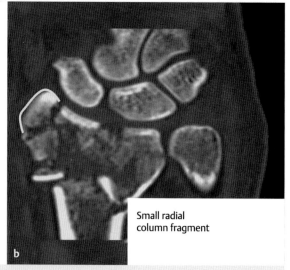

Small radial column fragment

b

Fig. 2.25 (a, b) Coronal computed tomography (CT) is useful for quantifying the size of the radial column fragment. This is important because standard volar plating may not stabilize a small radial column fragment even though it has important ligamentous attachments.

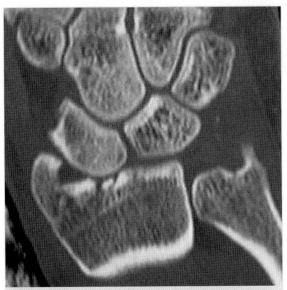

Fig. 2.26 Coronal computed tomography (CT) images can define central articular fragments.

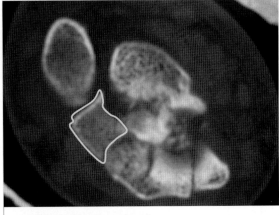

Dorsal ulnar split→ Sigmoid notch
DRUJ intra-articular #

Fig. 2.27 Axial computed tomography (CT) best demonstrates the sigmoid notch, dorsal ulnar fragment, and congruence of the distal radioulnar joint (DRUJ).

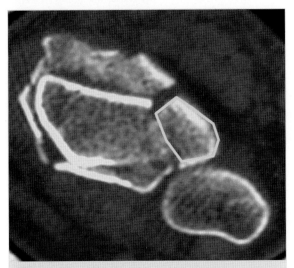

Fig. 2.28 Axial computed tomography (CT) also shows the volar ulnar critical corner fragment.

May be missed by volar plate unless very particular about positioning

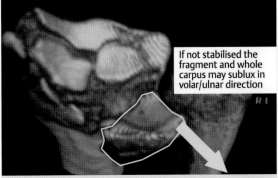

If not stabilised the fragment and whole carpus may sublux in volar/ulnar direction

Fig. 2.29 On-face three-dimensional computed tomography (3D-CT) reconstruction with the subtraction of the carpus can give a unique appreciation of articular fragments and in this case, reveals the critical corner fragment that is associated with volar ulnar subluxation of the carpus.

clinically significant DRUJ instability; however, failure of the radius to track smoothly around the ulnar head through a full range of prosupination is concerning. It should be compared to the contralateral side.

2.13.5 Three-Dimensional Reconstructions

Generally, 3D reconstructions add little to the other imaging sequences; however, in complex articular fractures with multiple intra-articular fragments, the "on-face" view of the articular surface with the carpus subtracted can provide an improved spatial appreciation of the fracture pattern (▶Fig. 2.29).

2.14 Magnetic Resonance Imaging and Distal Radius Fractures

MRI can help diagnose concomitant soft tissue injuries such as the TFCC. It has been suggested as a tool to gauge anatomical reduction of DRFs,[48] though this is rarely undertaken and of questionable value after the implantation of metallic internal fixation devices.

This is an expensive method and adequate XRs suffice to evaluate reduction.

We do not recommend MRI as a routine part of the work-up for DRFs. It is likely that soft tissue and ligamentous injuries coexist in the setting of DRFs, and often acute hemorrhage, edema, and hemarthrosis will make interpretation difficult and increase the risk of false positives. Although these structures could be assessed by MRI, Lindau et al diagnosed scapholunate injuries, which are the second most common soft tissue injuries after TFCC in the setting of DRFs, using wrist arthroscopy, which is the gold standard to which MRI is compared.[49] They followed patients who had DRFs treated but no treatment of the arthroscopically documented ligament lesions for 13 to 15 years and found that there was no difference in subjective, clinical, or radiological outcomes whether an SL injury was present at the time of DRF.[50] They concluded that it is not necessary to treat these injuries when treating DRFs, although, in their series, there were no cases of Geissler grade 4 scapholunate dissociation.

2.15 Summary

The primary questions that need to be answered when assessing the imaging of a DRF are:
- What is an adequate reduction?
- Can an adequate reduction be achieved?
- If so, will it stay that way in a cast? (Stability, *does it need to be fixed?*)
- If internal fixation is undertaken, what fragments need to be stabilized? (*How should it be fixed?*)

2.15.1 Plain Radiographs

In addition to the well-established parameters, familiarity with the relatively new concepts of carpal facet horizon, AP distance, teardrop angle, and coronal plane translation is important.

Extra-articular Stability

This assessment should be made primarily on preinjury XRs. The literature is somewhat inconclusive on the definition of what constitutes an unstable fracture. There seems to be consistent agreement that age > 60 years is a significant negative prognostic factor. In relation to other factors, studies have been generally underpowered; however, there is a trend towards significance in relation to radial length/ulnar variance and in the absence of better data, it seems reasonable to continue to utilize the thresholds proposed by Lafontaine.[28]

Intra-articular Reduction

Notwithstanding Jupiter's 2009 critique of the Knirk and Jupiter paper, the paper still offers useful information.[37,42]

Subsequent papers build on the conclusions of that paper and if anything, more modern imaging techniques and assessments suggest that perhaps even 2 mm is a generous threshold. Given that imaging, arthroscopic techniques, and modern internal fixation options allow reliable restoration of articular congruity combined with early mobilization, it seems reasonable that in the absence of high-quality contradictory data, the most accurate joint reduction should be the current goal wherever possible.

2.15.2 Computed Tomography Scans

Each imaging plane is especially suited to particular fracture components. The radial column and intra-articular fragments are best characterized on the coronal images, the volar and dorsal shear fragments are best seen on the sagittal plane, and the dorsomedial fragment and DRUJ congruence are best demonstrated on the axial images.

2.15.3 Magnetic Resonance Imaging Scans

These are of limited utility in the acute setting due to hematoma and swelling, where arthroscopy potentially has more value, although the prognostic significance of either MRI or arthroscopically identified soft tissue injuries remains unclear.

References

[1] Levin LS, Rozell JC, Pulos N. Distal Radius Fractures in the Elderly. J Am Acad Orthop Surg 2017;25(3):179–187
[2] Ebinger T, Koehler DM, Dolan LA, McDonald K, Shah AS. Obesity Increases Complexity of Distal Radius Fracture in Fall From Standing Height. J Orthop Trauma 2016;30(8):450–455
[3] Wadsten MA, Buttazzoni GG, Sjödén GO, Kadum B, Sayed-Noor AS. Influence of Cortical Comminution and Intra-articular Involvement in Distal Radius Fractures on Clinical Outcome: A Prospective Multicenter Study. J Wrist Surg 2017;6(4):285–293
[4] Christersson A, Nysjö J, Berglund L, et al. Comparison of 2D radiography and a semi-automatic CT-based 3D method for measuring change in dorsal angulation over time in distal radius fractures. Skeletal Radiol 2016;45(6):763–769
[5] Casagrande DJ, Morris RP, Carayannopoulos NL, Buford WL. Relationship Between Ulnar Variance, Cortical Bone Density, and Load to Failure in the Distal Radius at the Typical Site of Fracture Initiation. J Hand Surg Am 2016;41(12):e461–e468
[6] Mishra PK, Nagar M, Gaur SC, Gupta A. Morphometry of distal end radius in the Indian population: A radiological study. Indian J Orthop 2016;50(6):610–615
[7] Medoff RJ. Essential radiographic evaluation for distal radius fractures. Hand Clin 2005;21(3):279–288
[8] Yang Z, Mann FA, Gilula LA, Haerr C, Larsen CF. Scaphopisocapitate alignment: criterion to establish a neutral lateral view of the wrist. Radiology 1997;205(3):865–869
[9] Larsen CF, Stigsby B, Lindequist S, Bellstrøm T, Mathiesen FK, Ipsen T. Observer variability in measurements of carpal bone angles on lateral wrist radiographs. J Hand Surg Am 1991;16(5):893–898
[10] Geissler WB, Clark JM. Arthroscopic Reduction and Fixation of Distal Radius and Ulnar Styloid Fractures. In: Tornetta P, Wiesel SW, eds. Operative Techniques in Orthopaedic Trauma Surgery, 2nd Edition. Philadelphia: Wolters Kluwer;2016:41–52

[11] O'Malley MP, Rodner C, Ritting A, et al. Radiographic interpretation of distal radius fractures: visual estimations versus digital measuring techniques. Hand (N Y) 2014;9(4):488–493

[12] Ross M, Di Mascio L, Peters S, Cockfield A, Taylor F, Couzens G. Defining residual radial translation of distal radius fractures: a potential cause of distal radioulnar joint instability. J Wrist Surg 2014;3(1):22–29

[13] Ross M, Heiss-Dunlop W. Volar angle stable plating for distal radius fractures. In: Slutsky DJ, ed. Principles and Practice of Wrist Surgery. 2nd ed. Philadelphia: Elsevier; 2010:126–139

[14] Trehan SK, Orbay JL, Wolfe SW. Coronal shift of distal radius fractures: influence of the distal interosseous membrane on distal radioulnar joint instability. J Hand Surg Am 2015;40(1):159–162

[15] Ross M, Allen L, Couzens GB. Correction of Residual Radial Translation of the Distal Fragment in Distal Radius Fracture Open Reduction. J Hand Surg Am 2015;40(12):2465–2470

[16] Broadbent MR, Stevenson I, Maceachern C, Johnstone AJ. Investigation of radiolunate relations in normal and fractured wrists. Hand Surg 2009;14(2–3):105–112

[17] Koh KH, Lee HI, Lim KS, Seo JS, Park MJ. Effect of wrist position on the measurement of carpal indices on the lateral radiograph. J Hand Surg Eur Vol 2013;38(5):530–541

[18] Lee KW, Bae JY, Seo DK, Kim SB, Lee HI. Measurement of Carpal Alignment Indices Using 3-Dimensional Computed Tomography. J Hand Surg Am 2018;43(8):771.e1–771.e7

[19] Weil NL, El Moumni M, Rubinstein SM, Krijnen P, Termaat MF, Schipper IB. Routine follow-up radiographs for distal radius fractures are seldom clinically substantiated. Arch Orthop Trauma Surg 2017;137(9):1187–1191

[20] Daniele L, McLean A, Cocks N, Kalamaras M, Bindra R, Ezekiel Tan SL. Anatomic Variation in Volar Tilt of the Scaphoid and Lunate Facet of the Distal Radius. J Hand Surg Am 2016;41(11):e399–e404

[21] Rikli DA, Regazzoni P. Fractures of the distal end of the radius treated by internal fixation and early function. A preliminary report of 20 cases. J Bone Joint Surg Br 1996;78(4):588–592

[22] Melone CP Jr. Distal radius fractures: patterns of articular fragmentation. Orthop Clin North Am 1993;24(2):239–253

[23] Melone CP Jr. Articular fractures of the distal radius. Orthop Clin North Am 1984;15(2):217–236

[24] Bain GI, Alexander JJ, Eng K, Durrant A, Zumstein MA. Ligament origins are preserved in distal radial intraarticular two-part fractures: a computed tomography-based study. J Wrist Surg 2013;2(3):255–262

[25] Stirling E, Jeffer, y J, Johnson N, Dias J. Are radiographic measurements of the displacement of a distal radial fracture reliable and reproducible? Bone Joint J 2016;98-B(8):1069–1073

[26] Watson NJ, Asadollahi S, Parrish F, Ridgway J, Tran P, Keating JL. Reliability of radiographic measurements for acute distal radius fractures. BMC Med Imaging 2016;16(1):44

[27] Slutsky DJ. Predicting the outcome of distal radius fractures. Hand Clin 2005;21(3):289–294

[28] Lafontaine M, Hardy D, Delince P. Stability assessment of distal radius fractures. Injury 1989;20(4):208–210

[29] Nesbitt KS, Failla JM, Les C. Assessment of instability factors in adult distal radius fractures. J Hand Surg Am 2004;29(6):1128–1138

[30] Cai L, Zhu S, Du S, et al. The relationship between radiographic parameters and clinical outcome of distal radius fractures in elderly patients. Orthop Traumatol Surg Res 2015;101(7):827–831

[31] Batra S, Gupta A. The effect of fracture-related factors on the functional outcome at 1 year in distal radius fractures. Injury 2002;33(6):499–502

[32] Altissimi M, Antenucci R, Fiacca C, Mancini GB. Long-term results of conservative treatment of fractures of the distal radius. Clin Orthop Relat Res 1986;(206):202–210

[33] Mackenney PJ, McQueen MM, Elton R. Prediction of instability in distal radial fractures. J Bone Joint Surg Am 2006;88(9):1944–1951

[34] Walenkamp MM, Aydin S, Mulders MA, Goslings JC, Schep NW. Predictors of unstable distal radius fractures: a systematic review and meta-analysis. J Hand Surg Eur Vol 2016;41(5):501–515

[35] Basha MAA, Ismail AAA, Imam AHF. Does radiography still have a significant diagnostic role in evaluation of acute traumatic wrist injuries? A prospective comparative study. Emerg Radiol 2018;25(2):129–138

[36] Knirk JL, Jupiter JB. Intra-articular fractures of the distal end of the radius in young adults. J Bone Joint Surg Am 1986;68(5):647–659

[37] Haus BM, Jupiter JB. Intra-articular fractures of the distal end of the radius in young adults: reexamined as evidence-based and outcomes medicine. J Bone Joint Surg Am 2009;91(12):2984–2991

[38] Altissimi M, Mancini GB, Ciaffoloni E, Pucci G. Comminuted articular fractures of the distal radius. Results of conservative treatment. Ital J Orthop Traumatol 1991;17(1):117–123

[39] Catalano LW III, Cole RJ, Gelberman RH, Evanoff BA, Gilula LA, Borrelli J Jr. Displaced intra-articular fractures of the distal aspect of the radius. Long-term results in young adults after open reduction and internal fixation. J Bone Joint Surg Am 1997;79(9):1290–1302

[40] Fernandez JJ, Gruen GS, Herndon JH. Outcome of distal radius fractures using the short form 36 health survey. Clin Orthop Relat Res 1997;(341):36–41

[41] Loesaus J, Wobbe I, Stahlberg E, Barkhausen J, Goltz JP. Reliability of the pronator quadratus fat pad sign to predict the severity of distal radius fractures. World J Radiol 2017;9(9):359–364

[42] Jupiter JB, Fernandez DL. Comparative classification for fractures of the distal end of the radius. J Hand Surg Am 1997;22(4):563–571

[43] Grunz JP, Gietzen CH, Schmitt R, Prommersberger KJ. [Distal radius fractures: Update on imaging.] Radiologe 2018;58(2):159–174

[44] Ma Y, Yin Q, Rui Y, Gu S, Yang Y. Image classification for Die-punch fracture of intermediate column of the distal radius. Radiol Med (Torino) 2017;122(12):928–933

[45] Neubauer J, Benndorf M, Reidelbach C, et al. Comparison of Diagnostic Accuracy of Radiation Dose-Equivalent Radiography, Multidetector Computed Tomography and Cone Beam Computed Tomography for Fractures of Adult Cadaveric Wrists. PLoS One 2016;11(10):e0164859

[46] van Leerdam RH, Wijffels MME, Reijnierse M, Stomp W, Krijnen P, Schipper IB. The value of computed tomography in detecting distal radioulnar joint instability after a distal radius fracture. J Hand Surg Eur Vol 2017;42(5):501–506

[47] Dario P, Matteo G, Carolina C, et al. Is it really necessary to restore radial anatomic parameters after distal radius fractures? Injury 2014;45(Suppl 6):S21–S26

[48] Medlock G, Wohlgemut JM, Stevenson IM, Johnstone AJ. Magnetic resonance imaging investigation of radio-lunate relations: use in assessing distal radial fracture reduction. J Hand Surg Eur Vol 2017;42(3):271–274

[49] Schmitt R, Christopoulos G, Meier R, et al. [Direct MR arthrography of the wrist in comparison with arthroscopy: a prospective study on 125 patients] RoFo Fortschr Geb Rontgenstr Nuklearmed 2003;175(7):911–919

[50] Mrkonjic A, Lindau T, Geijer M, Tägil M. Arthroscopically diagnosed scapholunate ligament injuries associated with distal radial fractures: a 13- to 15-year follow-up. J Hand Surg Am 2015;40(6):1077–1082

3 Patient–Accident–Fracture Classification of Acute Distal Radius Fractures in Adults

Guillaume Herzberg, Thais Galissard, Marion Burnier

Abstract

The patient–accident–fracture (PAF) classification of acute distal radius fractures (DRF) in adults was designed because there is not yet enough evidence in the literature to support the use of any classification systems in this particular field.

It was the author's opinion that there was a need for the identification of more homogeneous groups of patients with DRF. Although the pathology remains a keystone factor, the extent of pretherapeutic radiological work-up and treatment options would match in priority the health status and functional needs of the patient.

The authors propose an innovative method to analyze and stratify acute DRF in adults. A one-page user-friendly chart includes criteria related to the patient (P), the energy of the accident (A), and the pathology of the fracture (F), including associated osseous/ligamentous ulnar and carpal lesions.

The preliminary results of the prospective use of the PAF chart in 1,650 consecutive adult patients (16 to 102 y) with unilateral acute DRF from a single academic upper extremity-specialized orthopaedic unit are presented.

A total of six homogeneous groups of patients is described. The relevance of this classification regarding the pretherapeutic radiological work-up and treatment options is discussed on an expert opinion basis. Specific studies of these groups may provide the guidelines that are currently lacking regarding the management of DRF.

Keywords: acute distal radius fracture, classification, epidemiology, pathology, radiological work-up

3.1 Introduction

There is not enough evidence in the literature to support the use of any classification system for distal radius fractures (DRF) in adults.[1–3]

However, there is a need for identification of more homogeneous groups of patients with DRF so that the extent of pretherapeutic radiological work-up and the choice of treatment would best match the needs of the patient.[4]

The purpose of this prospective epidemiological study based on 1,650 patients (1,650 wrists) was: (1) to propose a simple practical method allowing for a comprehensive analysis of DRF at the acute stage and (2) to identify from our preliminary results several homogeneous groups of patients within a wide array of acute DRF from an academic upper extremity-specialized orthopaedic center.

3.2 Material and Methods

From September 2008 to May 2018, a total of 1,650 consecutive patients presenting at our academic upper extremity-specialized surgery unit with acute unilateral DRF were included in a prospective epidemiological study. Criteria related to the patient, the accident, and the fracture type with associated injuries were included in a one-page chart that was previously described (▶ Fig. 3.1).[5]

3.2.1 Patient

Beside his/her age and gender, each patient was characterized by his/her general health status (normal 3, with comorbidities 2, or dependent 1). We arbitrarily defined by an interview at the acute stage the functional needs of the patient as maximum 3, intermediate 2, or minimal 1. All possible combination of general health status (1 to 3) and functional needs (1 to 3) could be encountered. Only patients "1–1," "2–2," or "3–3" were included in the present study.

3.2.2 Accident

The amount of energy of the accident may be an indirect predictor of the magnitude of the pathology of DRF, especially in terms of associated bony and/or ligamentous injuries. We defined high-energy accidents as 3 (such a fall from a roof or motorcycle high-velocity accident), medium-energy accidents as 2 (such as fall while playing tennis), and low energy accident as 1 (such as a simple fall). Polytraumatized and polyinjured patients were individualized from monoinjured patients because the treatment of DRF may not be a priority in the former.

3.2.3 Fracture

Distal Radius Fracture

The open or closed nature of the DRF and the presence of an acute associated carpal tunnel syndrome were recorded as well as the main Association for Osteosynthesis (AO) classification type "A," "B," or "C." In addition, several anatomical factors that could have an influence on the prognosis and treatment such as distal radius comminution, distal fracture line, impaction, and cartilage defect were included.[2,6]

A total of four extra-articular displacement criteria were defined on the initial PA views (Fig. 3.1). The radial inclination was defined by three classes around a "1" category where the radial inclination was considered

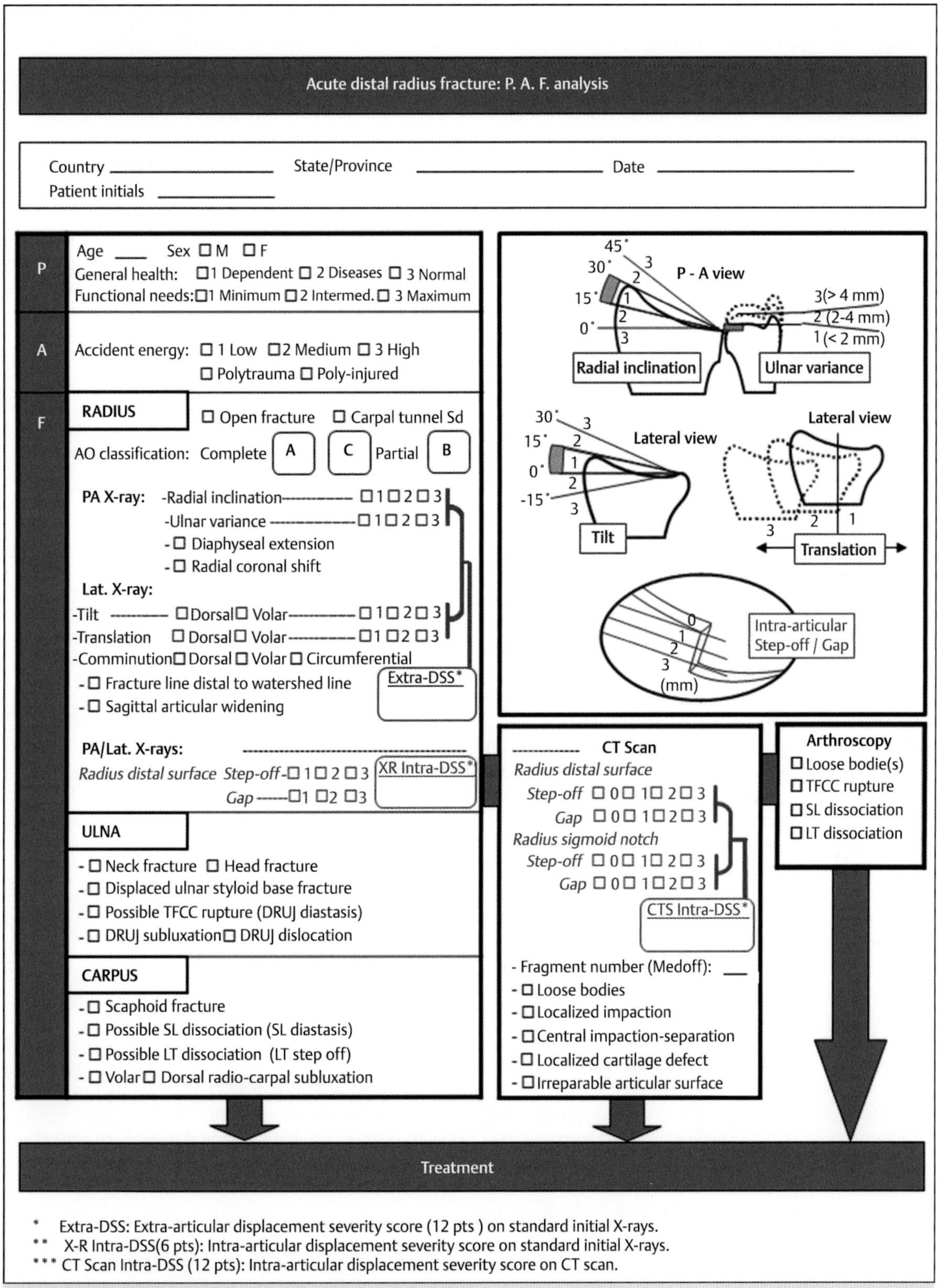

Acute distal radius fracture: P. A. F. analysis

Country _____ State/Province _____ Date _____
Patient initials _____

P
Age ____ Sex ☐ M ☐ F
General health: ☐ 1 Dependent ☐ 2 Diseases ☐ 3 Normal
Functional needs: ☐ 1 Minimum ☐ 2 Intermed. ☐ 3 Maximum

A
Accident energy: ☐ 1 Low ☐ 2 Medium ☐ 3 High
☐ Polytrauma ☐ Poly-injured

F
RADIUS   ☐ Open fracture   ☐ Carpal tunnel Sd

AO classification: Complete [A] [C] Partial [B]

PA X-ray: -Radial inclination———— ☐ 1 ☐ 2 ☐ 3
-Ulnar variance ————— ☐ 1 ☐ 2 ☐ 3
- ☐ Diaphyseal extension
- ☐ Radial coronal shift

Lat. X-ray:
-Tilt ———— ☐ Dorsal ☐ Volar———— ☐ 1 ☐ 2 ☐ 3
-Translation ☐ Dorsal ☐ Volar———— ☐ 1 ☐ 2 ☐ 3
-Comminution ☐ Dorsal ☐ Volar ☐ Circumferential
- ☐ Fracture line distal to watershed line | Extra-DSS* |
- ☐ Sagittal articular widening

PA/Lat. X-rays: -----------------------------
Radius distal surface Step-off ☐ 1 ☐ 2 ☐ 3 | XR Intra-DSS* |
Gap ——— ☐ 1 ☐ 2 ☐ 3

ULNA
- ☐ Neck fracture ☐ Head fracture
- ☐ Displaced ulnar styloid base fracture
- ☐ Possible TFCC rupture (DRUJ diastasis)
- ☐ DRUJ subluxation ☐ DRUJ dislocation

CARPUS
- ☐ Scaphoid fracture
- ☐ Possible SL dissociation (SL diastasis)
- ☐ Possible LT dissociation (LT step off)
- ☐ Volar ☐ Dorsal radio-carpal subluxation

P - A view
Radial inclination   Ulnar variance
45° 30° 15° 0° | 3 2 1 2 3 | 3 (> 4 mm) 2 (2-4 mm) 1 (< 2 mm)

Lateral view   Lateral view
Tilt   Translation
30° 15° 0° -15° | 3 2 1 2 3 | 3 2 1

Intra-articular Step-off / Gap
0 1 2 3 (mm)

----------- CT Scan
Radius distal surface
Step-off ☐ 0 ☐ 1 ☐ 2 ☐ 3
Gap ☐ 0 ☐ 1 ☐ 2 ☐ 3
Radius sigmoid notch
Step-off ☐ 0 ☐ 1 ☐ 2 ☐ 3
Gap ☐ 0 ☐ 1 ☐ 2 ☐ 3
| CTS Intra-DSS* |

- Fragment number (Medoff): ___
- ☐ Loose bodies
- ☐ Localized impaction
- ☐ Central impaction-separation
- ☐ Localized cartilage defect
- ☐ Irreparable articular surface

Arthroscopy
☐ Loose bodie(s)
☐ TFCC rupture
☐ SL dissociation
☐ LT dissociation

Treatment

* Extra-DSS: Extra-articular displacement severity score (12 pts) on standard initial X-rays.
** X-R Intra-DSS(6 pts): Intra-articular displacement severity score on standard initial X-rays.
*** CT Scan Intra-DSS (12 pts): Intra-articular displacement severity score on CT scan.

Fig. 3.1 Patient–accident–fracture classification chart. (*Source:* Reproduced from Herzberg G, Izem Y, Al Saati M, Plotard F. PAF analysis of acute distal radius fractures in adults. Preliminary results. Chirurgie de la main 2010;29:231–235. Copyright © 2010 Elsevier Masson SAS. All rights reserved.)

as within normal limits (15–30°). Radial shortening was defined within three classes of ulnar variance, class 1 (less than 2 mm of positive ulnar variance) being considered as acceptable. The presence or absence of proximal diaphyseal irradiation of the fracture line was recorded. Radial translation (or radial shift) of the radius epiphysis with respect to the radius diaphysis was recorded.

Another four extra-articular displacement criteria were defined on the initial lateral view. The tilt of the distal radius in a dorsal or volar direction was recorded within three classes around an acceptable "1" class (0–15°). Anterior or posterior translation of the distal radius epiphysis with respect to the diaphysis was recorded within three classes around a "1" nontranslated position. Anterior, posterior, or circumferential comminution was recorded as it is a major prognosis factor in DRF.[6,7] Articular sagittal widening was also recorded as it has recently proven to be simple standard X-ray criteria suggesting a severe involvement of the articular radiocarpal aspect of the distal radius, which should be refined by a computed tomography (CT) scan.

An extra-articular displacement severity (EDS) score was defined as the sum of radial inclination, ulnar variance, dorsal or volar radial tilt, and sagittal translation figures. This score was comprised between 4 (acceptable displacement) and 12 (maximal distal radius epiphyseal displacement). An EDS of 5 to 8 defined a displaced DRF, whereas an EDS of 9 to 12 defined a severely displaced DRF according to extra-articular criteria.

Within the intra-articular group of DRF, four criteria were defined from the initial standard X-rays or emergency CT scan if available. The radiocarpal and distal radioulnar joint (DRUJ) articular step-off and gaps were defined as three classes. The step-off and gap of the sigmoid notch of the distal radius could only be defined from transverse CT scan slices. A step-off of less than 1 mm (class 1) was considered as acceptable. Step-off of 2 mm (class 2) or 3 mm or more (class 3) characterized significant or major intra-articular displacements. A gap of less than 1 mm (class 1) was considered as acceptable. Gaps of 2 mm (class 2) or 3 mm or more (class 3) characterized significant or major intra-articular displacements.

When only standard radiographs were available, a simple 6 points intra-articular radiocarpal displacement severity score was defined as the addition of the step-off and gap classes at the radiocarpal level.

When a CT scan was available, a 12 points intra-articular displacement severity (CT-IDS) score was defined as the sum of the radiocarpal and sigmoid notch step-off and gap classes at both radiocarpal and sigmoid notch spots. The CT-IDS was comprised between 4 (acceptable displacement) and 12 (maximal intra-articular displacement). A CT-IDS of 5 to 8 defined a displaced intra-articular DRF, whereas a CT-IDS of 9 to 12 defined a severely displaced intra-articular DRF.

Transverse CT scan slices were used to record the number of major fragments according to Medoff classification.[8] The presence of localized impaction, central impaction

separation, or complete destruction of the radial distal surface was recorded. If applicable, arthroscopic findings (osteoarticular loose bodies, triangular fibrocartilage complex [TFCC], and scapholunate or lunotriquetral ligaments tears) were recorded.

Associated Ulnar Head and Distal Radioulnar Joint Lesions

Fractures of the neck/head of the ulna were included as binary criteria. Displaced fractures of the base of the ulnar styloid were recorded. Fractures of the tip of the ulnar styloid were not considered. DRUJ diastasis, subluxations, or dislocations were recorded.

Associated Carpal Injuries

Associated fractures of the scaphoid were recorded as well as any radiological suspicion of scapholunate injury (mainly increase of the scapholunate gap on PA radiographs and increase of the normal scapholunate angle on lateral radiographs). Any rupture of Gilula proximal line at the lunotriquetral interval was recorded as a possible associated lunotriquetral dissociation. The presence of volar of dorsal radiocarpal subluxation was recorded.

3.3 Results and Discussion

Within 1,650 patients with 1,650 unilateral acute DRF, a total of 1,485 patients fitted into "1–1," "2–2," or "3–3" categories according to general health and functional needs. Only 10% of the patients did not fit into the "1–1," "2–2," or "3–3" categories, which was remarkable. To provide a stronger message, only the 1,485 "1–1," "2–2," or "3–3" patients were considered. The distribution of "1–1," "2–2," or "3–3" patients were, respectively, 6, 29, and 65%.

Among the 1,485 patients, 61% were female. The ages ranged from 16 to 102 years with a mean of 56 years. We identified six homogeneous groups of patients with DRF. For each category, we propose our opinion about the relevance of the group definition regarding the treatment options. This discussion is subjective. However, it seems obvious that an arthroscopically assisted treatment is not indicated in a 90-year-old female presenting with an intra-articular severely displaced DRF. Defining the groups below helps focusing on a limited number of treatments for each category. Further studies may thus compare more focused treatments in more homogeneous groups.

3.3.1 Patients 1–1 (Dependent, Minimal Functional Needs) with AO Type "A" or "C" Fractures

We found 95 patients (95% female) within this group (6%). The average age of this group was 83 years. The distribution of extra "A" versus intra-articular "C" DRF was almost equivalent, that is, respectively, 47 versus 53%. There were no "B" fractures in this group.

It is our opinion that this group warrants simple management. No CT scan is needed and the treatment may be the same irrespective of the extra- or intra-articular nature of the fracture. In our opinion, the two main options may be below-elbow casting in a functional position in most cases or volar plating in case of high extra-articular displacement score. Studies comparing these two treatments in this specific group of patients may provide the guidelines that are currently lacking.

3.3.2 Patients 2–2 (Independent Patients with Comorbidities, Intermediate Functional Needs) with AO Type "A" Extra-articular Fractures

We found 146 patients (86% female) within this group (10%). The average age of this group was 77 years. A total of 48% of wrists in this group displayed a severe ulnar shortening and 62% displayed a severe extra-articular displacement index (9 or higher). Circumferential comminution was present in 29% and radial translation of the radius epiphysis was present in 45%.

As these patients are independent with extra-articular fractures, all efforts should be made at restoring normal or subnormal extra-articular indices, especially a class 1 ulnar variance so as to minimize the risk of a secondary ulnocarpal impingement.

Our opinion is that volar plating would be the best method to restore the ulnar variance.

The volar plating would be difficult in many cases in this group when circumferential comminution is present. Moreover, the surgeon should be prepared to add a lateral plating to maintain the correction of the radial translation of the epiphysis, which was frequently observed in this group (45%). Studies comparing these treatments according to these parameters in this specific group of patients may provide the guidelines that are currently lacking.

3.3.3 Patients 2–2 (Independent Patients with Comorbidities, Intermediate Functional Needs) with AO Type "C" Intra-articular Fractures

We found 280 patients (83% female) within this group (19%). The average age of this group was 75 years.

A total of 58% of wrists in this group displayed a severe ulnar shortening and 61% displayed a severe extra-articular displacement index (9 or higher). Circumferential comminution was present in 50% and radial

translation of the radius epiphysis was present in 37%. A severe intra-articular radiocarpal displacement index (5 or higher) was present in 58% and a severe intra-articular CT scan displacement index (9 or higher) was present in 52% of the 128 cases where a CT scan was performed to fully understand the displacement. The articular fracture was found to be irreparable in 27% of these 128 cases.

As these patients are independent at home, it is our opinion that all efforts should be made at providing them with a distal radius that would be as anatomical as possible. Volar plating would be the best option. However volar plating may be sometimes technically difficult in this group of patients and complications may be expected.[9] If the fracture is considered as irreparable, that is, not amenable to reliable open reduction internal fixation (ORIF), the use of a primary hemiarthroplasty may be discussed.[10–13] Studies comparing these treatments according to PAF anatomical parameters in this specific group of patients may provide the guidelines that are currently lacking.

3.3.4 Patients 3–3 (Patient with Normal General Health Status and Maximal Functional Needs) with AO Type "A" Extra-articular Fractures

We found 245 patients (64% female) within this group (18%). The average age of this group was 45 years.

It is obvious that the patients in this group are much more active than patients of the previous groups. It is our opinion that they all deserve an ORIF that would be as anatomical as possible. Given the extra-articular nature of the fracture and the better bone quality than in the previous groups, the technique of reduction and fixation may be depending on the surgeon's preference. Our opinion is that volar plating would be the best guarantee against shortening or rotational malunions. Despite the extra-articular nature of the injury, arthroscopy may be a useful adjunct to diagnose a foveal avulsion of the TFCC. Marked radial translation and DRUJ diastasis are important clues to the diagnosis of associated TFCC injury in an extra-articular fracture. Follow-up studies should be set up to compare the results of various treatment within this subgroup of patients.

3.3.5 Patients 3–3 (Patient with Normal General Health Status and Maximal Functional Needs) with AO Type "C" Intra-articular Fractures

We found 606 patients (46% female) within this group (41%). The average age of this group was the same as in the previous group (45 y).

The problem in this group is the extent of intra-articular involvement. It is the group that would sometimes be the most difficult to reduce and/or fix. A preoperative CT scan with three-dimensional (3D) reconstructions and subtractions should be a prerequisite to fully understand the fragments and displacements because the result of ORIF should be as anatomically as possible.

A total of 44% of wrists in this group displayed a severe ulnar shortening and 50% displayed a severe extra-articular displacement index (9 or higher). Circumferential comminution was present in 34% and radial translation of the radius epiphysis was present in 25%. A severe intra-articular CT scan displacement index (9 or higher) was present in 38% of the 502 cases where a CT scan was performed to fully understand the displacement. The articular fracture was found to be irreparable in 10% of these 502 cases.

If the fracture is considered as reparable, it is our opinion that ORIF should be the rule, most often (but not always) with volar plating. Arthroscopic assistance may be a useful adjunct to better control the articular reduction and to diagnose the associated ligamentous injuries.[14,15]

If the fracture is considered as irreparable, that is, not amenable to reliable ORIF because of severe articular comminution with loss of articular fragments, the use of a primary or secondary radioscapholunate fusion may be a reasonable alternative to ORIF.[4,16] Studies comparing these treatments according to PAF anatomical parameters in this specific group of patients may provide the guidelines that are currently lacking.

3.3.6 Patients 3–3 (Patient with Normal General Health Status and Maximal Functional Needs) with AO Type "B" Partial Articular Fractures

We found 92 patients (88% male) within this group (6%). The average age of this group (34 y) was very different from the previous groups. This study suggests that the AO partial articular "B" fractures are a very specific group in terms of general health, functional needs, age, and gender of the patients. Anatomically, these fractures are a transitional pattern to fracture-dislocations. In our opinion, these fractures deserve a sophisticated work-up, including CT scan with 3D reconstruction. Moreover, we think that the use of arthroscopy to optimize the articular reduction and check the associated ligamentous injuries should be as frequent as possible. Specific studies of this group may provide the guidelines that are currently lacking.

3.4 Conclusion

The authors present the preliminary results of the first DRF classification study that includes on a systematic basis the patient's general health and functional needs in addition to the pathology of the fracture. The combination of patient's and accident's characteristics with the main AO fracture types along with ulnar and carpal associated injuries provided a new look at the distribution and stratification of acute DRF. A total of six homogeneous groups of patients could be defined. Further studies are necessary to compare the results of focused treatments in each category.

References

[1] Handoll HHG, Madhok R. WITHDRAWN: Surgical interventions for treating distal radial fractures in adults. Cochrane Database Syst Rev 2009(3):CD003209
[2] Koval KJ, Harrast JJ, Anglen JO, Weinstein JN. Fractures of the distal part of the radius. The evolution of practice over time. Where's the evidence? J Bone Joint Surg Am 2008;90(9):1855–1861
[3] Lichtman DM, Bindra RR, Boyer MI, et al. Treatment of distal radius fractures. J Am Acad Orthop Surg 2010;18(3):180–189
[4] Herzberg G, Izem Y, Al Saati M, Plotard F. "PAF" analysis of acute distal radius fractures in adults. Preliminary results. Chir Main 2010;29(4):231–235
[5] Herzberg G. Acute Distal Radius Fracture: PAF Analysis. J Wrist Surg 2012;1(1):81–82
[6] Fernandez DL, Jupiter JB. Fractures of the Distal Radius. 2nd ed. New York: Springer; 2002
[7] Laulan J, Marteau E, Bacle G. Le système de classification MEU des fractures de l'extrémité distale du radius. Intérêts pronostique et thérapeutique d'une analyse indépendante des différents paramètres de la fracture. Hand Surg Rehabil 2016;35S:S28–S33
[8] Medoff RJ. Essential radiographic evaluation for distal radius fractures. Hand Clin 2005;21(3):279–288
[9] Arora R, Lutz M, Deml C, Krappinger D, Haug L, Gabl M. A prospective randomized trial comparing nonoperative treatment with volar locking plate fixation for displaced and unstable distal radial fractures in patients sixty-five years of age and older. J Bone Joint Surg Am 2011;93(23):2146–2153
[10] Herzberg G, Burnier M, Marc A, Izem Y. Primary Wrist Hemiarthroplasty for Irreparable Distal Radius Fracture in the Independent Elderly. J Wrist Surg 2015;4(3):156–163
[11] Ichihara S, Díaz JJ, Peterson B, Facca S, Bodin F, Liverneaux P. Distal Radius Isoelastic Resurfacing Prosthesis: A Preliminary Report. J Wrist Surg 2015;4(3):150–155
[12] Roux JL. Treatment of intra-articular fractures of the distal radius by wrist prosthesis. Orthop Traumatol Surg Res 2011:S46–S53
[13] Vergnenègre G, Mabit C, Charissoux J-L, Arnaud JP, Marcheix PS. Treatment of comminuted distal radius fractures by resurfacing prosthesis in elderly patients. Chir Main 2014;33(2):112–117
[14] Del Piñal F. Technical tips for (dry) arthroscopic reduction and internal fixation of distal radius fractures. J Hand Surg Am 2011;36(10):1694–1705
[15] Herzberg G. Intra-articular fracture of the distal radius: arthroscopic-assisted reduction. J Hand Surg Am 2010;35(9):1517–1519
[16] Freeland AE, Sud V, Jemison DM. Early wrist arthrodesis for irreparable intra-articular distal radial fractures. Hand Surg 2000;5(2):113–118

4 Distal Radius Fracture: The Evidence

Tracy Webber, Tamara D. Rozental

Abstract

Distal radius fractures are common injuries and, as such, a large number of studies focusing on both nonoperative and operative treatment have been published. A review of level one studies reveals that nonoperative management can be performed in either a cast or functional brace with equivalent results. The decision on whether to proceed with operative treatment remains controversial. In terms of surgical management, open reduction internal fixation (ORIF), closed reduction and pinning (CRPP), and external fixation produce similar results at 1 year although an earlier return to function favors ORIF with a volar plate. Treating surgeons should evaluate patients with fragility fractures for underlying osteoporosis and initiate treatment when appropriate.

Keywords: evidence-based distal radius fractures, cast

4.1 Introduction

Distal radius fractures (DRFs) are the most common fracture of the upper extremity, accounting for 2% of all emergency room visits and one-sixth of all fractures. There are more than 600,000 DRFs in the United States annually.[1] Furthermore, the overall incidence of DRFs has been increasing. DRFs have a bimodal age distribution, affecting young people with high-energy injuries and older patients with osteoporotic fractures. Given the common nature of DRF, there is a wide spectrum of existing literature examining the treatment and outcomes of these injuries. High-quality, randomized studies, however, are rare. This chapter reviews the existing evidence guiding the surgical management of DRF.

The Canadian task force originally described levels of evidence in 1979. They developed a system of grading evidence to optimize internal validity based on the study's level of bias.[2] Randomized controlled trials (RCTs) and meta-analyses of RCTs are considered level 1 evidence. This review focuses on level 1 studies examining the treatment of DRF.

4.2 Methods

We reviewed the 2009 American Academy of Orthopaedic Surgeons (AAOS) Guidelines on the Treatment of Distal Radius Fractures[3] and included all RCTs that were deemed high-quality studies. We next searched PubMed for newer RCTs published after the clinical guidelines were released. Keywords used included distal radius, radius, fracture, open reduction internal fixation (ORIF), external fixation, operative, nonoperative, percutaneous pinning, osteoporosis, therapy, and RCT. All studies reviewed were published after 1996, included at least 30 patients, and were published in the English language.

4.3 Nonoperative Fracture Treatment

Nonoperative treatment remains the most common method of treatment of DRFs.[1] When treating patients conservatively, fractures can be managed in a splint, cast, or functional brace. Splints can be removed for hygiene but provide less support. Functional braces provide circumferential support but require active motion producing muscle contractions to function correctly.[4]

To investigate the optimal method of immobilization for nondisplaced DRFs, O'Connor performed an RCT of 66 patients randomized to removable splint versus casting. Patients with nondisplaced DRFs had better outcomes when treated in a removable splint versus a cast when comparing patient satisfaction, complications related to the cast, functional assessment, and range of motion (ROM) at 6 weeks. However, at 12 weeks, their functional assessment and ROM were no longer significantly different.[5]

Tumia et al randomized 339 displaced and nondisplaced DRFs into treatment with a traditional plaster casts versus Colles prefabricated fracture braces after reduction. There were similar results in both study arms in regard to maintenance of fracture reduction and pain scores. The fracture brace group had better early grip strength at 5 weeks for both manipulated and nonmanipulated fractures. There was no difference in functional outcome between treatment groups.[6] DRFs that have satisfactory reduction either with or without manipulation can thus be treated in a plaster cast or a functional brace.

4.4 Surgery versus Immobilization for Displaced Distal Radius Fracture

The first decision in managing a displaced DRF is determining whether the patient should be treated conservatively or operatively. Normal radiographic parameters of acceptable reduction include 23° of radial inclination, 12 mm of radial height, and 11° of volar angulation. Measuring these radiographic parameters has been found to be reliable and reproducible.[7] The 2009 AAOS clinical guidelines suggested operative fixation for fractures with a postreduction radial shortening greater than 3 mm, dorsal tilt greater than 10°, or greater than 2 mm of intra-articular step-off. Although radiographic criteria exist,[3] there is a continuous debate in the literature on which patients benefit the most from operative management.

McQueen evaluated patients with displaced DRF initially treated with closed reduction. They randomized 120 patients to 4 groups: rereduction and casting, ORIF with a single K-wire and a corticocancellous iliac crest bone graft placed dorsally, spanning external fixation, and a hinged spanning external fixation with early wrist ROM. They found no difference in patient outcome (activities of daily living [ADL], grip strength, and ROM) between the groups although the ORIF arm had superior radiographic results. Carpal malalignment, defined as displacement on the lateral view of the longitudinal axis of the capitate in reference to the longitudinal axis of the radius, was associated with worse ROM, grip strength, and pinch strength, but the overall carpal malalignment was not significantly different between groups.[8] Although this study is well designed and executed, with four study arms, the techniques and technology of ORIF have evolved, leading us to question the current clinical relevance of the results.

Several studies have compared outcomes for displaced DRFs treated with casting versus external fixation. Young randomized 85 displaced DRFs to reduction and casting versus reduction and external fixation. At 7 years postinjury, there was no difference in functional outcome and patient satisfaction between groups. Radiographic malunion was significantly higher in the casted group but this did not correlate with functional outcome.[9] Kreder et al randomized 113 patients with displaced extra-articular fractures to casting versus external fixation with supplemental K-wires. There was a trend towards better function, clinical and radiographic outcomes in the operative group; however, this was not statistically significant. They found no difference in ROM, grip strength, or pinch strength between groups.[10]

Together, these studies suggest that similar functional outcomes can be obtained with surgical and nonsurgical management. However, the groups are heterogeneous and conclusions are difficult to generalize. As such, the decision as to whether to proceed with surgery or not should be shared between the patients and the treating physician.

4.5 The Management of Elderly Patients

DRFs often occur in elderly patients from a fall from a standing height. For the purpose of this chapter, we define elderly as patients older than 60 years. Underlying decreases in bone mineral density (BMD) puts them at higher risk for these low-energy fractures. Their demands and fracture morphology differ from younger patients with high-energy injuries. As such, the optimal treatment of DRFs in the elderly deserves special mention.

Two studies have compared casting to closed reduction percutaneous pinning (CRPP) of displaced extra-articular fractures in patients over the age of 60. A randomized controlled study of 60 patients over 65 years of age with displaced extra-articular DRFs (greater than 20° of dorsal angulation and 5-mm shortening) found no difference in Mayo wrist scores, quality of life, healing time, or complications in those treated with casting versus CRPP. Radiographic outcomes were significantly better in the CRPP group.[11] A similar study performed by Azzopardi et al randomized 57 patients over the age of 60 years with unstable extra-articular DRFs to closed reduction and casting in the operating room versus CRPP. They also reported an improvement in radiographic alignment but no difference in functional outcomes (pain, ROM, grip strength, and ADL). The CRPP group did have improved ulnar deviation, although this was of uncertain significance.[12]

When determining how to optimize the function of elderly patients, it is important to consider ORIF in addition to casting and CRPP. ORIF allows earlier return to activities, which may improve patient function. Arora randomized 73 patients over 65 years of age to ORIF versus casting. The operative group had significantly better radiographic parameters and grip strength. However, there was no difference in ROM or pain at any time point. They also found that functional outcomes were better at 6 and 12 weeks in the operative group but there was no significant difference at 6 and 12 months.[13]

In summary, nonoperative and operative management of DRF in patients over the age of 60 appears to have similar outcomes at 1 year. Operative treatment results in better radiographic alignment and may allow an earlier return of function. As our aging population becomes more active, it is important to individualize treatment for these patients when choosing operative versus nonoperative fracture management.

4.6 Operative Treatment for Displaced Distal Radius Fracture: Method of Fixation

Operative treatment is designed to restore anatomic alignment and maximize a patient's functional outcomes. Multiple options exist ranging from external fixation (bridging versus nonbridging), CRPP, a combination of external fixation with CRPP, and ORIF via multiple different surgical approaches.

4.6.1 Bridging versus Nonbridging External Fixation

External fixation can be used as a temporizing treatment or as definitive fixation. When placing an external fixator, the construct can span the wrist joint, achieving distal fixation in the metacarpals or it can be a nonbridging external fixator, allowing wrist ROM. McQueen et al randomized 60 patients to nonbridging and bridging external fixation and found that patients with nonbridging external fixators had significantly greater grip strength and flexion as well as better maintenance of volar tilt and carpal alignment at 6 weeks, 3 months, 6 months, and 1 year.[14] However, in another RCT of 60 patients, Krisnan found that there was no difference between bridging external fixation and nonbridging external fixator for intra-articular DRFs when comparing postoperative ROM, grip strength, and complications.[15] Although these two studies investigate the same question, they support different conclusions.

4.6.2 Closed Reduction Percutaneous Pinning versus Open Reduction Internal Fixation

CRPP for DRFs has been performed for almost a century with excellent results. ORIF using plate fixation has been gaining in popularity, particularly since the advent of volar plating.

An RCT of 180 patients found no difference in ROM, grip strength, pinch strength, or restoration of radiographic parameters at 2 years postoperatively in patients who underwent ORIF with a dorsal approach versus CRPP.[16] Volar locking plates (VLP) were introduced in 2001 and have had a large impact on the management of displaced DRF. In some parts of the world, this is now the most common approach in the surgical treatment of these injuries.[1] Rozental performed a two-institution RCT comparing ORIF with VLP to CRPP with a specific emphasis on early functional outcomes. They found that patients treated with VLP had significantly improved outcome by disabilities of the arm, shoulder, and hand (DASH) score at 6, 9, and 12 weeks postoperatively as well as significantly improved wrist ROM at 6 and 9 weeks. There was no difference in ROM or functional outcome at 1 year postoperatively. Patients treated with VLP reported better satisfaction with their treatment than patients managed by CRPP.[17] Since then, several RCTs have been performed with similar findings. A large RCT involving 461 patients across 18 trauma centers in the United Kingdom reported no difference in the patient-rated wrist evaluation in the VLP and CRPP groups at 3, 6, or 12 months. Additionally, they did not find a clinically relevant difference in the quality of life at these time points.[18]

Two recent meta-analyses of 7 RCTs including 875 fractures examined the outcomes in patients treated with VLPs versus CRPP. Chaudhry et al concluded that patients treated with VLPs had slightly better function than those treated with CRPP at 3 and 12 months postoperatively. However, at both of these time points, there was less than 10-point difference on DASH, a predetermined value demonstrated to be a clinically significant difference. At 3 months, those treated with VLP had improved flexion and supination, but at 1 year, there was no difference. The authors reported that superficial wound infection requiring oral antibiotics was more common in CRPP group.[19] In analyzing the same seven RCTs, Zong et al concluded that patients with VLPs had significantly improved grip strength, wrist flexion, and supination at 6 months compared to CRPP. They also noted that ORIF with VLP had statistically significantly lower DASH and less postoperative complications including postoperative infections when compared to CRPP.[20]

In conclusion, both VLP and CRPP are viable options in the treatment of displaced DRF although VLP may allow an earlier improvement in function.

4.6.3 Closed Reduction Percutaneous Pinning versus External Fixation

CRPP and external fixation both allow stabilization of DRFs with minimal soft tissue dissection. Harley et al randomized 50 patients with unstable DRFs to CRPP versus external fixation: clinically, there was no significant difference between the treatment groups in ROM, DASH scores, or grip strength.[21] Both techniques thus appear equivalent in the management of these injuries.

4.6.4 Open Reduction Internal Fixation versus External Fixation

Multiple authors have compared DRFs treated with ORIF to external fixation. In 77 patients randomized to ORIF versus external fixation with supplemental CRPP, there was some early improved ROM with volar ORIF at 3 months, but by 6 months and 1 year, the differences diminished. ORIF resulted in better wrist extension and pronation. The external fixation group required twice as many occupational therapy (OT) sessions to achieve these similar outcomes (43 vs. 20). Radiographic outcomes, DASH, pain scores, or grip strength were similar at all time points.[22] Xu randomized 30 patients to ORIF versus external fixation and concluded that there were no significant differences in clinical (ROM, grip strength, and outcome scores) or radiographic (parameters and signs of osteoarthritis [OA]) outcomes at 6, 12, or 24 months.[23] For 75 complex intra-articular DRFs randomized to ORIF versus external fixation with supplemental CRPP, there was no significant difference in fracture reduction radiographically; however, clinical results and grip strength were significantly better at 6 months in the ORIF group.[24] Leung evaluated outcomes at 2 years postoperatively in 144 intra-articular DRFs randomized to ORIF versus external fixation; ORIF had significantly better clinic results and fewer radiographic signs of arthritis at 2 years.[25]

Williksen followed 111 patients for 5 years after randomization to VLP versus external fixation with or without K-wires augmentation. There was no significant difference in Mayo wrist score, visual analog scale (VAS), or QuickDASH at 5 years although the VLP group had better supination and radial deviation. However, the subset with OA C2 fractures[26] had better clinical outcomes when treated with VLP, suggesting more unstable fractures may do better with more stable fixation.[27]

To investigate optimal plating technique, Wei randomized 46 patients into three different fixation techniques: VLP, radial column plating, and external fixation. There was no difference between study arms with regards to DASH score, ROM, or pinch strength at 6 months or 1 year. However, at 3 months, patient outcomes and DASH scores were significantly better in the volarplating group.[28]

In a meta-analysis of 10 RCTs comparing VLF to external fixation, Xie concluded that VLP resulted in better supination at 3 months, lower DASH scores at 12 months, and radiographically improved volar tilt and radial inclination. Additionally, the VLP group had fewer minor surgical complications.[29]

Patients treated with ORIF versus external fixation for DRF thus tend to have better early clinical outcomes but these benefits decrease over time. After 1 year, the method of fixation seems to have little influence on patient outcome.

4.6.5 Implant Type

The type of plate fixation has also been investigated. A small RCT, including 32 patients treated with ORIF with metal versus bioresorbable implants, found no difference in reoperation rate, ROM, or DASH. However, the bioresorbable plates were more expensive with some concerning complications: failure of material, adverse tissue reaction/adhesions, swelling, tendon rupture, and 33% loss of reduction.[30]

4.6.6 Management of the Pronator Quadratus

When performing an ORIF of a DRF with a volar approach, the pronator quadratus (PQ) is routinely taken down to expose the fracture. Authors have evaluated the benefit of repairing the pronator muscle after ORIF. Haberle randomized 60 patients to PQ repair versus no repair and reported no difference in pronation strength, ROM, Mayo, or QuickDASH scores at 6 or 12 weeks between groups. The pronator repair group did have significantly decreased pain (VAS) at 6 weeks with 84 versus 62% of patients having a score between 0 and 2 in the repair versus no repair group, respectively; however, this difference was no longer significant at 12 weeks.[31] Tosti performed a similar trial of 60 patients and found that repairing the PQ after volar plating of a DRF did not significantly improve postoperative ROM, grip strength, DASH, or VAS at 1 year.[32] Repair of the PQ after VLP of DRFs does not seem to be necessary although none of these studies reported on long-term follow-up and the influence of PQ repair on potential tendon ruptures.

4.7 Postoperative Rehabilitation

Postinjury and postoperative OT have been the subject of multiple randomized studies. Ninety-four patients treated with ORIF were randomized to formal OT versus a home exercise plan prescribed by their surgeon. Formal OT did not result in any improvement in ROM or DASH score at 3 or 6 months postoperatively. Actually,

the group undergoing the home exercise plan had statistically significant improvement in extension, ulnar deviation, supination, and grip strength at 6 months postoperatively.[33] A systematic review of 7 RCTs including 358 patients showed no difference in home exercise plan versus a therapist-supervised program following DRF.[34] A Cochrane review of 26 RCT concluded that the current data is insufficient to determine the best form of rehabilitation for patients with DRFs.[35]

When to initiate motion following fixation is a balancing act between stable fixation and preventing stiffness. Allain randomizes 60 patients following trans-styloid K-wire fixation to casting for 1 week (and early ROM) versus 6 weeks of casting for DRFs. The early motion did not change ROM, grip strength, or radiographic loss of reduction.[36] The benefit of formal OT thus remains controversial.

4.8 Management of Complications

After DRFs, a subset of patients develops complex regional pain syndrome (CRPS) although this diagnosis remains controversial. It has been postulated that taking vitamin C postoperatively can reduce the risk of developing CRPS. Zollinger performed an RCT of 427 wrists and found that vitamin C reduces the risk of CRPS in wrist fractures from 10 to 2.4%. Testing different doses of vitamin C, they found 500 mg for 50 days was found to be lowest efficacious dose.[37] However, a more recent meta-analysis of three RCTs (including Zollinger work) found that vitamin C does not reduce the risk of CRPS in DRFs when compared to placebo.[38] Furthermore, surgeons are not in agreement about what constitutes a diagnosis of CRPS in this setting.[39] We cannot recommend for or against the use of vitamin C as prophylaxis against CRPS.

The use of external fixation and CRPP for treatment of fractures has been associated with pin site infections. In an attempt to minimize pin site infection, Egol investigated different types of pin care in a cohort of 120 patients. They found no difference in pin site infection whether pins were treated with weekly dry dressing changes, hydrogen peroxide daily, or chlorhexidine weekly. Pin site complications were 19%, although most were successfully treated with observation and antibiotics.[40]

4.9 Treatment for Osteoporosis

Over half of women have osteoporosis at the time of DRF.[41] A low-energy DRF confers a two to four times increased risk of a secondary fragility fracture.[42] Therefore, it is important to diagnose and treat underlying abnormalities in bone metabolism at the time of initial fracture treatment, while patients are under our care as a captive audience. Unfortunately, the management of osteoporosis is often overlooked.

Rozental conducted a prospective randomized intervention where patients were randomized to have a BMD examination ordered by the treating surgeon with results sent to the primary care physician (PCP) versus a letter sent to the patients' PCP outlining guidelines for osteoporosis screening. The patients randomized to receive BMD testing had two- to threefold greater rates of BMD testing, discussion of osteoporosis with their PCP, and initiation of osteoporosis therapy.[43] As the first-line physician treating osteoporotic fractures, ordering BMD testing increases the likelihood that the patient receives treatment. Additionally, Majumdar demonstrated via a RCT of 272 patients that a multifaceted intervention via patient information packets and a reminder phone call on the importance of diagnosis and treatment of osteoporosis in wrist fracture patients led to improved rates of osteoporosis testing and treatment.[44] Empowering our patients with education can help increase the rate of osteoporosis treatment after fragility fractures.

The timing of bisphosphonate treatment continues to be controversial. Gong has demonstrated that the initiation of bisphosphonate treatment in the acute phase of fracture healing does not impact bone healing or functional outcomes of patients. In his RCT of 50 women over the age of 50, patients were randomized to initiate bisphosphonates 2 weeks versus 3 months after VLP fixation of the distal radius. Patients had equivalent radiographic healing times and DASH scores.[45] In a more recent cohort, Shoji et al enrolled patients on and off bisphosphonate treatment at the time of injury and performed serial radiographic and clinical examinations. No differences were identified between groups. Therefore, we should not be hesitant to begin or continue bisphosphonate treatment in the setting of a fragility fracture of the DRF.

4.10 Conclusion

DRFs are common injuries and have been the focus of many high-quality studies. Based on the existing literature, we recommend immobilization in a cast or splint for nondisplaced injuries as equivalent modalities. We cannot definitely conclude whether displaced fractures should be treated with or without surgery and this decision should be shared between the patient and treating physician. When managing DRFs in an elderly population, similar functional outcomes are seen with nonoperative and operative treatment, although operative fixation may allow earlier return to activities. Risks and benefits of surgical treatment should be discussed with these patients by the physician when individualizing treatment plans.

In terms of operative management, CRPP, external fixation, and ORIF result in similar long-term outcomes although ORIF with a VLP may allow a faster return to function and improved early clinical outcomes. Repair of the PQ during ORIF with VLP does not appear to be necessary.

Postoperatively, patients can elect a self-directed rehabilitation program or formal OT with similar results. Early versus delayed ROM does not change outcomes. We do not routinely employ vitamin C as prophylaxis for CRPS. Lastly, we recommend all postmenopausal women and men over the age of 60 obtain a BMD by dual-energy X-ray absorptiometry after DRF and are systematically assessed for osteoporosis risk. Treatment for osteoporosis with bisphosphonates can be initiated while the fracture is healing.

References

[1] Nellans KW, Kowalski E, Chung KC. The epidemiology of distal radius fractures. Hand Clin 2012;28(2):113–125
[2] Burns PB, Rohrich RJ, Chung KC. The levels of evidence and their role in evidence-based medicine. Plast Reconstr Surg 2011;128(1):305–310
[3] Lichtman DM, Bindra RR, Boyer MI, et al. Treatment of distal radius fractures. J Am Acad Orthop Surg 2010;18(3):180–189
[4] Sarmiento A, Horowitch A, Aboulafia A, Vangsness CT Jr. Functional bracing for comminuted extra-articular fractures of the distal third of the humerus. J Bone Joint Surg Br 1990;72(2):283–287
[5] O'Connor D, Mullett H, Doyle M, Mofidi A, Kutty S, O'Sullivan M. Minimally displaced Colles' fractures: a prospective randomized trial of treatment with a wrist splint or a plaster cast. J Hand Surg [Br] 2003;28(1):50–53
[6] Tumia N, Wardlaw D, Hallett J, Deutman R, Mattsson SA, Sandén B. Aberdeen Colles' fracture brace as a treatment for Colles' fracture. A multicentre, prospective, randomised, controlled trial. J Bone Joint Surg Br 2003;85(1):78–82
[7] Stirling E, Jeffery J, Johnson N, Dias J. Are radiographic measurements of the displacement of a distal radial fracture reliable and reproducible? Bone Joint J 2016;98-B(8):1069–1073
[8] McQueen MM, Hajducka C, Court-Brown CM. Redisplaced unstable fractures of the distal radius: a prospective randomised comparison of four methods of treatment. J Bone Joint Surg Br 1996;78(3):404–409
[9] Young CF, Nanu AM, Checketts RG. Seven-year outcome following Colles' type distal radial fracture. A comparison of two treatment methods. J Hand Surg [Br] 2003;28(5):422–426
[10] Kreder HJ, Agel J, McKee MD, Schemitsch EH, Stephen D, Hanel DP. A randomized, controlled trial of distal radius fractures with metaphyseal displacement but without joint incongruity: closed reduction and casting versus closed reduction, spanning external fixation, and optional percutaneous K-wires. J Orthop Trauma 2006;20(2):115–121
[11] Wong TC, Chiu Y, Tsang WL, Leung WY, Yam SK, Yeung SH. Casting versus percutaneous pinning for extra-articular fractures of the distal radius in an elderly Chinese population: a prospective randomised controlled trial. J Hand Surg Eur Vol 2010;35(3):202–208
[12] Azzopardi T, Ehrendorfer S, Coulton T, Abela M. Unstable extra-articular fractures of the distal radius: a prospective, randomised study of immobilisation in a cast versus supplementary percutaneous pinning. J Bone Joint Surg Br 2005;87(6):837–840
[13] Arora R, Lutz M, Deml C, Krappinger D, Haug L, Gabl M. A prospective randomized trial comparing nonoperative treatment with volar locking plate fixation for displaced and unstable distal radial fractures in patients sixty-five years of age and older. J Bone Joint Surg Am 2011;93(23):2146–2153
[14] McQueen MM. Redisplaced unstable fractures of the distal radius. A randomised, prospective study of bridging versus non-bridging external fixation. J Bone Joint Surg Br 1998;80(4):665–669
[15] Krishnan J, Wigg AER, Walker RW, Slavotinek J. Intra-articular fractures of the distal radius: a prospective randomised controlled

trial comparing static bridging and dynamic non-bridging external fixation. J Hand Surg [Br] 2003;28(5):417–421

[16] Kreder HJ, Hanel DP, Agel J, et al. Indirect reduction and percutaneous fixation versus open reduction and internal fixation for displaced intra-articular fractures of the distal radius: a randomised, controlled trial. J Bone Joint Surg Br 2005;87(6):829–836

[17] Rozental TD, Blazar PE, Franko OI, Chacko AT, Earp BE, Day CS. Functional outcomes for unstable distal radial fractures treated with open reduction and internal fixation or closed reduction and percutaneous fixation. A prospective randomized trial. J Bone Joint Surg Am 2009;91(8):1837–1846

[18] Costa ML, Achten J, Parsons NR, et al; DRAFFT. Study Group. Percutaneous fixation with Kirschner wires versus volar locking plate fixation in adults with dorsally displaced fracture of distal radius: randomised controlled trial. BMJ 2014;349:g4807

[19] Chaudhry H, Kleinlugtenbelt YV, Mundi R, Ristevski B, Goslings JC, Bhandari M. Are Volar Locking Plates Superior to Percutaneous K-wires for Distal Radius Fractures? A Meta-analysis. Clin Orthop Relat Res 2015;473(9):3017–3027

[20] Zong SL, Kan SL, Su LX, Wang B. Meta-analysis for dorsally displaced distal radius fracture fixation: volar locking plate versus percutaneous Kirschner wires. J Orthop Surg Res 2015;10:108

[21] Harley BJ, Scharfenberger A, Beaupre LA, Jomha N, Weber DW. Augmented external fixation versus percutaneous pinning and casting for unstable fractures of the distal radius--a prospective randomized trial. J Hand Surg Am 2004;29(5):815–824

[22] Egol K, Walsh M, Tejwani N, McLaurin T, Wynn C, Paksima N. Bridging external fixation and supplementary Kirschner-wire fixation versus volar locked plating for unstable fractures of the distal radius: a randomised, prospective trial. J Bone Joint Surg Br 2008;90(9):1214–1221

[23] Xu GG, Chan SP, Puhaindran ME, Chew WY. Prospective randomised study of intra-articular fractures of the distal radius: comparison between external fixation and plate fixation. Ann Acad Med Singapore 2009;38(7):600–606

[24] Jeudy J, Steiger V, Boyer P, Cronier P, Bizot P, Massin P. Treatment of complex fractures of the distal radius: a prospective randomised comparison of external fixation 'versus' locked volar plating. Injury 2012;43(2):174–179

[25] Leung F, Tu YK, Chew WY, Chow SP. Comparison of external and percutaneous pin fixation with plate fixation for intra-articular distal radial fractures. A randomized study. J Bone Joint Surg Am 2008;90(1):16–22

[26] Murphy WM, Murphy WM, Colton CL et al. Muller AO classification of fractures. Davos, Switzerland: AO Publishing and AO International; 2006

[27] Williksen JH, Husby T, Hellund JC, Kvernmo HD, Rosales C, Frihagen F. External Fixation and Adjuvant Pins Versus Volar Locking Plate Fixation in Unstable Distal Radius Fractures: A Randomized, Controlled Study With a 5-Year Follow-Up. J Hand Surg Am 2015;40(7):1333–1340

[28] Wei DH, Raizman NM, Bottino CJ, Jobin CM, Strauch RJ, Rosenwasser MP. Unstable distal radial fractures treated with external fixation, a radial column plate, or a volar plate. A prospective randomized trial. J Bone Joint Surg Am 2009;91(7):1568–1577

[29] Xie X, Xie X, Qin H, Shen L, Zhang C. Comparison of internal and external fixation of distal radius fractures. Acta Orthop 2013;84(3):286–291

[30] van Manen CJ, Dekker ML, van Eerten PV, Rhemrev SJ, van Olden GD, van der Elst M. Bio-resorbable versus metal implants in wrist fractures: a randomised trial. Arch Orthop Trauma Surg 2008;128(12):1413–1417

[31] Häberle S, Sandmann GH, Deiler S, et al. Pronator quadratus repair after volar plating of distal radius fractures or not? Results of a prospective randomized trial. Eur J Med Res 2015;20:93

[32] Tosti R, Ilyas AM. Prospective evaluation of pronator quadratus repair following volar plate fixation of distal radius fractures. J Hand Surg Am 2013;38(9):1678–1684

[33] Souer JS, Buijze G, Ring D. A prospective randomized controlled trial comparing occupational therapy with independent exercises after volar plate fixation of a fracture of the distal part of the radius. J Bone Joint Surg Am 2011;93(19):1761–1766

[34] Valdes K, Naughton N, Michlovitz S. Therapist supervised clinic-based therapy versus instruction in a home program following distal radius fracture: a systematic review. J Hand Ther 2014;27(3):165–173, quiz 174

[35] Handoll HH, Elliott J. Rehabilitation for distal radial fractures in adults. Cochrane Database Syst Rev 2015;(9):CD003324

[36] Allain J, le Guilloux P, Le Mouël S, Goutallier D. Trans-styloid fixation of fractures of the distal radius. A prospective randomized comparison between 6- and 1-week postoperative immobilization in 60 fractures. Acta Orthop Scand 1999;70(2):119–123

[37] Zollinger PE, Tuinebreijer WE, Breederveld RS, Kreis RW. Can vitamin C prevent complex regional pain syndrome in patients with wrist fractures? A randomized, controlled, multicenter dose-response study. J Bone Joint Surg Am 2007;89(7):1424–1431

[38] Evaniew N, McCarthy C, Kleinlugtenbelt YV, Ghert M, Bhandari M. Vitamin C to Prevent Complex Regional Pain Syndrome in Patients With Distal Radius Fractures: A Meta-Analysis of Randomized Controlled Trials. J Orthop Trauma 2015;29(8):e235–e241

[39] Del Piñal F. Editorial. I have a dream … reflex sympathetic dystrophy (RSD or Complex Regional Pain Syndrome – CRPS I) does not exist. J Hand Surg Eur Vol 2013;38(6):595–597

[40] Egol KA, Paksima N, Puopolo S, Klugman J, Hiebert R, Koval KJ. Treatment of external fixation pins about the wrist: a prospective, randomized trial. J Bone Joint Surg Am 2006;88(2):349–354

[41] Reed MR, Murray JR, Abdy SE, Francis RM, McCaskie AW. The use of digital X-ray radiogrammetry and peripheral dual energy X-ray absorptiometry in patients attending fracture clinic after distal forearm fracture. Bone 2004;34(4):716–719

[42] Cuddihy MT, Gabriel SE, Crowson CS, O'Fallon WM, Melton LJ III. Forearm fractures as predictors of subsequent osteoporotic fractures. Osteoporos Int 1999;9(6):469–475

[43] Rozental TD, Makhni EC, Day CS, Bouxsein ML. Improving evaluation and treatment for osteoporosis following distal radial fractures. A prospective randomized intervention. J Bone Joint Surg Am 2008;90(5):953–961

[44] Majumdar SR, Johnson JA, McAlister FA, et al. Multifaceted intervention to improve diagnosis and treatment of osteoporosis in patients with recent wrist fracture: a randomized controlled trial. CMAJ 2008;178(5):569–575

[45] Gong HS, Song CH, Lee YH, Rhee SH, Lee HJ, Baek GH. Early initiation of bisphosphonate does not affect healing and outcomes of volar plate fixation of osteoporotic distal radial fractures. J Bone Joint Surg Am 2012;94(19):1729–1736

5 Orthopaedic Treatment: When?

David Warwick, Oliver Townsend

Abstract

Although there are many ways to treat distal radius fractures (DRFs), the majority of DRFs can be managed nonoperatively. The distal radius can tolerate quite marked displacement without significant impact on function. Furthermore, symptomatic arthritis of the wrist is very uncommon following DRFs, even in the presence of joint line displacement and radiological features of arthritis.

So when should we operate? The evidence for surgery is less compelling than some surgeons imagine. The literature is flawed and recommendations or guidelines for treatment are inconsistent and difficult to generalize to an individual patient.

In patients over 65, there is consistent evidence that surgery does not influence the outcome, as lower functional demands mean malunion is better tolerated, and poorer bone quality increases the risk of fixation failure. Younger patients with higher demands are more likely to benefit from greater anatomical alignment. Although the risk of complications is higher with surgery, nonoperative management is certainly not without risk; choosing the "correct" treatment from the many options is not always easy and requires careful risk–benefit analysis.

The author's philosophy is as follows: Every case is different and the patient must be involved in the decision-making. Current common radiological "indications" for surgery (dorsal tilt and ulnar shortening) are insufficient, and other important radiological parameters should also be considered (radial, dorsal, and palmar translation). Even more than radiology, patient factors must be considered. Unstable fractures may benefit from early stabilization, though corrective osteotomy or delayed plate fixation may not affect the final outcome; therefore, attempting nonoperative management first may be beneficial. If the patient needs earlier mobilization and return to function, where a few weeks will make a difference, early surgery may be of benefit.

Keywords: distal radius fracture, nonoperative, malalignment, unstable, translation, functional outcome

5.1 *When* the Evidence and Benefits of Nonoperative Treatment Have Been Considered

5.1.1 Why Surgery Is Not Usually Needed

Surgery might be fun, fulfilling, exciting, and lucrative but it is also expensive, time-consuming, and potentially dangerous. We should remember that the great majority of distal radius fractures (DRFs) do not need surgical treatment. New techniques do not necessarily offer an advantage. We should always resist the temptation to perform surgery that will probably not improve patients' outcomes or that would put them at unnecessary risk of harm. The evidence for surgery is by no means as compelling as some proponents might imagine.[1] Indeed, the distal radius seems biologically designed to survive injury.[2]

There is scant evidence that radiology correlates strongly with outcome and most fractures will fare perfectly well even if they heal with modest displacement.[3,4,5,6] Furthermore, even after surgery, function does not seem to correlate well with the radiographic appearance.[7] Several studies show that fractures with modest displacement (intra- or extra-articular) do not predispose to symptomatic arthritis,[8,9,10,11,12] and there is consistent evidence that surgery for those over 65 does not influence outcome.[1,13,14,15] Surgery is expensive, particularly with modern implants,[16] and of course hazardous; any operation can harm patients and make them worse than nonoperative care.[17,18,19]

5.1.2 Nonoperative Treatment Is Usually Effective

An undisplaced stable crack through the distal radius will heal uneventfully with just 3 weeks in a cast.[20,21]

For a displaced fracture, manipulation under a local or regional anesthesia and then plaster are usually adequate; X-rays should be taken at the end of the first and second week to ensure that it has not slipped. If particularly unstable, X-rays into the third week are justified.[22,23] If the fracture does slip, gentle manipulation and replaster will suffice for many.

5.1.3 Surgery Carries Risk

Anesthetic complications are exceedingly unusual. Risks include an allergy to local anesthesia, neurological damage with an axillary block, and a cardiovascular event with a general anesthetic.

Volar plate fixation has a material risk. In a systematic review of 33 articles and 1,817 cases, Bentohami et al found a 16.5% complication rate: 8.8% minor (e.g., superficial infection, complex regional pain syndrome (CRPS), tendon irritation, and neuritis) and 7.7% major (e.g., hardware failure, deep infection, and tendon rupture).[17] Kirschner wires (K-wires) are even more hazardous than plates with 26 to 28% suffering a complication, including pin track infection, carpal tunnel syndrome due to fragment migration, and corrective osteotomy for malunion.[24,25] In a literature review, Diaz-Garcia et al found complications requiring surgery in 11% of those having volar plates and 1% in those having a plaster cast.[14]

5.1.4 Risks of Nonoperative Intervention

The patient and surgeon must also be aware that nonoperative care is not without risk.[26] Risks include:
- Tight plaster cast—predisposes to CRPS.[27,28]
- Poor fitting cast to include metacarpophalangeal (MP) joint—MP contracture.
- Excessive flexion—carpal tunnel syndrome.
- Loss of position and thus an avoidable unsatisfactory outcome.
- Losing opportunity for early simple fixation, requiring later complex osteotomy and fixation.
- Extensor pollicis longus rupture.

5.2 *When* the Literature Recommendations Have Been Considered

5.2.1 Drawbacks of the Literature

The recommendations or guidelines for treatment are inconsistent. This reflects the conflict between surgical experience and insufficient literature. Randomized trials are rarely translatable to clinical practice because of marked heterogeneity, exclusion criteria, and debatable outcome measures. Hence, apparently compelling studies comparing wires and plates[29] can be reasonably criticized.[30]

Furthermore, guidelines tend to be based on simple parameters of dorsal tilt and ulnar shortening; they do not capture more subtle but probably equally important measurements such as radial, dorsal, and palmar translation.

5.2.2 Authors' Recommendations

Some authors propose their own guidelines for surgery. See ▶ Table 5.1.

5.2.3 Consensus Review

Many authors and professional bodies have produced recommendations on indications for surgery. For example, the Danish Health and Medicines Authority and the American Academy of Orthopaedic Surgeons (AAOS) have produced clinical practice guidelines after a thorough literature review and expert panel consensus (▶ Table 5.1).[31,32] What is notable is the lack of consensus on the parameters for which surgery is indicated. The AAOS were only able to recommend their recommendations with "moderate" strength (▶ Table 5.1) due to a lack of compelling strong evidence[32]; others, including Green's textbook and the British Orthopaedic Association, decline to make specific recommendations for parameters indicating surgery, instead advising clinical discretion upon consideration of the individual patient and factors influencing fracture stability.[33,34]

5.3 *When* Age Has Been Considered

5.3.1 Older Age

Age is an important consideration. As patients get older, they have lower demands and therefore tolerate malunion better. They are also at higher risk of fixation failure due to osteoporosis. The AAOS practice guidelines could not conclusively recommend surgery for those over 55.[32]

Table 5.1 Parameters for which surgery is recommended

	Expert opinion and systematic review	Dorsal tilt (°)	Shortening	Radial inclination (°)	Step-off
American Association of Orthopaedic Surgeons[32]	Expert opinion and literature review	>10	>3 mm	–	>2 mm
Danish Health and Medicines Authority[31]	Expert opinion and literature review	>10	>2 mm	–	>2 mm
Ilyas and Jupiter[35]	Author opinion	>15	</=5 mm	<15	2 mm
Lidstrom[3]	Author opinion	>15	>5 mm	–	>2 mm
Orthobullets[36]		> 5° and within 20° of contralateral side	>5 mm	–	>2 mm
Green's Operative Hand Surgery (textbook)[33]	Expert opinion and literature review	No specific recommendations	No specific recommendations	No specific recommendations	No specific recommendations
British Orthopaedic Association Standards for Trauma[34]	NICE and BSSH guidelines	"Consider"	–	–	"Consider"

Abbreviations: BSSH, British Society for Surgery of the Hand; NICE, National Institute for Health and Care Excellence.

Researchers consistently fail to find benefit for operating on those over 60 or 65 with regards to functional outcome regardless of radiological anatomy.[6,14,37]

5.3.2 Younger Age

Those of a younger age with higher demands might be more aware of the physiological consequences of altered radiological anatomy. Gliatis et al suggest that function (measured with the patient evaluation measure) is less likely to be acceptable with a dorsal angulation of >10° in younger patients (median age 35, all below 49)[38]; Grewal and MacDermid found that there was a correlation between radiological position and outcome following extra-articular DRFs, but the strength of that correlation decreased with age and was not measurable over the age of 65.[13] These authors found that over the age of 65, 8 patients with malaligned fractures (malalignment defined as dorsal angulation >10°, radial inclination <15°, or positive ulnar variance ≥3 mm) would need corrective surgery to avoid one bad outcome (defined by poor disabilities of the arm, shoulder, and hand [DASH] score), whereas under the age of 65, only two patients would need surgery for one to benefit.[13]

5.4 *When* There Is a Predictable Risk of Poor Outcome

5.4.1 Exclusion Bias

As discussed above, the literature cannot be readily applied to an individual patient. Finsen and colleagues found in a series of 260 patients treated nonoperatively that although function correlated with anatomy, the magnitude was very small with only 11% of the variability in outcome being explained by the combination of ulnar variance, dorsal angulation, and radial inclination.[5] However, this series, as in other nonoperative series, will not include those in whom the surgeon has detected other variables such as high demand, intra-articular displacement, propensity to slip, marked displacement or joint subluxation such that these have been treated surgically and thus excluded from the apparently favorable outcome. The same argument can apply to randomized trials comparing wires, plasters, or plates.

5.4.2 Distal Radioulnar Joint Incongruity

Volar tilt or dorsal tilt will alter congruity of the distal radioulnar joint (DRUJ). It is difficult to predict the threshold of tilt at which fractures will lose rotation if left untreated because different patients are likely to be affected differently, depending on the relative concavity or flatness of the sigmoid notch. Nevertheless, abnormal volar or dorsal tilt will affect rotation.[39,40]

Rotation will also be affected by radial translation of the distal radius[41] as well as by dorsal/palmar *translation*. These parameters are not captured in the usual radiological functional studies discussed above. While computed tomography scans are not routinely performed, obvious incongruity on the transverse images would be a prompt to surgical reduction.

In clinical practice, it is commonly observed that loss of rotation with a malunited DRF will cause substantial disability and will usually respond well to corrective osteotomy of the radius. As the tilt is corrected, rotation returns (unless there is secondary capsular contracture, which may also need releasing).

5.4.3 Adaptive Midcarpal Malalignment

If the distal radius heals with marked dorsal or volar tilt, then the midcarpal joint will compensate to align the hand axially with the carpus. This can theoretically lead to midcarpal pain and weakness as well as altered joint forces. The literature is sparse on this point, but one's experience from patients who present some time after injury for a corrective osteotomy shows that malunion with midcarpal malalignment can be problematic. Thus, again it seems sensible to correct obvious midcarpal malalignment by nonoperative or operative means.

5.4.4 Positive Ulnar Variance

Shortening of the radius will inevitably cause impaction of the ulnar head into the lunotriquetral joint. The threshold at which this causes pain and reduced function will vary but most sources agree at 3 to 5 mm in younger patients. In the elderly, there is a lower risk.

Reducing the radial length is easy but maintenance can be difficult with osteopenic bone; plaster cast and even K-wires may not be reliable. A volar locking plate (VLP) is perhaps most suitable if indicated (and the surgeon must be cautious about invading some elderly patients). For some very impacted fractures, a distraction device (external fixator or internal bridging plate) might even be considered (again with due circumspection balancing the potential complications, cost and lack of clear evidence of benefit).

5.4.5 Fracture Dislocation

Not captured by the plethora of radiology outcomes papers because they are usually treated operatively, a transverse shear fracture into the distal radius articular surface with volar (Barton) or dorsal subluxation of the carpus is highly unstable and will lead to a poor outcome unless treated meticulously. Control by nonoperative means is challenging and if resources are available, surgery is usually preferred.

5.5 *When* There Is a Predictable Risk of Instability

5.5.1 Instability

While it is true that most fractures can and should be managed nonoperatively, cast immobilization requires not just the skill of a well-molded cast[42] but also regular radiological review for at least 14 days and into the third week for very unstable fractures.

If a fracture slips, then it can be remanipulated but if the fracture is unstable, then further slipping is likely, especially with increasing age.[43] Therefore, for particularly unstable fractures, to avoid repeated X-rays and displacement into a predictably unfavorable position, earlier stabilization may be chosen. A trial of nonoperative management is justified as volar plate fixation delayed for up to 30 days does not appear to affect outcome.[44]

5.5.2 Prediction of Instability

Various methods have been used to predict failure of cast immobilization.

Lafontaine Criteria

Lafontaine and colleagues proposed that if three or more of five criteria were present prior to reduction, then the fracture would likely lose position in a cast.[45]
- Dorsal angulation >20°.
- Dorsal comminution.
- Intra-articular involvement.
- Associated ulnar fracture.
- Age 60+ years.

McQueen Formula

A formula was devised to predict malunion.[46] The criteria are:
- Age.
- Dorsal comminution (prereduction).
- Ulnar variance (prereduction).
- Ability to perform own grocery shopping (= independence).

The formula is then derived as:

Probability of Malunion
= (0.04 × age) − 0.8 (if independent)
+ 0.53 (if dorsal comminution)
+ (0.09 × ulnar variance at presentation)
− 1.65

Volar Hook

Martina and colleagues validated these methods in 168 patients in predicting radial height, ulnar variance, and radial tilt but not dorsal/volar tilt or midcarpal malalignment. They found that the latter could be maintained by hooking of the volar cortex in the initial reduction.[47] Age was the most significant factor of all in slipping of the position (albeit without evidence that the loss of position actually matters with advanced age).

5.6 *When* There Is a Predictable Risk of Symptomatic Arthritis

5.6.1 Does Arthritis Really Matter in the Hand and Wrist?

Concave surfaces in the hand and wrist fare better than we might imagine when there is a displaced intra-articular fracture. The joint surfaces spread apart then fill with scar and thus will tolerate incongruity. The hand does not carry as much impact or load as the lower limb. Even if arthritis develops, we know from our clinical experience of joints elsewhere (thumb carpometacarpal joint, scaphotrapeziotrapezoidal joint, proximal interphalangeal joints, and radioscaphoid joint) that advanced radiological change can, and probably usually does, exist without significant symptoms.

5.6.2 How Often Does a Hand Surgeon Actually See Arthritis after a Distal Radius Fracture?

On reflection, a hand surgeon might realize that patients never present with symptomatic wrist arthritis many years after a DRF. It is simply not a part of routine practice to fuse or replace a wrist 10 or 20 years after a fracture. If we do operate for persisting or developing symptoms after a DRF, then it is usually in the first year or so when the unresolving consequences of ulnocarpal impaction or carpal malalignment are apparent. See Chapter 5.9.3: Rescuing a Wrong Decision with Corrective Osteotomy.

5.6.3 Literature Evidence

The risk of arthritis is low with modestly displaced fractures: the orthopaedic mantra that joint line displacement leads to arthritis has not been established for the DRF. Long-term studies all find symptomatic arthritis to be very uncommon.[4,8,9,10,11]

Even a 2-mm gap, once thought to be relevant,[48] appears on reflection not as significant.[49] While intra-articular malunion does result in accelerated progression

Table 5.2 Options for treatment of distal radius fractures

Nonoperative	Closed reduction and fixation	Open reduction and internal fixation	Other
Bandage	K-wires	Simple plates	Arthroscopic reduction and fixation
Velcro and metal splint	External fixator (static and dynamic)	Volar locking plates	
Plaster cast	Intramedullary nail	Fragment-specific plates (e.g., volar rim, dorsoulnar corner, etc.)	
	Pins and plaster	Internal bridge plate	

Abbreviation: K-wires, Kirschner wires.

to radiographic features of post-traumatic arthritis, long-term postoperative outcome data shows little correlation with functional outcome and patient satisfaction.[50]

5.7 *When* the Appropriate Method Is Available

There are many ways to treat a DRF; see ▶ Table 5.2 for available methods.

The more complex methods will not be available in some economic circumstances; even if they are, some methods are technically very complex and the patient may be served better by a simple technique unless the surgical expertise is available to match the device. A more complex and expensive technique by no means guarantees a better result.

5.8 *When* the Patient Understands the Options and the Risks

5.8.1 The Patient's Rights

In some countries, litigation is a major influence on healthcare delivery. Even if the lawyers are not prowling, the patients have an absolute right to be involved fully in deciding the most suitable treatment for them as an individual. Each patient will have own view on risk, cost, and acceptable outcome. The eventual treatment must always be personalized.

5.8.2 Honest Consent

Meticulous consent requires a full and balanced explanation of options and risks and outcomes. In addition, the information upon which to base informed consent, despite endless research, is itself uncertain. In the consent process, we must clearly share and document the uncertainty.

5.8.3 Personalized Treatment

A patient without insurance may well choose to have the simplest option of a plaster or percutaneous wires rather than be subjected to the expense of a glamorous implant with no evidence of superiority. A professional musician with a minimally displaced fracture may not want to risk the smallest chance of a tendon rupture with K-wires or a plate. A self-employed dentist might want to have a plate for a minimally displaced fracture so that he can return to practice within 2 weeks.

5.9 *When* the Patient Prefers to Have Urgent Surgery that May Not Be Needed rather than Wait for a Corrective Osteotomy

5.9.1 Natural History of Recovery after Distal Radius Fracture

When Does a Distal Radius Fracture Stop Recovering?

Data on the rate of recovery after DRF are sparse; yet patients want to know how long they need to wait after the injury before realizing their final outcome. These data would also help the surgeon advise on when to consider corrective osteotomy if the fracture has not recovered well enough. Clinical experience would suggest 6 to 12 months.

Ulnar Corner Pain

Ulnar corner pain is common after DRF, with causes to include impaction of the ulnar head, incongruity of the DRUJ, ulnar styloid fracture, triangular fibrocartilage complex perforation, and lunotriquetral rupture.

Ulnar pain tends to improve over time and should be observed for at least several months. A longitudinal study of outcome after DRF surgery found that of 140 patients with ulnar corner pain after DRF surgery, 16% had ulnar corner pain at 3 months, 8% at 6 months, and only 2% at 12 months.[51]

Functional Recovery

After nonoperative treatment, the majority of recovery occurs within 6 months with very little further improvement by 12 months.[52] A meta-analysis of 46 studies of patients treated for DRF with volar plate fixation found that function continues to improve for 12 months after fixation of DRF.[53]

5.9.2 Managing Uncertainty

The Grey Zone

The correct choice of treatment is not easy. There are many options and our knowledge base is incomplete. We should, therefore, recognize that there is a "grey zone" and sometimes we cannot decide whether to treat early or wait for the natural history to emerge. Surgeons must learn to manage this type of conflict, which is a constant part of their professional life.[54]

Pearl of Wisdom

Reproduced below is some advice provided by the author to the International Federation of Societies for Surgery of the Hand Ezine in 2016[55]:

Sometimes we face a dilemma when advising a patient with a displaced DRF. Should we offer surgery or should we not?

Of course, we monitor the fracture for the first 10 to 14 days. Some fractures are so displaced initially, or displace so rapidly after an initial closed reduction in the emergency room, that surgical stabilization seems obvious. Not to do so would predictably lead to a poor result. However, what amount of angulation/shortening can be accepted? We know that in fact, patients with extra-articular radius fractures (and indeed intra-articular as well) can recover well regardless of the final anatomical position,[5] especially in older and lower demand patients. Thus, surgery for anatomical perfection is by no means always needed. We also know that volar plate fixation is not without risk—16% get a complication[17] and is an expensive intervention. Finally, we also know that distal radius osteotomy for an extra-articular fracture is a reliable operation with good results when performed carefully, before secondary changes in the midcarpus and the DRUJ.

Therefore, if a patient has a fracture with 2 or 3 mm of shortening and/or 10 to 15° of dorsal tilt at the 2-week X-ray, do we accept or do we operate? If the patient is left alone and then goes on to a symptomatic malunion, they will be dissatisfied and may even litigate. However, supposing a volar plate is inflicted on them and the patients then had a tendon rupture or infection, they might be equally dissatisfied that surgery was given with scant evidence of benefit.

It is always wise to avoid unnecessary surgery—expensive and hazardous. Therefore, I try and frame the discussion with the patient as follows:

If we operate now for this mildly displaced fracture, there is a 100% chance of a precipitous operation now for your fracture for which there is only a 20% chance of really needing an operation (osteotomy) in the future were you to have waited instead. But if we avoid surgery now, and wait and see instead, there is only a 20% chance of you needing an operation in the future; that operation (osteotomy) is almost the same as surgery now—a cut at the front of the wrist and a metal plate but perhaps with a small incision from the edge of the hip for some bone graft or perhaps some artificial material in the gap.

5.9.3 Rescuing a Wrong Decision with Corrective Osteotomy

When to Make the Decision

A patient will have almost reached the final outcome by 6 to 12 months and if that is unsatisfactory, and if the malalignment is suitable for an osteotomy, then the expected benefits and the potential risks of that intervention can then be discussed.

Results of Osteotomy

Patients may wisely choose to wait to see their own outcome rather than to have urgent treatment. If they then find that they are in the small proportion who do not fare well with a modestly displaced radiological configuration, then they will be reassured to know that the results of a later osteotomy can be very satisfactory and probably not different from primary surgery. This was shown in a review of ulnar shortening osteotomy[56] and in several studies of radial corrective osteotomy.[57,58,59]

5.10 *When* the Patient Wants Early Return of Function

A fracture treated by volar plate fixation will have earlier restoration of function if mobilized immediately rather than at 5 weeks.[60] K-wire fixation or plaster cast fixation do not allow early mobilization. Early return to function and avoiding a cast is very important for many patients—the self-employed, the carer, the traveler, and the musician. While randomized studies of various techniques examine function at 3 months or even a year and may find little or no difference, the lost early weeks are not captured.[30] Meta-analysis of seven studies comparing VLP and K-wires showed a small advantage for plates in DASH at 3 and 12 months although not reaching a minimal clinically important difference of 10 points; supination and flexion had small improvements until 3 months but then equalized.[61] Two of the included studies had earlier comparisons. Karantana et al found a significant advantage for plates over wires with regard to function and driving at 6 weeks, which had evaporated by 3 months.[62] Rozental compared DASH at 6 weeks and found a score of 27 in the plate group compared with 53 in the wire group.[25] Arora and colleagues found a similar advantage for plates over plaster in patients over 65 in the first 6 to 12 weeks but not by 6 months.[26]

Thus, if a patient wants or needs early return to function, where a few weeks make a big difference, then surgery (subject of course to understanding of risks and benefits) is an option they may choose; if surgery is offered in this context, then volar plates without postoperative immobilization would have an advantage over K-wires.

5.11 *When* Cost-Benefit Analysis Supports Surgery

All health economies are strained by the costs of health care. Doctors are custodians of healthcare resources. If money is spent on one intervention that will mean less money is available for another intervention.

Health economics is a complex topic. On face value, treatment in plaster is cheaper than surgery, and treatment with wires is cheaper than treatment with plates.[16,63] Such studies should be interpreted with caution. The studies are only as valid as the sampling. If a study only included a very small proportion of those eligible,[29] then it is quite possible that those who would have chosen to benefit from the potential early recovery of function with VLP would not have chosen a study that might inflict wires or plaster upon them and thus excluded themselves. The patients chosen for the comparative study may have been older and thus not so likely to benefit from quicker return to work. These studies do not include the personal benefit to the self-employed of early return to work or the return to taxpaying status of other workers, which might readily offset the cost of the plate over wires. Moreover, while plaster or wires are cheaper than a plate, they incur the costs of repeated follow-up, plaster change, radiology to exclude slippage, and eventual surgery for those who do slip. They also incur the cost of hospital transport and parking as well as a considerable burden on the family and social support. The patient themselves may be a primary caregiver and therefore even a few weeks earlier return to driving and independence may reduce the family's social cost that would otherwise be inflated with plaster or K-wire treatment.

Only when all these factors are fully weighed, the real cost-effectiveness can be calculated.

5.12 Conclusion

When deciding whether to manage a DRF operatively, there are a number of important considerations to take into account. The majority of DRFs do not require surgical management and can be adequately managed conservatively with excellent outcomes. When the patient is over 65, conservative management results in no significant difference in functional outcome compared with operative management even in the presence of radiological deformity, as reduced functional demands mean this is well tolerated. When faced with young patients with higher functional demands and unstable fractures, surgery can produce superior outcomes, especially in the short term.

The authors' philosophy is as follows: Every case is different and the patient must be involved in the decision-making. Current common radiological "indications" for surgery (dorsal tilt and ulnar shortening) are insufficient, and other important radiological parameters should also be considered (radial, dorsal, and palmar translation). Even more than radiology, patient factors must be considered. Unstable fractures may benefit from early stabilization, though corrective osteotomy or delayed plate fixation may not affect the final outcome; therefore, attempting nonoperative management first may be beneficial. If the patient needs earlier mobilization and return to function, where a few weeks will make a difference, then early surgery may be of benefit.

References

[1] Diaz-Garcia RJ, Chung KC. Common myths and evidence in the management of distal radius fractures. Hand Clin 2012;28(2):127–133
[2] Uzoigwe C, Johnson N. Wrist function in malunion: Is the distal radius designed to retain function in the face of fracture? Ann R Coll Surg Engl 2016;98(7):442–445
[3] Lidstrom A. Fractures of the distal end of the radius. A clinical and statistical study of end results. Acta Orthop Scand Suppl 1959;41:1–118
[4] Warwick D, Field J, Prothero D, Gibson A, Bannister GC. Function ten years after Colles' fracture. Clin Orthop Relat Res 1993;(295):270–274
[5] Finsen V, Rod O, Rød K, Rajabi B, Alm-Paulsen PS, Russwurm H. The relationship between displacement and clinical outcome after distal radius (Colles') fracture. J Hand Surg Eur Vol 2013;38(2):116–126
[6] Song J, Yu AX, Li ZH. Comparison of conservative and operative treatment for distal radius fracture: a meta-analysis of randomized controlled trials. Int J Clin Exp Med 2015;8(10):17023–17035
[7] Plant CE, Parsons NR, Costa ML. Do radiological and functional outcomes correlate for fractures of the distal radius? Bone Joint J 2017;99-B(3):376–382
[8] Kopylov P, Johnell O, Redlund-Johnell I, Bengner U. Fractures of the distal end of the radius in young adults: a 30-year follow-up. J Hand Surg [Br] 1993;18(1):45–49
[9] Goldfarb CA, Rudzki JR, Catalano LW, Hughes M, Borrelli J Jr. Fifteen-year outcome of displaced intra-articular fractures of the distal radius. J Hand Surg Am 2006;31(4):633–639
[10] Lutz M, Arora R, Smekal V, et al. [Long-term results following ORIF of dorsal dislocated distal intraarticular radius fractures] Handchir Mikrochir Plast Chir 2007;39(1):54–59
[11] Forward DP, Davis TRC, Sithole JS. Do young patients with malunited fractures of the distal radius inevitably develop symptomatic post-traumatic osteoarthritis? JBJS 2008;90B:629–637
[12] Haus BM, Jupiter JB. Intra-articular fractures of the distal end of the radius in young adults: reexamined as evidence-based and outcomes medicine. J Bone Joint Surg Am 2009;91(12):2984–2991
[13] Grewal R, MacDermid JC. The risk of adverse outcomes in extra-articular distal radius fractures is increased with malalignment in

patients of all ages but mitigated in older patients. J Hand Surg Am 2007;32(7):962–970

[14] Diaz-Garcia RJ, Oda T, Shauver MJ, Chung KC. A systematic review of outcomes and complications of treating unstable distal radius fractures in the elderly. J Hand Surg Am 2011;36(5): 824-8-35.e2

[15] Chen Y, Chen X, Li Z, Yan H, Zhou F, Gao W. Safety and Efficacy of Operative Versus Nonsurgical Management of Distal Radius Fractures in Elderly Patients: A Systematic Review and Meta-analysis. J Hand Surg Am 2016;41(3):404–413

[16] Pang EQ, Truntzer J, Baker L, Harris AHS, Gardner MJ, Kamal RN. Cost minimization analysis of the treatment of distal radial fractures in the elderly. Bone Joint J 2018;100-B(2):205–211

[17] Bentohami A, de Burlet K, de Korte N, van den Bekerom MP, Goslings JC, Schep NW. Complications following volar locking plate fixation for distal radial fractures: a systematic review. J Hand Surg Eur Vol 2014;39(7):745–754

[18] Lutz K, Yeoh KM, MacDermid JC, Symonette C, Grewal R. Complications associated with operative versus nonsurgical treatment of distal radius fractures in patients aged 65 years and older. J Hand Surg Am 2014;39(7):1280–1286

[19] Azzi AJ, Aldekhayel S, Boehm KS, Zadeh T. Tendon rupture and tenosynovitis following distal radius fractures: a systematic review. Plast Reconstr Surg 2017;139:717–724

[20] Jensen MR, Andersen KH, Jensen CH. Management of undisplaced or minimally displaced Colles' fracture: One or three weeks of immobilization. J Orthop Sci 1997;2(6):424–427

[21] Vang Hansen F, Staunstrup H, Mikkelsen S. A comparison of 3 and 5 weeks immobilization for older type 1 and 2 Colles' fractures. J Hand Surg [Br] 1998;23(3):400–401

[22] Lichtman DM, Bindra RR, Boyer MI, et al; American Academy of Orthopaedic Surgeons. American Academy of Orthopaedic Surgeons clinical practice guideline on: the treatment of distal radius fractures. J Bone Joint Surg Am 2011;93(8):775–778

[23] Wadsten MA, Sjödén GO, Buttazzoni GG, Buttazzoni C, Englund E, Sayed-Noor AS. The influence of late displacement in distal radius fractures on function, grip strength, range of motion and quality of life. J Hand Surg Eur Vol 2018;43(2):131–136

[24] McFadyen I, Field J, McCann P, Ward J, Nicol S, Curwen C. Should unstable extra-articular distal radial fractures be treated with fixed-angle volar-locked plates or percutaneous Kirschner wires? A prospective randomised controlled trial. Injury 2011;42(2):162–166

[25] Rozental TD, Blazar PE, Franko OI, Chacko AT, Earp BE, Day CS. Functional outcomes for unstable distal radial fractures treated with open reduction and internal fixation or closed reduction and percutaneous fixation. A prospective randomized trial. J Bone Joint Surg Am 2009;91(8):1837–1846

[26] Arora R, Lutz M, Deml C, Krappinger D, Haug L, Gabl M. A prospective randomized trial comparing nonoperative treatment with volar locking plate fixation for displaced and unstable distal radial fractures in patients sixty-five years of age and older. J Bone Joint Surg Am 2011;93(23):2146–2153

[27] Field J, Protheroe DL, Atkins RM. Algodystrophy after Colles fractures is associated with secondary tightness of casts. J Bone Joint Surg Br 1994;76(6):901–905

[28] Gillespie S, Cowell F, Cheung G, Brown D. Can we reduce the incidence of complex regional pain syndrome type I in distal radius fractures? The Liverpool experience. Hand Ther 2016;21(4):123–130

[29] Costa ML, Achten J, Parsons NR, et al; DRAFFT Study Group. Percutaneous fixation with Kirschner wires versus volar locking plate fixation in adults with dorsally displaced fracture of distal radius: randomised controlled trial. BMJ 2014;349:g4807

[30] Fullilove S, Gozzard C. Dorsally displaced fractures of the distal radius: a critical appraisal of the DRAFFT (distal radius acute fracture fixation trial) study. Bone Joint J 2016;98-B(3):298–300

[31] Danish Health Authority. National clinical guidance on the treatment of distal radial fractures. 2016. https://www.sst.dk/en/publications/2014/~/media/22E568AA633C49A9A0A128D5FD-C4D8B7.ashx. Accessed April 19, 2018

[32] American Association of Orthopedic Surgeons. The treatment of distal radius fractures: Guideline and evidence report. 2009. https://www.aaos.org/research/guidelines/drfguideline.pdf. Accessed April 19, 2018

[33] Wolfe SW, Hotchkiss RN, Kozin SH, Pederson WC, Cohen MS, eds. Green's Operative Hand Surgery, Seventh Edition. Chapter 15. Philadelphia, PA: Elsevier; 2017

[34] British Orthopaedic Association. British Orthopaedic Association Audit Standards for Trauma (BOAST): The management of distal radial fractures. 2017. https://www.boa.ac.uk/wp-content/uploads/2017/12/BOAST-Management-of-Distal-Radial-Fractures.pdf. Accessed April 19, 2018

[35] Ilyas AM, Jupiter JB. Distal radius fractures- classification and indication. Hand Clin 2010;26(1):37–42

[36] Orthobullets. https://www.orthobullets.com/trauma/1027/distal-radius-fractures. Accessed April 19, 2018

[37] Wong TC, Chiu Y, Tsang WL, Leung WY, Yam SK, Yeung SH. Casting versus percutaneous pinning for extra-articular fractures of the distal radius in an elderly Chinese population: a prospective randomised controlled trial. J Hand Surg Eur Vol 2010;35(3):202–208

[38] Gliatis JD, Plessas SJ, Davis TR. Outcome of distal radial fractures in young adults. J Hand Surg [Br] 2000;25(6):535–543

[39] Nishiwaki M, Welsh MF, Gammon B, Ferreira LM, Johnson JA, King GJ. Effect of Volarly Angulated Distal Radius Fractures on Forearm Rotation and Distal Radioulnar Joint Kinematics. J Hand Surg Am 2015;40(11):2236–2242

[40] Xing SG, Chen YR, Xie RG, Tang JB. In Vivo Contact Characteristics of Distal Radioulnar Joint With Malunited Distal Radius During Wrist Motion. J Hand Surg Am 2015;40(11):2243–2248

[41] Ross M, Allen L, Couzens GB. Correction of Residual Radial Translation of the Distal Fragment in Distal Radius Fracture Open Reduction. J Hand Surg Am 2015;40(12):2465–2470

[42] Charnley J. The Colles' Fracture. In: The Closed Treatment of Common Fractures. 4th ed. Cambridge: Cambridge University Press; 2003:128–142

[43] McQueen MM, Hajducka C, Court-Brown CM. Redisplaced unstable fractures of the distal radius: a prospective randomised comparison of four methods of treatment. J Bone Joint Surg Br 1996;78(3):404–409

[44] Weil YA, Mosheiff R, Firman S, Liebergall M, Khoury A. Outcome of delayed primary internal fixation of distal radius fractures: a comparative study. Injury 2014;45(6):960–964

[45] Lafontaine M, Hardy D, Delince P. Stability assessment of distal radius fractures. Injury 1989;20(4):208–210

[46] Mackenney PJ, McQueen MM, Elton R. Prediction of instability in distal radial fractures. J Bone Joint Surg Am 2006;88(9):1944–1951

[47] LaMartina J, Jawa A, Stucken C, Merlin G, Tornetta P III. Predicting alignment after closed reduction and casting of distal radius fractures. J Hand Surg Am 2015;40(5):934–939

[48] Knirk JL, Jupiter JB. Intra-articular fractures of the distal end of the radius in young adults. J Bone Joint Surg Am 1986;68(5):647–659

[49] Haus BM, Jupiter JB. Intra-articular fractures of the distal end of the radius in young adults: reexamined as evidence-based and outcomes medicine. J Bone Joint Surg Am 2009;91(12):2984–2991

[50] Catalano LW III, Cole RJ, Gelberman RH, Evanoff BA, Gilula LA, Borrelli J Jr. Displaced intra-articular fractures of the distal aspect of the radius. Long-term results in young adults after open reduction and internal fixation. J Bone Joint Surg Am 1997;79(9):1290–1302

[51] Kim JK, Kim DJ, Yun Y. Natural history and factors associated with ulnar-sided wrist pain in distal radial fractures treated by plate fixation. J Hand Surg Eur Vol 2016;41(7):727–731

[52] Dewan N, MacDermid JC, Grewal R, Beattie K. Recovery patterns over 4 years after distal radius fracture: Descriptive changes in fracture-specific pain/disability, fall risk factors, bone mineral density, and general health status. J Hand Ther 2018;31(4):451–464

[53] Stinton SB, Graham PL, Moloney NA, Maclachlan LR, Edgar DW, Pappas E. Longitudinal recovery following distal radial fractures managed with volar plate fixation. Bone Joint J 2017;99-B(12): 1665–1676

[54] Warwick D. Montgomery and wrist fractures- what should we tell the patient? Journal of Trauma and Orthopaedics 2016;4:44–46

[55] Warwick D. Pearls of wisdom. International Federation of Societies for Surgery of the Hand 2016;22:48–49

[56] Kamal RN, Leversedge FJ. Ulnar shortening osteotomy for distal radius malunion. J Wrist Surg 2014;3(3):181–186

[57] Mulders MA, d'Ailly PN, Cleffken BI, Schep NW. Corrective osteotomy is an effective method of treating distal radius malunions with good long-term functional results. Injury 2017;48(3):731–737

[58] Opel S, Konan S, Sorene E. Corrective distal radius osteotomy following fracture malunion using a fixed-angle volar locking plate. J Hand Surg Eur Vol 2014;39(4):431–435

[59] Pillukat T, Gradl G, Mühldorfer-Fodor M, Prommersberger KJ. [Malunion of the distal radius - long-term results after extraarticular corrective osteotomy] Handchir Mikrochir Plast Chir 2014;46(1):18–25

[60] Quadlbauer S, Pezzei C, Jurkowitsch J, et al. Early Rehabilitation of Distal Radius Fractures Stabilized by Volar Locking Plate: A Prospective Randomized Pilot Study. J Wrist Surg 2017;6(2):102–112

[61] Chaudhry H, Kleinlugtenbelt YV, Mundi R, Ristevski B, Goslings JC, Bhandari M. Are Volar Locking Plates Superior to Percutaneous K-wires for Distal Radius Fractures? A Meta-analysis. Clin Orthop Relat Res 2015;473(9):3017–3027

[62] Karantana A, Downing ND, Forward DP, et al. Surgical treatment of distal radial fractures with a volar locking plate versus conventional percutaneous methods: a randomized controlled trial. J Bone Joint Surg Am 2013;95(19):1737–1744

[63] Tubeuf S, Yu G, Achten J, et al. Cost effectiveness of treatment with percutaneous Kirschner wires versus volar locking plate for adult patients with a dorsally displaced fracture of the distal radius: analysis from the DRAFFT trial. Bone Joint J 2015;97-B(8):1082–1089

6 Is There a Role for External Fixation with or without Kirschner Wires?

Frédéric Schuind

Abstract

The best indication of distal radius external fixation is the highly comminuted fracture, operated shortly after the accident. Other good indications are open, contaminated distal radius fracture and the unstable polytrauma patient ("damage control" principle). Volar marginal Barton-type fractures are better treated by plate. Radiometacarpal external fixation, with pins inserted in the radius and second metacarpal diaphyses and half-frame fixation, relies on transarticular distraction to reduce the fracture and to maintain its reduction. An excellent or good reduction is obtained in 93.5% of the cases, though minor bone settling frequently occurs. Sometimes a step-off is observed on postoperative CT scan, justifying the subsequent implantation of a volar plate, keeping the fixator for length and alignment of the radius. The main drawback of external fixation is the bone and skin reactions to the percutaneous pins. The recovery of function is slower than after plate fixation, but, after 1 year, the functional results are equivalent. Overall, there are less major complications after external fixation, there is no volar scar, and no necessity to remove an internal implant.

Keywords: distal radius fractures, distraction, external fixation, external fixateur, soft tissue defects radius, infection radius

6.1 Introduction

The traditional care of distal radius fractures is closed reduction and cast immobilization. In unstable fractures, this treatment leads to an unacceptable rate of secondary displacement, up to 60%.[1] According to Lafontaine et al,[2] the factors of instability include dorsal tilt > 20°, dorsal comminution, intra-articular radiocarpal involvement, associated fracture of the ulna, and age over 60. In subsequent studies, age has been reported to be the main factor of instability.[3,4] Most unstable fractures are, therefore, nowadays operated in an effort to prevent symptomatic malunion. During many years, external fixation has been considered the technique of choice, but for the last 15 years, locked volar plate has become the standard. External fixation has fallen out of favor because of significant drawbacks, including the risk of infection at pin sites, postoperative complex regional pain syndrome (CRPS), poor tolerance of the external frame by the patients, and the higher risk of redisplacement. Some of these criticisms are well established (infections at pin–skin sites); others are more beliefs than facts, as demonstrated in comparative studies and meta-analyses.[5,6,7,8,9,10,11,12,13,14,15,16,17,18,19,20] In fact, there is no clear evidence that locked plate fixation is a better technique. The initial functional results are better after plate fixation, but after 1 year, there is almost no difference; the rate of reoperation is higher after plate fixation, mainly for tendon complications—not seen after external fixation. Considering not only the functional results but also the rate and seriousness of their complications, neither external fixation nor palmar plating has demonstrated an obvious benefit over nonoperative methods or simple pinning techniques, especially in geriatric patients.[21,22,23,24,25,26]

6.2 Indications and Contraindications

External fixation can be used to treat most distal radius fractures. In our opinion, the best indication is the highly comminuted fracture, operated immediately after the accident (▶Fig. 6.1). Of course, external fixation is the technique of choice in the infrequent open, contaminated distal radius fracture (▶Fig. 6.2), and in the unstable polytrauma patient, following the principle of "damage control."[27] Relative indications also include the patient unwilling to undergo open reduction and internal fixation of his/her distal radius fracture, and the rare cases of general (allergy to metals and coagulation problems—an external fixator can be implanted without discontinuing anticoagulant therapy) or local contraindications to open surgery and plate fixation. External fixation is not a good technique to fix volar marginal Barton-type fractures, better treated by a volar plate, nor pediatric distal radius fractures, where pinning remains the golden standard. Another relative contraindication to external fixation is the severely immunocompromised patient when pin infection may represent a serious risk. Some patients also refuse an external frame, a rare situation in our experience.

6.3 Surgical Techniques

External fixation is a "keep it simple and safe" method. The classical technique is the implantation of pins in the diaphysis of the radius and of the second (or sometimes third) metacarpal bone ("radiometacarpal external fixation"), "bridging" the wrist joints.[28,29,30] The method relies on transarticular distraction to reduce the fracture and to maintain its reduction. It is usually assumed that the fracture fragments are pulled in place by the intact ligaments ("ligamentotaxis").[31] Having observed that transarticular distraction also allows to reduce fragments devoid of ligament insertion, we have suggested another explanation of the mechanism of reduction, a decrease of the intra-articular pressure during distraction with a suction effect on the small articular fragments.[32] This mechanism can occur only in very recent fractures. The fixator is, therefore, ideally applied

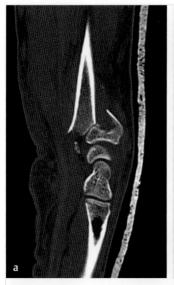
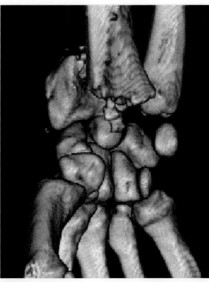

Fig. 6.1 (a, b) Comminuted distal radius fracture treated by distraction bridging radiometacarpal external fixation.

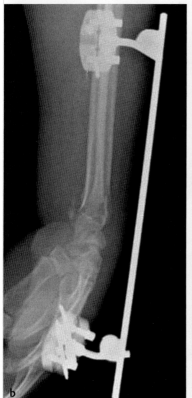
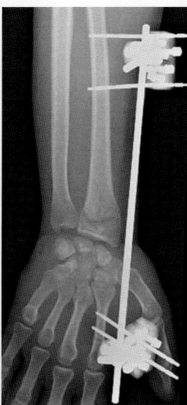

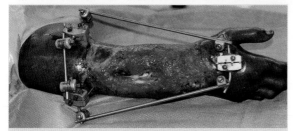

Fig. 6.2 A 70-year-old woman transferred from Africa after traditional treatment of an open forearm and distal radius fracture. Obvious contraindication to internal fixation techniques.

within 72 hours of the fracture; after this delay, it is more difficult to obtain by simple reduction, a good reduction of an articular fracture. Radiometacarpal external fixation can be implanted using different types of mountings. At our university clinic, we have chosen the Stryker Trauma Hoffmann II device. Two 3-mm Apex pins are implanted in the middle third of the radius and two identical pins in the diaphysis of the second metacarpal bone. A simple half-frame is then constructed, allowing maintenance of the position of closed reduction of the fracture, which is usually obtained by axial traction, and some palmar flexion and ulnar inclination (▶Fig. 6.1, ▶Fig. 6.3). If necessary, additional Kirschner

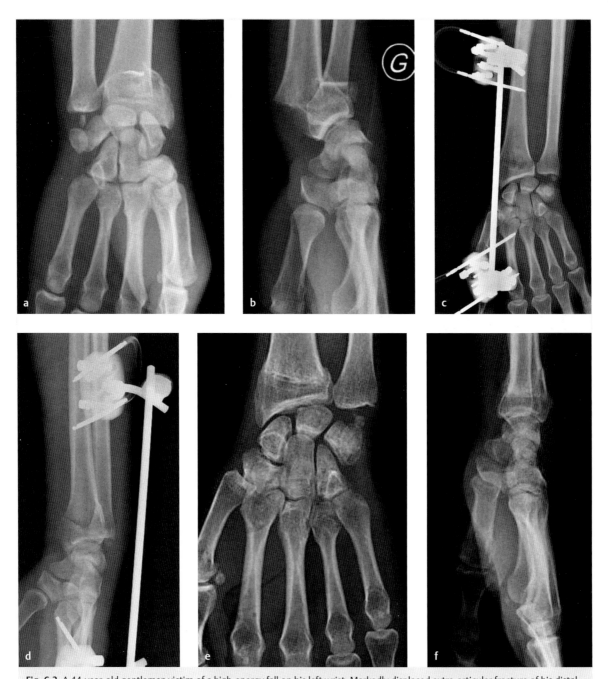

Fig. 6.3 A 44-year-old gentleman victim of a high-energy fall on his left wrist. Markedly displaced extra-articular fracture of his distal radius with associated fracture of the ulnar styloid (Frykman VI **[a, b]**). Acute dysesthesias in median nerve dermatoma. Emergency reduction and radiometacarpal external fixation **(c, d)**. Rapid disappearance of all neurologic symptoms without carpal tunnel decompression. Removal of the fixator after 6 weeks. At 6 months, the patient has no pain and has recovered almost full wrist joint amplitudes and 89% grasping strength, as compared to the right dominant side. Note however on the X-rays done after removal of the fixator at 3 months **(e, f)**, some shortening of the radius causing a positive ulnar variance. This bone settling, not present on the immediate postoperative radiograms **(c, d)**, could possibly have been prevented by additional Kirschner-wire (K-wire) fixation.

wires (K-wires) are pinned in epiphyseal fragments, if the reduction obtained by distraction is not sufficient or to provide additional stability[33,34] (▶ Fig. 6.4). We never open the fracture to insert a bone graft or a bone substitute.[35] Control imaging is obtained after the operation. About 3 weeks later, the external fixation rod is unlocked and the wrist straightened to a neutral position, releasing the transarticular distraction. The relocked fixator remains in place for another 3 to 4 weeks, before removal of the pins at the outpatient clinic or in day surgery. Physiotherapy is then instituted, if not already started during fixator time until good motion of wrist and fingers is recovered.

Beside this classical method of external fixation, other techniques are available. We do not use dynamic

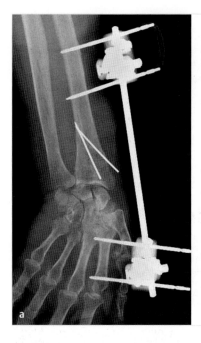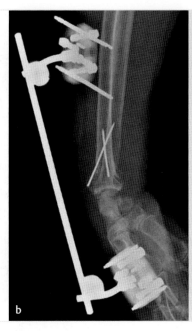

Fig. 6.4 (a, b) An 83-year-old osteoporotic woman victim of a low-energy closed Frykman IV fracture of her right distal radius. Osteosynthesis by radiometacarpal external fixation with additional Kirschner wires (K-wires). Good function after fracture healing, though the K-wires did not prevent some radius shortening at final follow-up. The wires could have been folded at their extremity to prevent migration.

external fixation that could promote earlier recovery of wrist function with the risk of loss of fracture reduction.[36,37] Some authors use external fixation as a neutralizing osteosynthesis, after closed or arthroscopic reduction and pinning of the bone fragments: this method has been named "augmented external fixation."[34] McQueen has popularized radioradial external fixation to treat simple extra-articular fractures.[38] Pins are then implanted only in the radius, a first group in the distal diaphysis, proximal to the fracture line, and the second group in the distal radius epiphysis, distally to the fracture. The reduction is obtained by direct manipulation of the fracture fragments. Hoel and Liverneaux recently proposed another external fixation method using K-wires directly implanted in the fracture fragments, fixed by an external connector (HK2 technique).[39]

6.4 Prevention of Redisplacement

The justification of operative bone fixation of a distal radius fracture, whatever the chosen method, is to maintain a satisfactory reduction until the fracture has healed. Like all other methods of osteosynthesis of distal radius fractures, including plate fixation,[40] redisplacement may occur under external fixation (▶ Fig. 6.3). We have specifically studied this complication in a retrospective series of 35 cases and have reported a rate of secondary displacement of 48.5%. However, this loss of reduction concerned primarily palmar tilt and was moderate. No patient with intra-articular fracture lines ended up with a gap or step-off of over 2 mm. We noted that 41.2% of the losses of reduction occurred within the first weeks, before wrist straightening, and 47.2% after, before fixator removal.[41] It is possible—but still needs to be demonstrated—that adding one or two K-wires to the fixator construction could prevent these early losses of

reduction, a practice that we have not implemented at our clinic. Adding K-wires, while increasing the stability of the osteosynthesis,[34] is not without added morbidity. Several papers have pointed out the potentially very serious complications of K-wires.[42,43,44,45] Contrarily to external fixation pins, K-wires are implanted in the distal radius epiphysis fragments; therefore, an infection may have catastrophic consequences. In addition, K-wires may irritate tendons and superficial nerves, potentially causing tendon attrition/rupture and/or neuroma. Migration of the pins is also possible. Of course, if external fixation is used as a neutralization osteosynthesis, the reduction of the fracture relies only on the K-wires fixing the bone fragments, usually implanted before the fixator.

6.5 Prevention of Other Complications of External Fixation

Beside secondary displacement, the most frequent complication of external fixation is the infection of the pins. Specific preventive pin–skin exit care, preferably done by the patient him-/herself, is recommended. If an infection occurs, it is usually because of poor patient's hygiene and is easily managed by better local disinfection and oral antibiotics. A neuroma of the sensory branch of the radial nerve may be the consequence of inappropriate insertion of the radius pins. As for all operations at the hand and wrist, good knowledge of anatomy is mandatory. CRPS can be a devastating complication after treatment of a distal radius fracture. The prevention is, in addition to vitamin C, early active finger motion, which can be difficult if the wrist is fixed in marked flexion and ulnar inclination, a dangerous position to be avoided if possible. We also feel it important to avoid overdistraction and to release the tension applied by the fixator on the wrist, after 3 weeks. Another rare complication of external fixation is the fracture of an osteoporotic second metacarpal after pin insertion.

In our clinic, external fixation has been well tolerated by the patients, even in the geriatric group. We have conducted a prospective randomized study comparing external fixation and plate fixation for the treatment of comminuted articular fractures of the distal radius. The patients were informed of the random selection of the methods of treatment. Those who refused the study chose in majority external fixation, to avoid a palmar scar at the distal forearm (pictures of a fixator and of the scar after plate fixation were provided in the informed consent form) and a possible second operation for plate removal, preferring 6 weeks of external fixation (unpublished data).

6.6 Results

Using external fixation, we have achieved good or anatomical fracture reduction in 93.5% of the treated distal radius fractures.[29] Over the years, we have become more and more exigent with the quality of reduction, and now almost systematically perform a postoperative CT scan in young, active patients, even with an apparently good reduction on postoperative radiograms. In the infrequent cases of a persistent step-off, even of less than 2 mm, a reoperation is decided, implanting a volar plate but keeping the fixator, which restored the general radius length and alignment, and this technique greatly facilitates the subsequent internal osteosynthesis (▶ Fig. 6.5).

Regarding complications, we reported in our initial series of 225 cases fracture of the second metacarpal at the site of pin implantation in 1.6%, carpal tunnel syndrome in 2.6%, neuroma on a sensory branch of the radial nerve in 2.1%, secondary displacement with significant loss of the initial reduction in 2.1%, pin infection in 12.8%, and CRPS in 0.5%. There was not a single case of tendon rupture, nonunion, or osteomyelitis, despite 8% open fractures.[29] Tendon complications are quite frequent after plate osteosynthesis.[46]

Tips and Tricks

Planning the operation:
- Do not hesitate to obtain a computed tomography (CT) scan to better understand the fracture lines.
- No necessity to discontinue anticoagulant therapy.
- If you rely on distraction to reduce the fracture, operate as soon as possible (within 72 h) or you will not get a good reduction, particularly of the articular fragments.

External fixation application:
- The operation needs the same rules of asepsis as open reduction and internal fixation, though prophylactic antibiotherapy is probably not necessary.
- Avoid the superficial nerves and tendons by carefully choosing the pin site insertion (radius: posterolateral middle third of the diaphysis).
- Make sufficient stab wounds for pin insertion and dissect the soft tissues to the bone—pin infection is usually related to localized soft tissue necrosis at the site of pin insertion, in conjunction with poor hygiene of the patient.
- Insert 3-mm self-drilling self-tapping pins (if you choose 4-mm pins, the risk of bone fracture at the site of pin insertion becomes significant).
- To improve the stability of the mounting, try to separate the pins as much as possible so that they will be fixed at both extremities of the clamp.
- The pins should be solidly anchored in both cortices of the bone—check manually the quality of pin fixation and with the C-arm if they are bicortical.
- A simple half-frame is sufficient for most fractures, to be locked after reduction of the fracture under C-arm control.
- Before locking the clamps, check that the rod is not too close to the skin, allowing for some swelling in the first postoperative days.
- Check at the end of the procedure if the distal radioulnar joint is stable, if not consider fixing the ulnar styloid or repairing the distal radioulnar ligaments.[47]
- Cover the pin–skin exit sites by a light dry dressing.

Prevention of pin infection:
- Removal of crusts by the patient himself and alcoolization twice a day until skin healing.
- Hygiene of the fixator, the patient is allowed to shower.
- In case of pin infection, local care and oral antibiotics; do not remove the fixator for infection before fracture healing.

Follow-up:
- Obtain postoperative posteroanterior and profile X-rays and if necessary a CT scan to check the precise reduction of the articular bone fragments.
- Elevate the hand (preferably by suspending the fixator) to decrease the post-traumatic edema as quickly as possible.
- Encourage the patient to move his fingers and elbow to prevent stiffness; if necessary, prescribe physiotherapy.
- Release the transarticular distraction at 3 wk and redress the fixator, keeping the device for another 3 wk.
- Remove the fixator in day clinic at 42 postoperative days or 1 or 2 wk later.
- No necessity thereafter of a splint.
- Prescribe physiotherapy and active remobilization of the wrist and fingers.
- Control radiograms after fixator removal, at 3 and 6 mo; if possible, follow-up the patient for 1 y.

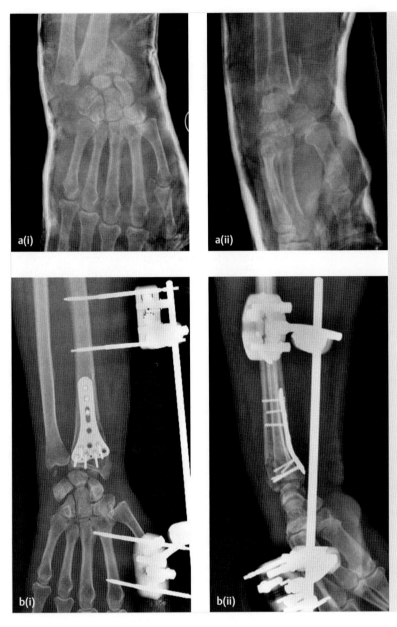

Fig. 6.5 (a, b) Insufficient reduction of a distal radius fracture by radiometacarpal external fixation. The fixator was kept, providing the general alignment, and in a second operation a few days later, a plate was added, allowing finally an anatomical reduction. Given the fracture comminution, such a perfect reduction would have been quite difficult to achieve using only a plate. The fixator was removed 2 weeks later, keeping, of course, the plate in place.

6.7 Conclusion

Radiometacarpal external fixation is an established method to treat most unstable distal radius fractures in adults, except volar marginal Barton-type fractures, better treated by volar plating. The best indications of distraction bridging external fixation are comminuted articular fracture, operated within the first posttraumatic days. Such fractures are difficult to fix by palmar plates. Unfortunately, the poor organization of many operation facilities for the management of traumatology and the referral to specialized hand surgeons is at the origin of delays in the treatment of distal radius fractures, and then the only option remains open reduction and internal fixation. As with all other osteosynthesis techniques, secondary displacements occur after external

fixation, possibly prevented by the insertion of K-wires in the epiphysis. The main drawbacks of external fixation are the bone and skin reactions to the percutaneous pins, which are more a serious inconvenience than a major complication.

An anatomical reduction is not always obtained after distraction bridging external fixation, even with the additional use of K-wires. Sometimes the control radiograms seem satisfactory but a step-off is observed on the postoperative CT scan. This may justify a reoperation, implanting a palmar plate but keeping, at least initially, the fixator for the length and alignment of the radius.

Theoretically, radioradial or dynamic external fixation could allow earlier functional recovery, similar to what is seen after implantation of a volar plate, but this has not been clearly demonstrated.[48]

References

[1] Gartland JJ Jr, Werley CW. Evaluation of healed Colles' fractures. J Bone Joint Surg Am 1951;33-A(4):895–907

[2] Lafontaine M, Delincé P, Hardy D, Simons M. L'instabilité des fractures de l'extrémité inférieure du radius: à propos d'une série de 167 cas. Acta Orthop Belg 1989;55(2):203–216

[3] Leone J, Bhandari M, Adili A, McKenzie S, Moro JK, Dunlop RB. Predictors of early and late instability following conservative treatment of extra-articular distal radius fractures. Arch Orthop Trauma Surg 2004;124(1):38–41

[4] Nesbitt KS, Failla JM, Les C. Assessment of instability factors in adult distal radius fractures. J Hand Surg Am 2004;29(6):1128–1138

[5] Bentohami A, de Burlet K, de Korte N, van den Bekerom MP, Goslings JC, Schep NW. Complications following volar locking plate fixation for distal radial fractures: a systematic review. J Hand Surg Eur Vol 2014;39(7):745–754

[6] Chaudhry H, Kleinlugtenbelt YV, Mundi R, Ristevski B, Goslings JC, Bhandari M. Are volar locking plates superior to percutaneous K-wires for distal radius fractures? A meta-analysis. Clin Orthop Relat Res 2015;473(9):3017–3027

[7] Egol K, Walsh M, Tejwani N, McLaurin T, Wynn C, Paksima N. Bridging external fixation and supplementary Kirschner-wire fixation versus volar locked plating for unstable fractures of the distal radius: a randomised, prospective trial. J Bone Joint Surg Br 2008;90(9):1214–1221

[8] Esposito J, Schemitsch EH, Saccone M, Sternheim A, Kuzyk PR. External fixation versus open reduction with plate fixation for distal radius fractures: a meta-analysis of randomised controlled trials. Injury 2013;44(4):409–416

[9] Gouk CJC, Bindra RR, Tarrant DJ, Thomas MJE. Volar locking plate fixation versus external fixation of distal radius fractures: a meta-analysis. J Hand Surg Eur Vol 2018;43(9):954–960

[10] Leung F, Tu YK, Chew WY, Chow SP. Comparison of external and percutaneous pin fixation with plate fixation for intra-articular distal radial fractures. A randomized study. J Bone Joint Surg Am 2008;90(1):16–22

[11] Li-hai Z, Ya-nan W, Zhi M, et al. Volar locking plate versus external fixation for the treatment of unstable distal radial fractures: a meta-analysis of randomized controlled trials. J Surg Res 2015;193(1):324–333

[12] Saving J. External fixation versus volar plate fixation for unstable distal radial fractures. A 3-year follow-up of a randomized controlled trial. J Hand Surg Am 2017;42:S39–S40

[13] Stockmans F, Libberecht KM, Vanhaecke J, et al. Prospective study comparing external fixation and volar locking plating of distal radius fractures. New Orleans, LA: American Academy of Orthopaedic Surgeons (AAOS) Congress; 2010

[14] Walenkamp MM, Bentohami A, Beerekamp MS, et al. Functional outcome in patients with unstable distal radius fractures, volar locking plate versus external fixation: a meta-analysis. Strateg Trauma Limb Reconstr 2013;8(2):67–75

[15] Wang D, Shan L, Zhou JL. Locking plate versus external fixation for type C distal radius fractures: A meta-analysis of randomized controlled trials. Chin J Traumatol 2018;21(2):113–117

[16] Wei DH, Raizman NM, Bottino CJ, Jobin CM, Strauch RJ, Rosenwasser MP. Unstable distal radial fractures treated with external fixation, a radial column plate, or a volar plate. A prospective randomized trial. J Bone Joint Surg Am 2009;91(7):1568–1577

[17] Wei DH, Poolman RW, Bhandari M, Wolfe VM, Rosenwasser MP. External fixation versus internal fixation for unstable distal radius fractures: a systematic review and meta-analysis of comparative clinical trials. J Orthop Trauma 2012;26(7):386–394

[18] Wilcke MK, Abbaszadegan H, Adolphson PY. Wrist function recovers more rapidly after volar locked plating than after external fixation but the outcomes are similar after 1 year. Acta Orthop 2011;82(1):76–81

[19] Xie X, Xie X, Qin H, Shen L, Zhang C. Comparison of internal and external fixation of distal radius fractures. Acta Orthop 2013;84(3):286–291

[20] Yuan ZZ, Yang Z, Liu Q, Liu YM. Complications following open reduction and internal fixation versus external fixation in treating unstable distal radius fractures: Grading the evidence through a meta-analysis. Orthop Traumatol Surg Res 2018;104(1):95–103

[21] Arora R, Lutz M, Deml C, Krappinger D, Haug L, Gabl M. A prospective randomized trial comparing nonoperative treatment with volar locking plate fixation for displaced and unstable distal radial fractures in patients sixty-five years of age and older. J Bone Joint Surg Am 2011;93(23):2146–2153

[22] Costa ML, Achten J, Parsons NR, et al; DRAFFT. Study Group. Percutaneous fixation with Kirschner wires versus volar locking plate fixation in adults with dorsally displaced fracture of distal radius: randomised controlled trial. BMJ 2014;349:g4807

[23] Handoll HH, Madhok R. Surgical interventions for treating distal radial fractures in adults. Cochrane Database Syst Rev 2003(3):CD003209

[24] Handoll HH, Huntley JS, Madhok R. External fixation versus conservative treatment for distal radial fractures in adults. Cochrane Database Syst Rev 2007(3):CD006194

[25] Koval KJ, Harrast JJ, Anglen JO, Weinstein JN. Fractures of the distal part of the radius. The evolution of practice over time. Where's the evidence? J Bone Joint Surg Am 2008;90(9):1855–1861

[26] Lutz K, Yeoh KM, MacDermid JC, Symonette C, Grewal R. Complications associated with operative versus nonsurgical treatment of distal radius fractures in patients aged 65 years and older. J Hand Surg Am 2014;39(7):1280–1286

[27] Aly A, Moungondo F, Cermak K, Schuind F. Complex open fractures-dislocations of the wrist. In: Garcia-Elias M, Mathoulin CH, eds. Articular Injury of the Wrist. Stuttgart: Thieme; 2014:139–150

[28] Rasquin C, Burny F, Andrianne Y, Quintin J. Traitement des fractures du poignet par fixation externe. Indications et résultats préliminaires. Acta Orthop Belg 1979;45:678–683

[29] Schuind F, Donkerwolcke M, Rasquin C, Burny F. External fixation of fractures of the distal radius: a study of 225 cases. J Hand Surg Am 1989;14(2 Pt 2):404–407

[30] Schuind F, El Kazzi W, Cermak K, Donkerwolcke M, Burny F. Fixation externe au poignet et à la main. Rev Med Brux 2011;32 (6, Suppl):S71–S75

[31] Vidal J, Buscayret C, Connes H, Melka J, Orst G. Guidelines for treatment of open fractures and infected pseudarthroses by external fixation. Clin Orthop Relat Res 1983(180):83–95

[32] Schuind FA, Cantraine FR, Fabeck L, Burny F. Radiocarpal articular pressures during the reduction of distal radius fractures. J Orthop Trauma 1997;11(4):295–299

[33] Williksen JH, Husby T, Hellund JC, Kvernmo HD, Rosales C, Frihagen F. External fixation and adjuvant pins versus volar locking plate fixation in unstable distal radius fractures. A randomized, controlled study with a 5-year follow-up. J Hand Surg Am 2015;40(7):1333–1340

[34] Wolfe SW, Swigart CR, Grauer J, Slade JF III, Panjabi MM. Augmented external fixation of distal radius fractures: a biomechanical analysis. J Hand Surg Am 1998;23(1):127–134

[35] Handoll HH, Watts AC. Bone grafts and bone substitutes for treating distal radial fractures in adults. Cochrane Database Syst Rev 2008(2):CD006836

[36] Asche G. Die dynamische Behandlung von handgelenksnahen und gelenksbeteiligten Speichenbrüchen mit einem neuartigen Bewegungsfixateur. Aktuelle Traumatol 1990;20(1):6–10

[37] Pennig DW. Dynamic external fixation of distal radius fractures. Hand Clin 1993;9(4):587–602

[38] McQueen MM. Non-spanning external fixation of the distal radius. Hand Clin 2005;21(3):375–380

[39] Maire N, Lebailly F, Zemirline A, Hariri A, Facca S, Liverneaux P. Prospective continuous study comparing intrafocal cross-pinning HK2(®) with a locking plate in distal radius fracture fixation. Chir Main 2013;32(1):17–24

[40] Gruber G, Gruber K, Giessauf C, et al. Volar plate fixation of AO type C2 and C3 distal radius fractures, a single-center study of 55 patients. J Orthop Trauma 2008;22(7):467–472

[41] Farah N, Nassar L, Farah Z, Schuind F. Secondary displacement of distal radius fractures treated by bridging external fixation. J Hand Surg Eur Vol 2014;39(4):423–428

[42] Hsu LP, Schwartz EG, Kalainov DM, Chen F, Makowiec RL. Complications of K-wire fixation in procedures involving the hand and wrist. J Hand Surg Am 2011;36(4):610–616

[43] Lakshmanan P, Dixit V, Reed MR, Sher JL. Infection rate of percutaneous Kirschner wire fixation for distal radius fractures. J Orthop Surg (Hong Kong) 2010;18(1):85–86

[44] Ridley TJ, Freking W, Erickson LO, Ward CM. Incidence of treatment for infection of buried versus exposed Kirschner wires in phalangeal, metacarpal, and distal radial fractures. J Hand Surg Am 2017;42(7):525–531

[45] van Leeuwen WF, van Hoorn BT, Chen N, Ring D. Kirschner wire pin site infection in hand and wrist fractures: incidence rate and risk factors. J Hand Surg Eur Vol 2016;41(9):990–994

[46] Azzi AJ, Aldekhayel S, Boehm KS, Zadeh T. Tendon rupture and tenosynovitis following internal fixation of distal radius fractures. A systematic review. Plast Reconstr Surg 2017;139(3):717e–724e

[47] Lindau T, Aspenberg P. The radioulnar joint in distal radial fractures. Acta Orthop Scand 2002;73(5):579–588

[48] Handoll HH, Huntley JS, Madhok R. Different methods of external fixation for treating distal radial fractures in adults. Cochrane Database Syst Rev 2008(1):CD006522

7 Volar Locking Plates: Basic Concepts

Hermann Krimmer

Abstract

Volar locking plates nowadays are mainly used for fixation of distal radius fractures. Multidirectional locking is preferable as it offers the possibility to place the screws according to the fracture type. The different locking mechanisms represent significant differences and should be known to the surgeon. Fracture-specific plate selection is best based on preoperative computed tomography scan. Complications by secondary dislocation are reduced by rigid fixation of the key fragments. To avoid irritation of the flexor tendons, plate prominence should be avoided and for protection of the extensor tendons, screw length must be precisely checked.

Keywords: radius fracture, volar locking plate, tendon rupture, watershed line, lunate facet

7.1 Introduction

In recent years, the treatment of distal radius fracture has seen a significant change in trend, moving away from conservative treatment towards surgical treatment. Secondary dislocation after an initially good reduction outcome, inadequate restoration of the articular surface after closed reduction in the case of intra-articular fractures, and a long period of wrist immobilization often lead to unsatisfactory outcomes. Using the osteosynthesis methods of Kirschner wire (K-wire) fixation and the external fixator, it was often impossible to achieve satisfactory anatomical reduction and long-term retention. The difficulty with plate osteosynthesis, especially in the case of a dorsal comminuted fracture zone and intra-articular fractures, was that in the distal comminuted fracture zone, standard screws are insecure and it was often necessary to perform a cancellous bone graft as well. In addition, it was not always possible to make plate design meet the requirements for accurate reduction and retention; therefore, there are often scar problems and misaligned healing.

Only upon introduction of fixed-angle plates and ultimately also multidirectional fixed-angle plates, it was possible to solve many of these problems.[1] Locking plates act as an internal fixator where the screws are locked in the plate and by that can stabilize comminuted areas till bony healing is present. Fixed-angle plates are always preferable for osteosynthesis of unstable distal radius fractures because, with this method, the risk of secondary dislocation of the fragments is much lower. Palmar fixed-angle plate osteosynthesis now represents the preferred method of osteosynthesis and allows long-term anatomical retention of the articular surface, especially in cases of intra-articular involvement. In the case of

fractures with a pronounced dorsal comminuted fracture zone or a dislocation that cannot be reduced from palmar, the development of special dorsal osteosynthesis plates has brought about considerable progress. Additionally, arthroscopically assisted fracture management with a direct view of the radius articular surface allows precisely examining the reduction.[2]

7.2 Locking Mechanisms

A distinction is made between *unidirectional* and *multidirectional* fixed-angle plates as well as between palmar and dorsal use thereof. In the case of unidirectional fixed angles, the direction of the screw is dictated by the plate. This is often adequate if plate position is optimal. However, if the plate has to be positioned far distal or far proximal on account of the fracture situation, there is a risk of an intra-articular screw position or suboptimal support of the articular surface because the screws can no longer be positioned subchondral.

With the multidirectional fixed-angle plate, the screws can be introduced in various directions with a lateral deviation of up to approximately 15° from the perpendicular position. This permits screw positioning that is customized, fracture-oriented, and adapted to plate position.[3]

There are three fundamentally different methods of locking the screw head with the plate.

Applying the principle of *material deformation*, a hard external thread in the region of the screw head cuts into the softer plate material. The drawback with this is that if the screw direction is adjusted, the screw head tends to take the path of least resistance and returns to the original direction. In addition, when the plate is removed, there is the problem of cold fusion between the screw head and the plate, which makes sometimes removal impossible or leads to breakage of the screw head.

Another method often used is to interlock the screw by engaging an *external thread* in the head section with an *internal thread* in the plate section. However, the disadvantage of this is that in the interlock, the screw head seeks the path of least resistance and thus counteracts the variability of screw direction.

A more recent method is *spherical head space locking* in which, during insertion of the screw head into the plate, friction grip occurs when resistance has been overcome; by that, a kind of wedging takes place between the screw head and the plate (▶ Fig. 7.1). This creates the advantage of infinite locking without the risk of any cold fusion. In addition, with this method, the plate design can be kept very flat and metal removal, when indicated, is possible without any problems.

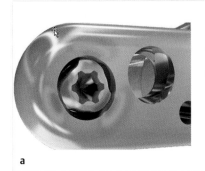
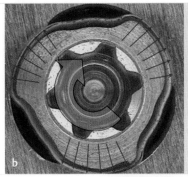

Fig. 7.1 (a) Spherical locking mechanism (b) locked by friction.

7.3 Indications

7.3.1 Plate Design and Plate Position

The historical shape of the palmar radius plate is represented by the traditional T-plate (▶Fig. 7.2). Later on, with the development of the multidirectional locking plates, the principles of two distal rows were established to provide better support of the articular surface, especially in case of severe comminution and osteoporosis (▶Fig. 7.3). Through the distal row, the screws can be placed exactly in the subchondral area, which represents the most stable part and through the proximal row, support of the dorsal aspect of the radius is possible (▶Fig. 7.4).

Secondary ruptures of the flexor tendons, especially the long thumb flexor tendon (flexor pollicis longus [FPL] tendon), are a feared complication. Prominent distal plate rims and projecting screw heads increase the risk of a rupture.[4] For this reason, plates were developed with a low-profile design as well as special plates that are recessed in the region of the FPL tendon, thus minimizing the secondary rupture risk.

With the recognition of the anatomical shape of the radius, the term *watershed line* was established as the distal border of plate position to avoid flexor tendon injuries.[5] Based on this concept, plates with watershed design were developed to allow far distal placement, especially for the so-called troublesome lunate facet fragments (▶Fig. 7.4). To support the lunate area far distal, the FPL design was created, which spares the floor of FPL tendon completely (▶Fig. 7.5). Limits for fracture plate fixation alone are seen in case of rim fractures, which require additionally fragment-specific fixation by small hook plates, tiny screws, or even tension band techniques, which is described in Chapter 12.[6]

The distal and palmar prominence of the plates is defined by *Soong line* (▶Fig. 7.6). Soong 0 describes an optimal plate position. In Soong 1, the distal plate end exhibits palmar prominence. In Soong 2, there is palmar and distal plate prominence, which requires absolutely hardware removal.[7,8]

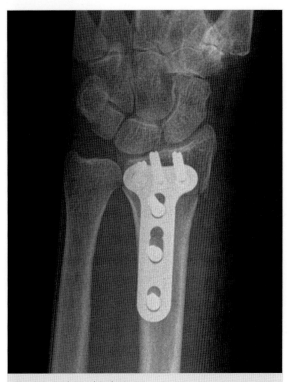

Fig. 7.2 Traditional T-plate.

7.3.2 Fracture-Specific Plate Selection

In the case of extra-articular fractures with a stable bone structure, conventional T-plates with just one distal row of screws appear to be adequate. However, with intra-articular or multifragment fractures, multidirectional fixed-angled plates should be used with two rows because then both the central and the dorsal articular surfaces can be optimally supported. Subchondral screw position is mandatory to provide maximum stability and to avoid secondary subsidence. If the radial styloid and the central articular surfaces are involved, conventional plate design can be used; however, for lunate facet fragments, plates with watershed design or FPL design are preferable.

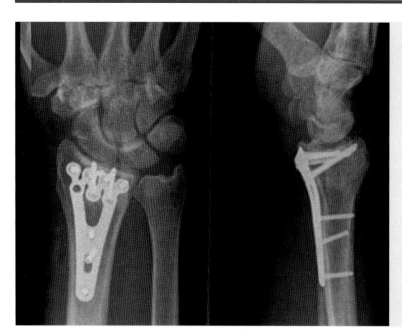

Fig. 7.3 Multidirectional locking plate with two rows.

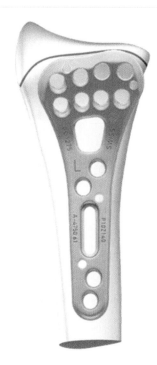

Fig. 7.4 Watershed plate design.

7.4 Surgical Technique

A longitudinal incision over the distal part of the flexor carpi radialis (FCR) tendon is followed by deep exposure between that tendon and the radial artery. After exposure of the pronator quadratus, this muscle is detached from the radius.

Intra-articular fractures where the styloid process is involved the distal insertion of the brachioradialis muscle should be detached from the radius subperiosteally if the latter prevents anatomical reduction due to its traction proximally. Ulnar-sided fractures, especially the lunate facet fragments, need a good exposure. For that, the distal release of the FCR tendon sheath allows retraction of the flexor tendons and the median nerve far ulnarly. The approach ulnar of the median nerve inherits an increased risk of scarring, leading to progressive nerve pain and should be reserved only for special fracture patterns. If carpal tunnel release due to compression neuropathy is necessary, one should never combine the incisions for the same reasons and use a separate incision as usual.

In the case of extension fractures, exposure of the fracture is followed by reduction with traction and counter-traction, ulnar duction, and palmar flexion, if necessary with pressure from dorsal. The reduction outcome can be subjected to temporary stabilization with a K-wire (1.4 or 1.6 mm) introduced percutaneously from the styloid process of the radius, possibly supplemented by one introduced from ulnar or additionally through special holes of the plate.

Die-punch fracture can be lifted up with K-wires through the plate or one can insert screws distally in the proximal direction and before locking, the direction is moved distally guided by the screwdriver in the screw head and then the screw is locked. Inspection of the reduction by fluoroscopy or arthroscopy is followed by placement and alignment of the plate proximal at the shaft region in the gliding hole with a cortical screw. After another fluoroscopic check and possibly correction of plate position, a second screw is placed proximally for stable fixation of the plate. Next one or two nonlocking screws are placed distally to catch the fragment against

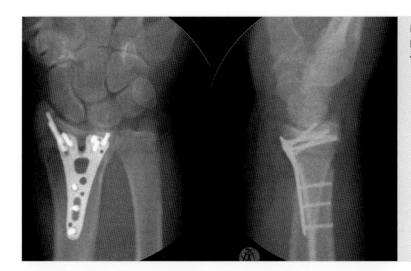

Fig. 7.5 Flexor pollicis longus (FPL) plate provides rigid support of the lunate facet avoiding the risk of tendon irritation.

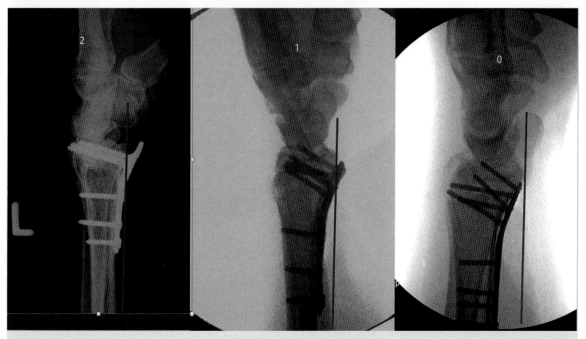

Fig. 7.6 Soong criteria.

the plate and after that for the other holes, locking screws are used. Screw direction in the distal row for subchondral placement should run parallel to the articular surface and from the proximal row into slight distal direction to support the dorsal rim. To check if there is any intra-articular position of a screw, fluoroscopic control parallel to the articular surface should be performed.

To avoid secondary extensor tendon ruptures, the selected distal screws should always be 2 mm shorter than measured. Biomechanically, this does not bring about any reduction instability.[9] It is absolutely essential to avoid extensor-side prominence of screws. In case of doubt, this can be examined by means of an X-ray

checkup with a horizontal beam (skyline view, dorsal horizontal view[10]). It is important to note that the distal radius towards dorsal has a triangular contour and on the lateral X-ray image, the dorsal rim can falsely suggest that the screw ends are in a subcortical position.

In exceptional cases, far distal positioning of the plate may be necessary to support a fragment that is located far distal. In such a case (Soong 2), early plate removal should be done at least after 6 months to avoid irritation and ruptures of the flexor tendons. Intraoperatively, this risk might be reduced by opening the carpal tunnel. In the case of a pronounced dorsal comminuted fracture zone or a dislocation that cannot be reduced from palmar, primary dorsal plate osteosynthesis may be indicated. If both sides are involved, one can start through a palmar approach followed by additional reduction from the dorsal aspect with temporary K-wire fixation and finally stabilization by palmar plate and screws. Only in exceptional cases, double plating is necessary (▶Fig. 7.7).

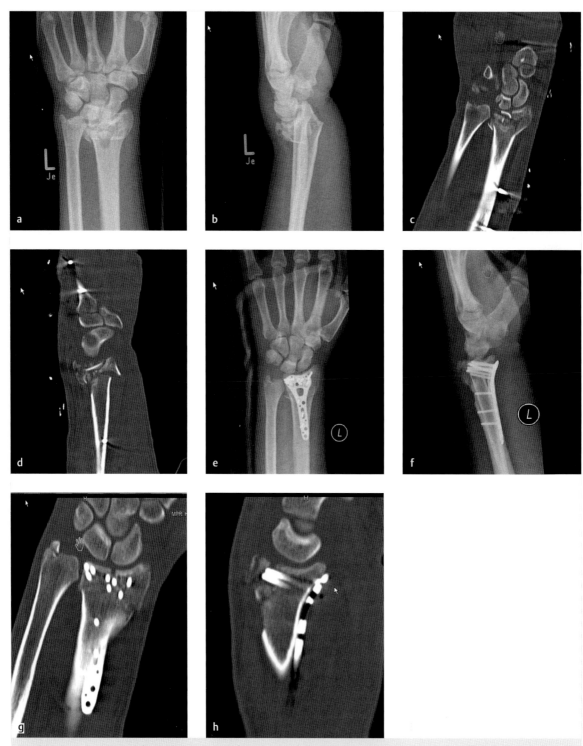

Fig. 7.7 Fracture treatment of severely comminuted fracture pattern. **(a, b)** Preoperative radiograph posteroanterior (PA) and lateral. **(c, d)** Coronal and sagittal computed tomography (CT) revealing die-punch fragment. **(e, f)** Postoperative PA and lateral radiograph following palmar plating by watershed plate design. **(g, h)** Postoperative coronal and sagittal CT demonstrating joint congruity.

7.5 Pitfalls

7.5.1 Tendon Ruptures

Flexor tendons respect the watershed line and the Soong criteria. Extensor tendons take the screws shorter at least 2 mm than measured in doubt check by skyline view.

7.5.2 Secondary Subsidence

Place the screws subchondral, look for proper fixation of the lunate facet fragments at least with two screws, check by postoperative CT scan, and go for early revision in case of failure.[11]

Tips and Tricks

- Analyze precisely the fracture pattern, especially by examining the initial trauma radiographs.
- CT scan should be performed routinely in case of intraarticular fractures.
- Look for the *key fragments* where the carpus dislocates volarly or dorsally; they absolutely need rigid fixation.
- Regard fracture-specific plate selection by selecting between conventional, watershed, and FPL design.
- Be aware of subchondral position of the distal screws to avoid secondary dislocation.
- Take the screws at least 2 mm shorter than measured.
- Check screw position parallel to the articular surface and length by the horizontal view.

References

[1] Orbay JL, Touhami A. Current concepts in volar fixed-angle fixation of unstable distal radius fractures. Clin Orthop Relat Res 2006;445(445):58–67
[2] del Piñal, F. Atlas of Distal Radius Fractures. New York, NY: Thieme Medical Publishers; 2018
[3] Mehrzad R, Kim DC. Complication Rate Comparing Variable Angle Distal Locking Plate to Fixed Angle Plate Fixation of Distal Radius Fractures. Ann Plast Surg 2016;77(6):623–625
[4] Soong M, van Leerdam R, Guitton TG, Got C, Katarincic J, Ring D. Fracture of the distal radius: risk factors for complications after locked volar plate fixation. J Hand Surg Am 2011;36(1):3–9
[5] Tanaka H, Hatta T, Sasajima K, Itoi E, Aizawa T. Comparative study of treatment for distal radius fractures with two different palmar locking plates. J Hand Surg Eur Vol 2016;41(5):536–542
[6] O'Shaughnessy MA, Shin AY, Kakar S. Volar Marginal Rim Fracture Fixation With Volar Fragment-Specific Hook Plate Fixation. J Hand Surg Am 2015;40(8):1563–1570
[7] Soong M, Earp BE, Bishop G, Leung A, Blazar P. Volar locking plate implant prominence and flexor tendon rupture. J Bone Joint Surg Am 2011;93(4):328–335
[8] Lutsky KF, Beredjiklian PK, Hioe S, Bilello J, Kim N, Matzon JL. Incidence of Hardware Removal Following Volar Plate Fixation of Distal Radius Fracture. J Hand Surg Am 2015;40(12):2410–2415
[9] Baumbach SF, Synek A, Traxler H, Mutschler W, Pahr D, Chevalier Y. The influence of distal screw length on the primary stability of volar plate osteosynthesis—a biomechanical study. J Orthop Surg Res 2015;10:139
[10] Joseph SJ, Harvey JN. The dorsal horizon view: detecting screw protrusion at the distal radius. J Hand Surg Am 2011;36(10):1691–1693
[11] Harness NG. Fixation Options for the Volar Lunate Facet Fracture: Thinking Outside the Box. J Wrist Surg 2016;5(1):9–16

8 Intramedullary Devices

Stephanie Malliaris, Scott Wolfe

Abstract

Intramedullary (IM) fixation can be an elegant and effective method for fixation of appropriately selected distal radius fractures. There are multiple types of IM fixation, including nails, pins, and an IM cage device. Surgical technique, results, and pitfalls/contraindications for each of these techniques are addressed.

Keywords: intramedullary fixation, distal radius fracture, intramedullary cage, intramedullary nail

8.1 Introduction

With the wide variety of distal radius fracture types, no single method of distal radius fracture treatment has demonstrated superior outcomes across all patients.[1] Choosing the appropriate method of fixation for any given fracture variant contributes to improved outcomes. Displaced and unstable fracture patterns require operative stabilization in active patients for optimal outcome. Volar locking plate (VLP) fixation for distal radius fracture has become popular over the last 15 years; however, the reported risk of complication ranges between 16 and 27%,[2,3] including tendon irritation or rupture, carpal tunnel syndrome, loss of reduction, hardware failure, nerve irritation, and complex regional pain syndrome.[2,3] Hardware removal rates in the first year are reported in 15 to 34% of patients.[4]

Complications of tendon and nerve irritation, hardware prominence, and need for hardware removal are not confined to volar plates; indeed, the complication rate of dorsal plating, including hardware removal and tendon complications, ranges between 15.4 and 50% in several series.[5,6,7] A meta-analysis of 12 studies that compare complications of volar and dorsal plating for distal radius fractures found no overall difference in the rate of complications, and an increased rate of neuropathy and carpal tunnel syndrome and decreased risk of tendinopathy in volar plating as compared to dorsal plating.[8]

Intramedullary (IM) fixation is common in both upper and lower extremity long bone fractures. IM fixation is successful in achieving restoration of bony anatomy, allowing early return to function, and minimizes soft tissue disruption through smaller incisions. Given the close proximity and dense collection of tendons and nerves to the distal radius, IM fixation poses an attractive alternative to conventional plating techniques.

There are several types of IM fixation that have been described for use in distal radius fracture fixation, including intramedullary nails (IMNs), cannulated pins, and an IM cage device. The Micronail (Wright Medical Technology, Inc., Arlington, TN) is a rigid IMN that is inserted through the radial styloid with three distal fixed-angle locking screws (▶Fig. 8.1).[9] A similar IMN system is the Targon DR (B. Braun, Melsungen, Germany) and previously the Sonoma WRx wrist fracture nail, which was previously available but as of this publication, currently off the market.[10,11]

The T-Pin (Union Surgical, LLC, Philadelphia, PA) is a cannulated, self-drilling, self-tapping threaded pin implant (▶Fig. 8.2).[12] The T-Pin is placed percutaneously

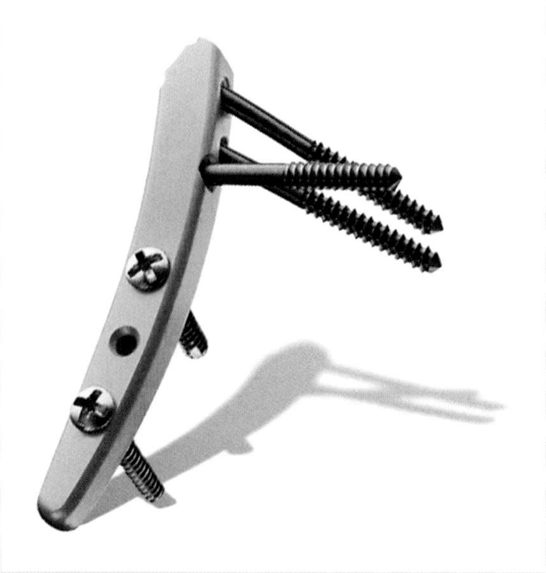

Fig. 8.1 The Micronail device has three fixed-angle distal locking screws and up to three proximal bicortical fixation screws.

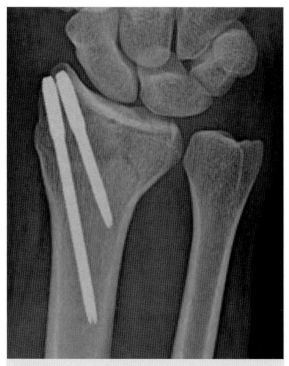

Fig. 8.2 Two T-Pins inserted through the radial styloid. (This image is provided courtesy of John S. Taras, MD.)

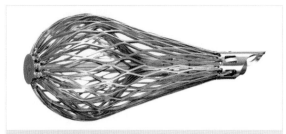

Fig. 8.3 Image of Conventus Distal Radius System (DRS) nitinol expandable cage implant. (*Source:* Conventus Orthopaedics, Maple Grove, MN.)

into the radial styloid of extra-articular distal radius fractures and provides a more rigid, fixed-angle solution than smooth Kirschner wires (K-wires).[13]

Recently, the Distal Radius System (DRS) Implant (Conventus Orthopedics, Maple Grove, MN) was introduced (▶ Fig. 8.3).[14] The DRS Implant is a nitinol expandable balloon-shaped scaffold implant that is placed immediately beneath the subchondral plate of the distal radius through a proximal hole in the dorsal or radial diaphysis. The implant is secured in place proximally with two diaphyseal screws. Individual fragment fixation is performed distally to fix articular fragments using percutaneous 2.7-mm cannulated screws (▶ Fig. 8.4). These cannulated screws gain locked fixation of the fracture fragments by threading through the four-ply nitinol cage.

Biomechanical studies have been performed to evaluate the stiffness of a number of different IM devices. The Targon DR was compared to the Synthes 2.4-mm titanium VLP with axial- and dorsal-eccentric loading as well as load to failure in an extra-articular dorsal wedge osteotomy model used to simulate an Association for Osteosynthesis (AO) A3 type fracture; the IMN was significantly stiffer with both axial- and dorsal-eccentric loading and had higher stability in load-to-failure testing.[15] The Conventus DRS IM scaffold implant was compared to two commercially available volar plates: the stiffness of the IM scaffold was not statistically different from the VLP but was significantly stiffer than a nonlocking stainless steel T-plate.[14] From a strictly mechanical perspective, IM constructs for distal radius fracture fixation appear to be at least equivalent to volar plate constructs.

8.2 Indications

The indications for IM fixation depend on the fracture type, the extent of soft tissue injury, and whether the fracture can be reduced either closed or percutaneously.[16] Impacted articular fractures, AO type C3 fractures, articular shear fractures or marginal rim fractures, and fractures with extensive metaphyseal/diaphyseal extension are generally contraindicated for IM fixation. Contraindications also include pediatric fractures with open physes,

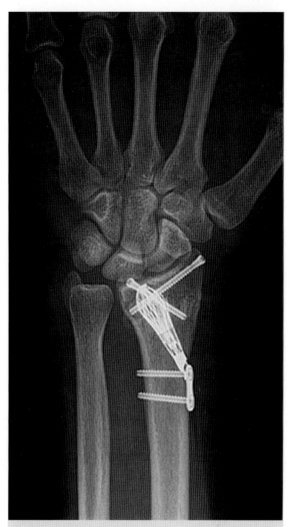

Fig. 8.4 Conventus Distal Radius System (DRS) Implant in place in the distal radius. Radial side approach for insertion of implant is used here. (Copyright © Scott Wolfe, MD)

open fractures with inadequate soft tissue coverage, and active or recent local infection.

Fracture indications vary to some extent by the type of IM implant. The main indications for the use of the T-Pin is an unstable nonarticular dorsally displaced distal radius fracture; it can also be used for simple displaced radial styloid fractures.[13] Some AO type B fractures can be treated with an IMN, a few examples of which are seen in three published series describing Micronail fixation in AO types B1 and B3 fractures.[16,17,18,19] Most of the treated fractures in the Micronail series are types A1, A2, A3, C1, and C2. Provided the fracture can be reduced closed, the IM cage device has the ability to fix more difficult and multifragmentary articular fractures using percutaneous locked articular screws. IM fixation has also been described for osteotomy and fixation of malunited distal radius fractures.[20]

8.3 Intramedullary Nail: Surgical Technique

The technique for insertion of the distal radius IMN (Micronail, Wright Medical Technologies, Arlington, TN) employs two limited incision approaches: one radial and one dorsal. The procedure is performed under general or regional anesthesia, and tourniquet control may be used at the surgeon's discretion.[21] Closed reduction is performed using standard techniques, and the fracture is provisionally fixed with a percutaneous 1.6-mm K-wire inserted through the dorsoulnar corner of the radius, and engaging the volar radial diaphyseal cortex proximal to the fracture site. In the event that an acceptable reduction cannot be attained, a dorsal 2-cm incision is made 1 cm proximal to Lister tubercle and a K-wire or Freer elevator is used to manipulate the articular fragment(s) into acceptable alignment. This same incision can be extended later for the proximal fixation. Temporary K-wire fixation should be placed as far ulnarly as possible to avoid interference with the IMN placement.

A 2- to 3-cm incision is made along the midsagittal axis of the radius over the radial styloid and blunt dissection carried out through subcutaneous tissue, identifying and protecting superficial radial sensory nerve branches. A subperiosteal interval between the first and second dorsal compartments is developed, and a long (at least 12-cm) 1.6-mm K-wire is introduced through the radial styloid, just a few millimeters proximal to the tip. A 6.1-mm cannulated starter drill is inserted through the starter drill/K-wire guide and over the guidewire, and a cortical window is opened. If necessary, a small rongeur can be used to open the window proximally to allow for insertion of the awl. The awl is inserted and directed into the IM canal across the reduced fracture, taking care to hug the radial cortex. After the awl, the canal across the fracture line is sequentially broached until a good proximal fill is achieved while ensuring that the fracture remains reduced. It is

necessary to ensure that the awl does not penetrate the radial cortex.[21]

The nail is sized, using the same size nail as the last broach, when the broach does not spin in the medullary canal. There are four sizes of nail available, and if there is a question, downsizing is recommended. The nail is trialed, the nail and insertion jig are assembled, and the nail is inserted. It is critical to ensure the nail is fully seated before proceeding. The insertion jig then remains in place for insertion of the three divergent fixed-angle locking subchondral screws.

After fluoroscopic confirmation of fracture reduction, proximal fixation with bicortical screws is performed. A 2-cm dorsal incision is made approximately 1 cm proximal to Lister tubercle. Careful dissection is performed down through the interval between the second and third dorsal compartments to the dorsal cortex of the radius. The aiming guide on the insertion jig is used, and two interlocking proximal screws are placed. The incisions are closed, and a volar wrist splint is placed. Injury and postoperative images are shown for a 58-year-old female patient who sustained a dorsally displaced distal radius fracture (▶Fig. 8.5, ▶Fig. 8.6). Five months postoperatively, she had experienced no complications and had recovered excellent range of motion (▶Fig. 8.7).

8.4 Intramedullary Nail: Outcomes

An early series of 10 patients with AO types A and C distal radius fractures were treated with the Micronail IM implant.[22] At an average of 21-month follow-up, all patients had regained full finger motion, with full extension and all fingertips able to touch the palm. At final follow-up, average wrist flexion was 67°, wrist extension was 71°, supination was 82°, and pronation was 85°. Final average disabilities of the arm, shoulder, and

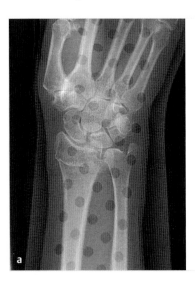 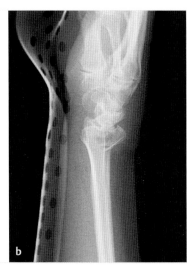

Fig. 8.5 (a) Anteroposterior (AP) and **(b)** lateral preoperative injury radiographs of the wrist in a 58-year-old female patient who sustained distal radius fracture in a ground-level fall. (These images are provided courtesy of Virak Tan, MD.)

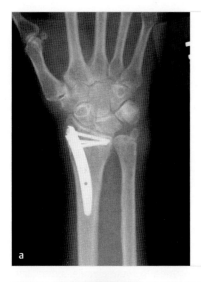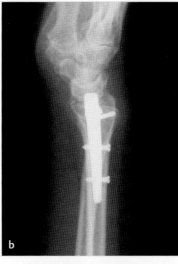

Fig. 8.6 (a) Anteroposterior (AP) and **(b)** lateral postoperative radiographs of the wrist of the same 58-year-old female patient with the dorsally displaced distal radius fracture, 5 months after closed reduction and internal fixation with Micronail. (These images are provided courtesy of Virak Tan, MD.)

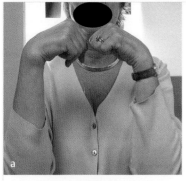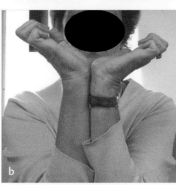
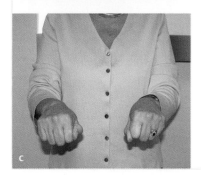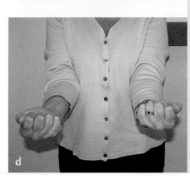

Fig. 8.7 Range of motion of bilateral wrists shown 5 months after closed reduction and internal fixation with Micronail, including **(a)** flexion, **(b)** extension, **(c)** pronation, and **(d)** supination. (These images is provided courtesy of Virak Tan, MD.)

hand (DASH) score was 2.7 after removal of one unrelated outlier. Two of 10 patients had > 5° of loss of reduction. The complications in this series included three cases of penetration of screws into the distal radioulnar joint (DRUJ), one causing DRUJ arthritis. None of these patients underwent hardware removal. A second larger retrospective study on prospectively collected data compared two groups of patients with distal radius fractures: 31 patients treated with the Micronail (AO type A, *n* = 18 patients; type B3, *n* = 1; and type C, *n* = 12) and 32 patients treated in a cast (AO type A, *n* = 19; type B1, *n* = 1; and type C, *n* = 12).[16] This series showed significantly increased flexion–extension arc (at 2-, 6-, and 12-mo follow-up) and significantly lower DASH scores at final (12 mo) follow-up in the IMN group, and the casting group had five

major and five minor delayed complications, while the IMN group had seven minor complications in the first 2 months (three patients had radial sensory neuritis, one CRPS, one trigger finger, and one finger stiffness) and no major or delayed complications, including no screw penetration to DRUJ and no need for hardware removal.

A number of other small studies report the outcomes of use in distal radius fracture fixation. A systematic review of IMN fixation by Hardman et al identified 14 studies involving 357 patients with a mean age of 63.7 years (standard deviation [SD] 11.3).[17] Eleven of the series used the Micronail, two used the Sonoma WRx, and one series reported results of the Targon DR. Functional scores, range of motion (ROM), grip strength, radiologic outcomes, and complications were evaluated. In 10 studies

(169 patients), DASH was reported with an aggregate mean of 6.33 (SD 8.45). Three studies (72 patients) used Mayo score with an aggregate mean of 93.17 (SD 7.66), and 2 studies (97 patients) used Gartland and Werley with an aggregate mean of 2.32 (SD 1.37). Radiological outcomes were reported in the studies (radial height was reported in 10 studies, volar tilt in 12, radial inclination in 12, and ulnar variance in 6) and were pooled together; the authors commented that radial height was the value restored closest to anatomical value (mean 8.98 mm; normal values 11–12 mm). ROM values were pooled and demonstrated an average 110 ± 17° of flexion/extension arc and 46 ± 11° of radioulnar deviation. Average pronosupination arc measured 139 ± 12°. Regarding complications, radial nerve irritation was the most common, at 11.4% (39 patients), and accounting for 58% of all complications. All of these cases were transient and resolved without further intervention. Only one case of device removal was reported, and the removal was at the patient's request. There were no cases of tendon rupture, and tendon irritation occurred in 0.88% (three patients).

8.5 T-Pin: Surgical Technique

This technique can be performed under general or regional anesthesia, with tourniquet control. Under fluoroscopic guidance, standard closed reduction of the fracture is performed, and if needed, a percutaneous 1.6-mm K-wire is used as a joystick to regain volar tilt. Alternatively, a Kapandji pinning technique can be used to temporarily secure the reduction while the T-Pin is placed (▶Fig. 8.8). Typically, if the bone stock is adequate, two T-Pins are placed through the radial styloid within a single 2-cm incision (▶Fig. 8.2). For isolated radial styloid fractures, a single pin can be used (▶Fig. 8.9). A less common location for guidewire/T-Pin placement is through the dorsal lip of the distal radius, also using a 2-cm incision.[13] After incision, the soft tissues are bluntly dissected, and the radial nerve is protected. At the incision over the radial styloid, the first dorsal compartment is routinely released to facilitate pin placement. Smooth 1-mm guidewires are inserted at the site of anticipated pin placement, and fluoroscopy is used to adjust placement. Guidewire advancement stops

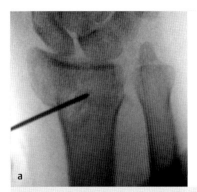
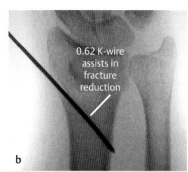
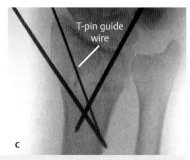

0.62 K-wire assists in fracture reduction

T-pin guide wire

Fig. 8.8 **(a)** Insertion prior to reduction and **(b)** placement of a 1.6-mm Kirschner wire (K-wire) used as a joystick for fracture reduction, and **(c)** temporary fracture reduction and T-Pin guidewire placement through the radial styloid. (These images are provided courtesy of John S. Taras, MD.)

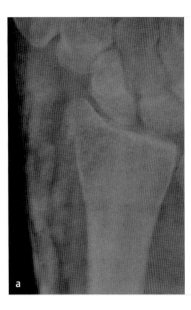
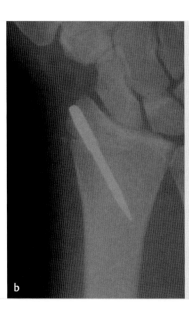

Fig. 8.9 **(a)** Preoperative and **(b)** postoperative AP fluoroscopic images of a radial styloid fracture treated with a single T-Pin. (These image is provided courtesy of John S. Taras, MD.)

when cortical contact is made. A cannulated measuring guide is applied along each guidewire, and the proper length pin is chosen. Pins from 40 to 70 mm are available in 5-mm increments. After measuring and prior to advancing the T-Pin over the guidewire, the guidewire is backed out 10 mm to avoid guidewire kinking or bending near the tip. The T-Pin is advanced until the trailing threads are nearly flush with the bone, and the split tissue protector opens to allow for removal and final seating of the pin, without having to remove the driver. The break-off driver mechanism is disengaged and the guidewire is removed, leaving only the T-Pin in place.[12,13,23] Fluoroscopy is used to assess reduction and fixation. Once complete, the Kapandji pins are removed if present, the tourniquet is released, the incision(s) are closed, and a volar splint is placed.

8.6 T-Pin: Outcomes

A series of 24 patients with AO types A2, A3, and B1 distal radius fractures treated with T-Pin fixation was reported with an average follow-up of 25 months. ROM was recorded but not reported. Radiographic outcomes were reported for volar tilt and radial height. Average preoperative volar tilt was 19.4° dorsal (range 12.0° volar to 38.7° dorsal) and average preoperative radial height was 4.3 mm (range −18.0 to 15.0 mm). The immediate and final radiographic volar tilt and radial height averages were not reported; however, it was noted that immediate and final postoperative radiographs were assessed and showed maintenance of reduction in all but one patient. DASH score was used to evaluate functional outcomes, and the average final DASH score was 4.3 (range 0–35). The patient with the DASH score of 35 required carpal tunnel release 6 months after surgery; this patient had no symptoms of carpal tunnel syndrome until 4 months after distal radius fracture operation. Regarding complications, one patient (4%) who was noted to have loss of radial height, however, grip strength and ROM were excellent and DASH score was 2.5, 2 years after surgery. One patient reported transient radial sensory neuritis, and one patient required carpal tunnel decompression. One patient requested elective hardware removal 6 months after the initial procedure, and one patient had hardware removal 3 years after the initial procedure because of tenderness and pain at the pin insertion site with ROM. This patient's symptoms resolved after pin removal, and the DASH score was 0 postoperatively.[23]

8.7 Distal Radius System Intramedullary Cage: Surgical Technique

The procedure is performed with the patient supine on a hand table. Tourniquet use is optional; alternatively, lidocaine 1% with epinephrine (1:100,000) can be infiltrated at the incision site. Closed or percutaneous reduction of the fracture is performed. The reduction is then provisionally held using parallel 1.6-mm Kirschner "caging" wires inserted obliquely from the dorsal rim to the volar diaphysis on the far radial and ulnar margins of the radius. The wires are placed so as not to interfere with reaming or the placement of the IM cage. A target wire is placed in a dorsal volar direction, starting near Lister tubercle, at the planned apex of the implant and immediately beneath the subchondral bone (▶ Fig. 8.10). A small or large implant is chosen based on a sizing template, which also specifies the site of the incision, which is 2.5 cm in length and may be made dorsally or radially at the surgeon's discretion. After incision, blunt dissection is performed down to bone, protecting the subcutaneous nerves. A custom self-retaining retractor is inserted, and a 2.5-mm side-cutting drill is used to perforate the dorsal cortex and then it is directed distally towards the target wire. A guidewire is inserted and overdrilled with a 5.0-mm drill (▶ Fig. 8.10). After confirmation with fluoroscopy, the cavity is prepared using a collapsible cannulated reamer, taking care to preserve endosteal cortical bone (▶ Fig. 8.11). This cavity prep tool is then collapsed and removed, and the implant is placed, expanded, and locked in position. A two-hole washer is then placed over the cortex and two cortical screws are placed to secure the washer and the implant (▶ Fig. 8.12).

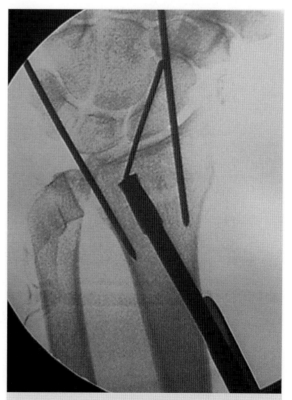

Fig. 8.10 Anteroposterior (AP) fluoroscopy image of the provisional reduction and guidewires in place and the cannulated drill in place. (Copyright © Scott Wolfe, MD)

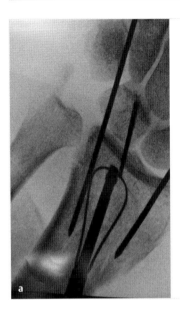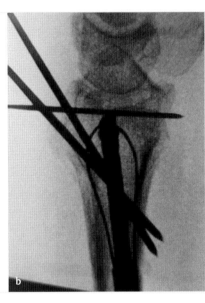

Fig. 8.11 (a) Anteroposterior (AP) and **(b)** lateral fluoroscopic images of the reamer in place, with the provisional wires and guidewire remaining in place. (Copyright © Scott Wolfe, MD)

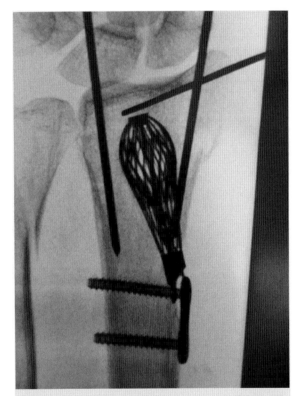

Fig. 8.12 Anteroposterior (AP) fluoroscopic image of the Distal Radius System (DRS) intramedullary (IM) cage expanded in place and proximally secured with a washer and two screws. Kirschner wire (K-wire) remain in place, prior to screw fixation. (Copyright © Scott Wolfe, MD)

The articular fragments are then maintained in their reduced position by using 2.7-mm cannulated screws inserted percutaneously, passing through the fragment and through all four layers of the expandable cage implant. The far cortex can be engaged at the surgeon's discretion, though there is likely no mechanical benefit to do so. There is a 270° arc that can be used for screw insertion, such that percutaneous or mini-incision placement of fixation screws can be placed in the radial styloid, dorsal cortex, dorsal ulnar fragment, or volar ulnar fragment. The two standard sites for screw placement are the radial styloid and the dorsoulnar corner positions. Following wire placement and fluoroscopic confirmation of engagement of all four leaves of the cage, the wire is measured and then overdrilled with cannulated drill through a protective soft tissue sleeve, followed by insertion of the cannulated fixation screw (▶ Fig. 8.13).

Once complete, the incisions are closed, and the patient is placed in a volar resting splint. Dressings are removed in several days and the patient is instructed to remove the splint for full active and active-assisted wrist ROM. Resistive exercises are held for 6 weeks or until healing is confirmed radiographically.

8.8 Distal Radius System Intramedullary Cage: Outcomes

Only two outcome studies have been published to date for the Conventus DRS IM cage implant.[24,25] The largest was a multicenter case series of 100 patients with the following distal radius fracture types: 27 patients with AO type A2; 38 patients with AO type A3; 6, 5, and 1 patients with AO types B1, B2, and B3, respectively; and 19 patients with AO type C1 and 5 patients with AO type C2. The patients were all treated with reduction and fixation using the DRS IM cage implant for distal radius fracture. In this study, ROM was measured as a percentage of the contralateral uninjured wrist. Wrist flexion and extension were on average 50% of normal at 2 weeks and 75% of normal at 12 weeks. Pronation and supination improved

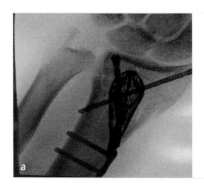 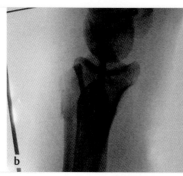

Fig. 8.13 (a) Anteroposterior (AP) and **(b)** lateral fluoroscopic images of the Distal Radius System (DRS) intramedullary (IM) cage and two cannulated screws securing distal fragments in place. (Copyright © Scott Wolfe, MD)

to 88% of normal at 2 weeks and 85% at 12 weeks. Radial and ulnar deviation approached 60% at 2 weeks and 78% by 12 weeks. There continued to be improvement up to 1 year but most of the recovery was achieved by 12 weeks. Excellent functional results were reported (mean DASH at 12 months was 9, and mean patient-rated wrist evaluation at 12 months was 11). There were five adverse events reported, including two patients with radial nerve irritation. One underwent neurolysis at 8 weeks, and both the patients' symptoms resolved by 12 weeks. Three patients developed pain from prominent screws during the healing period and underwent removal of the screws after the fracture had healed. The IM devices did not require removal, though removal instrumentation is available if required. The overall complication rate was 5%.[24]

8.9 Pitfalls and Contraindications

Overall, for IM implants, proper patient selection and recognition of the fracture type are important for successful treatment. With the smaller incisions, direct fracture fragment visualization is limited, and fluoroscopy is relied upon to evaluate the adequacy of reduction and hardware placement.

Shear fractures are generally contraindicated. The T-Pin device is not generally utilized for complex articular fractures. Micronail and DRS IM cage can be used for some articular fractures, including AO type C1 or C2 fractures. With the Conventus DRS IM cage, volar shear fractures and small articular rim fragments are challenging to reduce and fix anatomically, and as for all fixation systems, there is a learning curve. When drilling with the 5-mm cannulated drill, the surgeon should ensure as obtuse a drilling angle as possible, to direct the drill tip distally without penetrating or reaming the contralateral cortex. Fluoroscopy is used throughout the case to confirm the correct placement of wires, drills, reamer, cage, and screws. Careful dissection of the four to five interval should be done and the tendons of the fourth and fifth dorsal compartments retracted to expose the dorsal cortex safely.

Tips and Tricks

Micronail:
- Careful awl placement ensures smooth progression to nail placement.
- Ensure nail is well seated before placing distal locking screws—avoid radiocarpal and radioulnar joint penetration.

T-Pin:
- The guidewire will deflect off the inner cortices and bend, whereas the T-Pin will not; therefore, guidewire insertion should stop when cortical contact is made.
- Retract guidewire partially before completion of final T-pin insertion to avoid wire breakage or bending.

Distal Radius System Intramedullary Cage:
- Be careful to reduce any "coronal shift" of the articular fragment to increase the stability of the distal radioulnar joint.[26]
- Be sure the incision is in the dorsal midline when using the dorsal approach. If the entry hole is radial or ulnar of the midline, correct placement will be difficult.
- Increase incision size proximally as necessary to allow the 5-mm drill to "lay down" as much as possible and improve the angle of entry.
- Fractures that are initially volar displaced, especially with small articular fragments, may be challenging from the dorsal approach, as the drill may displace the articular fragment.
- Plan the starting position for the dorsoulnar wire to be 2–3 mm radial to the sigmoid notch to avoid articular penetration.

8.10 Conclusion

IM devices present a relatively new, effective, and safe option for distal radius fracture fixation. They offer the advantage of comparably rigid fixation with small incisions, decreased soft tissue disruption, and buried hardware. Published series demonstrate an excellent complication profile, including what may prove to be a lower rate of tendon rupture and hardware removal when compared to traditional internal fixation techniques. As with any newer technology, there is a learning curve for device application and limitations in terms of the complexity of fracture types that may be treated with IM devices.

As the different types of IM fixation for distal radius have evolved, the indications for this type of fixation are broadening. The cannulated pin implant is used for simple displaced extra-articular metaphyseal distal radius fractures and offers better bony purchase than smooth K-wires. The IMN implants offer improved fixed-angle subchondral support of the articular surface that may expand indications to more complicated fracture types. The IM cage implant with the percutaneous screw placement adds a level of fragment-specific fixation to the IM construct, achieving secure locked fixation of large fragments and expanded indications, to include a larger number of fracture fragments and articular fracture patterns.

Acknowledgment

The authors thank John S. Taras, MD, and Virak Tan, MD, for their contributions of images and expertise in techniques of IM fixation for distal radius fracture fixation.

References

[1] Chen Y, Chen X, Li Z, Yan H, Zhou F, Gao W. Safety and Efficacy of Operative Versus Nonsurgical Management of Distal Radius Fractures in Elderly Patients: A Systematic Review and Meta-analysis. J Hand Surg Am 2016;41(3):404–413

[2] Arora R, Lutz M, Hennerbichler A, Krappinger D, Espen D, Gabl M. Complications following internal fixation of unstable distal radius fracture with a palmar locking-plate. J Orthop Trauma 2007;21(5):316–322

[3] Berglund LM, Messer TM. Complications of volar plate fixation for managing distal radius fractures. J Am Acad Orthop Surg 2009;17(6):369–377

[4] Knight D, Hajducka C, Will E, McQueen M. Locked volar plating for unstable distal radial fractures: clinical and radiological outcomes. Injury 2010;41(2):184–189

[5] Disseldorp DJ, Hannemann PF, Poeze M, Brink PR. Dorsal or Volar Plate Fixation of the Distal Radius: Does the Complication Rate Help Us to Choose? J Wrist Surg 2016;5(3):202–210

[6] Ruch DS, Papadonikolakis A. Volar versus dorsal plating in the management of intra-articular distal radius fractures. J Hand Surg Am 2006;31(1):9–16

[7] Rein S, Schikore H, Schneiders W, Amlang M, Zwipp H. Results of dorsal or volar plate fixation of AO type C3 distal radius fractures: a retrospective study. J Hand Surg Am 2007;32(7):954–961

[8] Wei J, Yang TB, Luo W, Qin JB, Kong FJ. Complications following dorsal versus volar plate fixation of distal radius fracture: a meta-analysis. J Int Med Res 2013;41(2):265–275

[9] Tan V, Capo J, Warburton M. Distal radius fracture fixation with an intramedullary nail. Tech Hand Up Extrem Surg 2005;9(4):195–201

[10] Gradl G, Mielsch N, Wendt M, et al. Intramedullary nail versus volar plate fixation of extra-articular distal radius fractures. Two year results of a prospective randomized trial. Injury 2014;45 (Suppl 1):S3–S8

[11] Gunther SB, Lynch TL. Rigid internal fixation of displaced distal radius fractures. Orthopedics 2014;37(1):e34–e38

[12] Taras JS, Zambito KL, Abzug JM. T-Pin for distal radius fracture. Tech Hand Up Extrem Surg 2006;10(1):2–7

[13] Bilbrew L, Matthias R, Wright T. Cannulated Self-Drilling, Self-Tapping Pins for Displaced Extra-articular Distal Radius Fractures. J Hand Surg Am 2018;43(3):294.e1–294.e5

[14] van Kampen RJ, Thoreson AR, Knutson NJ, Hale JE, Moran SL. Comparison of a new intramedullary scaffold to volar plating for treatment of distal radius fractures. J Orthop Trauma 2013;27(9):535–541

[15] Burkhart KJ, Nowak TE, Gradl G, et al. Intramedullary nailing vs. palmar locked plating for unstable dorsally comminuted distal radius fractures: a biomechanical study. Clin Biomech (Bristol, Avon) 2010;25(8):771–775

[16] Tan V, Bratchenko W, Nourbakhsh A, Capo J. Comparative analysis of intramedullary nail fixation versus casting for treatment of distal radius fractures. J Hand Surg Am 2012;37(3):460–468.e1

[17] Hardman J, Al-Hadithy N, Hester T, Anakwe R. Systematic review of outcomes following fixed angle intramedullary fixation of distal radius fractures. Int Orthop 2015;39(12):2381–2387

[18] Safi A, Hart R, Těknědžjan B, Kozák T. Treatment of extra-articular and simple articular distal radial fractures with intramedullary nail versus volar locking plate. J Hand Surg Eur Vol 2013;38(7):774–779

[19] van Vugt R, Geerts RW, Werre AJ. Osteosynthesis of distal radius fractures with the Micronail. Eur J Trauma Emerg Surg 2010;36(5):471–476

[20] Ilyas AM, Reish MW, Beg TM, Thoder JJ. Treatment of distal radius malunions with an intramedullary nail. Tech Hand Up Extrem Surg 2009;13(1):30–33

[21] Ilyas AM. Intramedullary fixation of distal radius fractures. J Hand Surg Am 2009;34(2):341–346

[22] Ilyas AM, Thoder JJ. Intramedullary fixation of displaced distal radius fractures: a preliminary report. J Hand Surg Am 2008;33(10):1706–1715

[23] Taras JS, Saillant JC, Goljan P, McCabe LA. Distal Radius Fracture Fixation With the Specialized Threaded Pin Device. Orthopedics 2016;39(1):e98–e103

[24] Strassmair MK, Jonas M, Schäfer W, Palmer A. Distal Radial Fracture Management With an Intramedullary Cage and Fragment Fixation. J Hand Surg Am 2016;41(8):833–840

[25] Rancy SK, Malliaris SD, Bogner EA, Wolfe SW. Intramedullary Fixation of Distal Radius Fractures Using CAGE-DR Implant. J Wrist Surg 2018;7(5):358–365

[26] Trehan SK, Orbay JL, Wolfe SW. Coronal shift of distal radius fractures: influence of the distal interosseous membrane on distal radioulnar joint instability. J Hand Surg Am 2015;40(1):159–162

9 Mini Approaches

Gustavo Mantovani Ruggiero

Abstract

Minimally invasive surgery is a tendency in surgical fields, and it is no exception in distal radius fracture (DRF) surgery. Nowadays it is feasible to fix a DRF using a volar plate through a 10-mm incision. This chapter is focused on the current mini-approaches used for volar plate osteosynthesis on DRF, discussing its origins, indications, techniques, pitfalls, and limitations.

Keywords: minimal approach, mini-approach radius, scarring radius, distal radius fracture, minimal invasive surgery.

9.1 Introduction

Distal radius fractures (DRFs) treatment suffered a revolution in early 2000 with the upcoming of fixed-angle volar plates and the extended volar approach.[1] The promising results, moreover on complex fractures, allowing anatomical reduction and faster mobilization, showed a remarkable difference to other traditional methods.[2]

The use of arthroscopy during DRF surgery made clear the quantity and quality of associated injuries,[3,4] permitting a better treatment of those injuries and judgment about the better postoperative immobilization protocol.

The flexor carpi radialis (FCR) extended approach demonstrated excellent results on the treatment of complex DRF, showing a capacity of anatomical reduction not seen before by the previous reduction and fixation methods. Nevertheless, the relevance of complications increased as much as the use of technique became more popular, leading to evolution of dissection technique and implant fixation.[5] The study of complications on the use of volar locking plates on DRF had shown the capital mistakes on dissection, reduction, and plate/screws position.[6,7] Tips and tricks to avoid flexor tendons rupture were described, like local soft tissues flaps[8] and pronator-sparing techniques.[9,10]

The complications reported around this technique, and the potential benefit of a more conservative postoperative immobilization protocol, awaken a new discussion, opposing the extended volar approach to minimally invasive techniques, moreover percutaneous pinning.[11,12,13]

Regarding the simple extra-articular DRF, there are important questions: Is that necessary an aggressive extended surgical approach, to provide anatomical reduction and rigid fixation, for a simple DRF we traditionally treat by percutaneous Kirschner wires (K-wires)? Is the benefit of prompt mobilization after surgery worthy the disadvantages of more aggressive surgical approach? What is the economic impact facing a more expensive fixation method to a longer recovery and more expensive

rehabilitation protocol? Is a conservative treatment or percutaneous pinning for DRF, with 6 weeks in a cast exempt of complications? How relevant may be to an elder or younger patient to provide his independence for daily life activities (DLA) right after surgery? Literature stressed all these questions with papers comparing results with plates and percutaneous pinning, with variable results, some defending the plate fixation, and others showing a similar result in a long-term follow-up.[11,12] Nevertheless, this debate leads many surgeons and researchers to pursue new fixation solutions able to provide rigid stability using less aggressive approaches. Several new solutions were described like nonbridged external fixators and different innovative intramedullary fixed-angle devices (▶Fig. 9.1). The results of the intramedullary locking devices are good and comparable to the volar locking plates and other percutaneous methods.[14,15,16,17] Drawbacks are the higher costs of the implants and the longer learning curve necessary to master an entirely new technique and instruments. In parallel, a simple solution for this question was to use the same well-known volar plates, but by minimally invasive approaches, with less soft tissue dissection and smaller skin incisions.[2]

This chapter will focus on the minimally invasive plate osteosynthesis (MIPO) techniques using volar locking plates on DRF, as we perceive the volar plates as more practical and available implant worldwide, and the actual gold standard on DRF treatment.

9.2 Volar Minimally Invasive Plate Osteosynthesis History

There was always a quest in surgery specialties for minimal aggression. The surgical treatment of DRF should not be different.

First descriptions mentioning mini approaches for DRF reduction and fixation using plates are from 2000[18] and 2001.[19] Those papers were the first to mention the concept of "minimally invasive approach," and gathered a combination of different techniques with less aggressive surgical exposure for reduction and fixation. Basically, the authors used K-wires combined with small nonlocking mini plates to achieve the fixation[18] and arthroscopic assistance for articular reduction[19] in some cases. This concept was updated later with the popularization of DRF volar locking plates on 2005 when the technique described was basically a "bridge" approach with two longitudinal incisions to spare the pronator quadratus (PQ) muscle.[20] The skin incision size was not the relevant issue because the two incisions size together was bigger than a single traditional

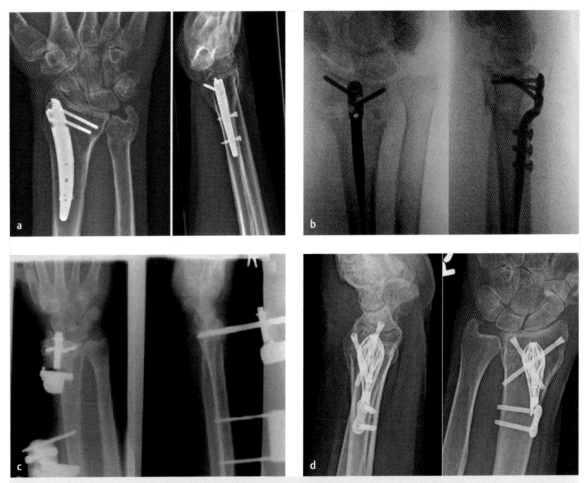

Fig. 9.1 Different minimally invasive fixation methods for distal radius fracture (DRF) with fixed-angle stability. **(a)** Micronail (Wright Medical, Memphis, TN, USA). **(b)** Minimally invasive Dorsal Nail-Plate (Hand Innovations, Miami, FL, USA). **(c)** External fixation in nonbridging assembly. **(d)** Conventus Cage–DR (Conventus Orthopaedics, Maple Grove, MN, USA).

FCR volar skin incision. The major concern on this technique was the potential benefit in not disrupting the PQ muscle, as a factor for painless postoperative, less scar formation, less contracture, and better functional outcome.[9] Several authors also described PQ-sparing techniques using traditional open approach and its influence on clinical outcome.[10]

Soon, the concept of PQ-sparing approach and double skin incisions, evolved to one single small skin incision, longitudinal to the FCR, is widely spread by the Strasbourg group in several reports and publications.[21,22,23] This group was the greater promoter of this technique, evolving its indications and efficiency along the years, applying not only to simple extra-articular fractures but also to more complex fractures and even to malunions corrections.[24] This experience leads to the development of new specific implants, obtaining the smaller skin incision description.[25]

In 2011, a Japanese group described the experience on MIPO technique with another double-incision approach, using a transverse incision distally and a longitudinal incision proximally.[26] This group claimed a better cosmetic result since distal skin scar was hidden by the proximal wrist crease. However, the size of skin incisions was considerable big for a mini approach (30 mm for the distal incision and 20 mm for the proximal incision, according to paper pictures), and the distal transverse scar could promote a stigma of suicidal attempt when becomes hypertrophic and more visible.

Parallel to those, in 2010, our team started our own MIPO technique, using the PQ sparing concept and double incisions: a small transverse skin incision distally (20 mm) and a punctual incision proximally (5 mm). This technique may be found on Internet videos published by the chapter author.

After all, two major lines of MIPO techniques evolved and got new promoters: single longitudinal incision and double transverse incision, leading to the creation of new special volar plates setups adapted to each technique's pitfalls and benefits.

9.3 Indications

Initially, the major indication for MIPO technique was the extra-articular reducible DRF: the classical Colles fracture, usually treated by closed reduction and percutaneous K-wires. This fracture, with low-energy trauma mechanism, was rarely involved with severe associated ligament injuries, affecting elder patients, to whom the prompt recover for DLA is very important.

Thus, offering a minimally invasive procedure, equivalent in morbidity and risks to K-wires percutaneous fixation, that could provide a "cast-free" postoperative recovery, is a great benefit for those patients.

Thus, extra-articular and unstable DRF (Association for Osteosynthesis [AO] type A3) is the main indication for MIPO techniques because of two important aspects: reducibility of the fracture by closed maneuvers and low probability of associated injuries (▶ Fig. 9.2). The fracture must be reducible because the mini approach does not provide a large exposure of fracture site and makes difficult to manipulate bone fragments to perform a laborious open reduction maneuver. The absence of associated injuries is relevant because the main benefit of the technique compared to percutaneous pinning is to allow the prompt mobilization of the wrist and let the patient be without a cast after the surgery. If there is a ligament injury that requires 4 to 6 weeks of wrist immobilization, there will be no greater benefit on MIPO compared to percutaneous K-wires.

The indications may also include nondisplaced and stable fractures (AO type A2) where conservative treatment is possible, in special on the group of younger and productive patients. On those cases, where the immobilization is a relevant social and economic problem, MIPO technique may provide a good solution. We had some patients in our series on these conditions, working as private drivers, surgeons, dentists, and other liberal professions (▶ Fig. 9.3).

After a good learning curve and familiarity with MIPO approach, one can increase the possibilities to more complex fractures and include articular fractures, preferable the simple articular fractures (AO

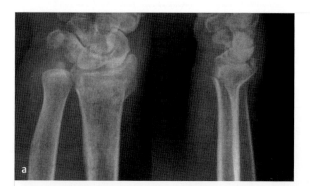
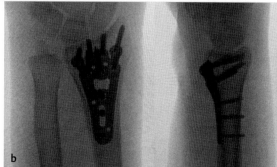
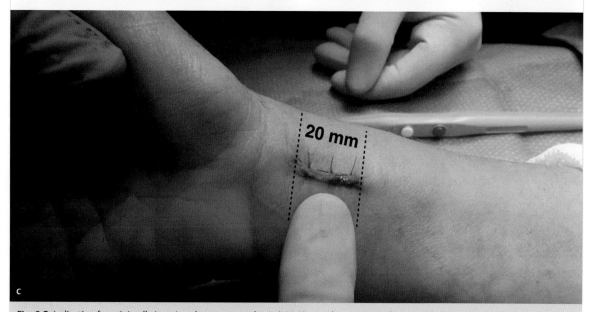

Fig. 9.2 Indication for minimally invasive plate osteosynthesis (MIPO): simple extra-articular unstable fractures. **(a)** Initial X-rays showing Association for Osteosynthesis (AO) type A3 distal radius fracture (DRF). **(b)** Intraoperative fluoroscopy with final fixation. **(c)** Final skin aspect with longitudinal MIPO technique.

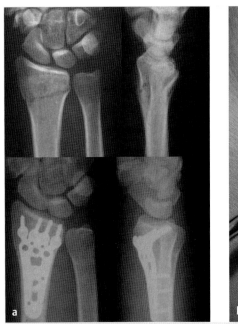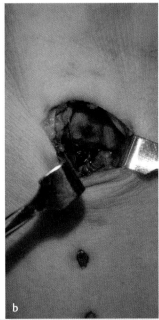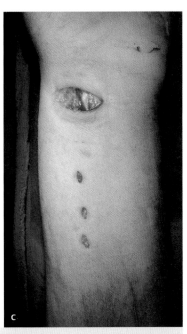

Fig. 9.3 Indication for minimally invasive plate osteosynthesis (MIPO): stable and nondisplaced fracture on a patient profile that requires immediate mobilization. **(a)** Initial X-rays showing an extra-articular stable fracture, Association for Osteosynthesis (AO) type A2 distal radius fracture (DRF), and the final fixation. **(b)** Intraoperative aspect of the distal mini approach using transverse incision MIPO technique. **(c)** Global aspect of the mini approaches for distal and proximal fixation.

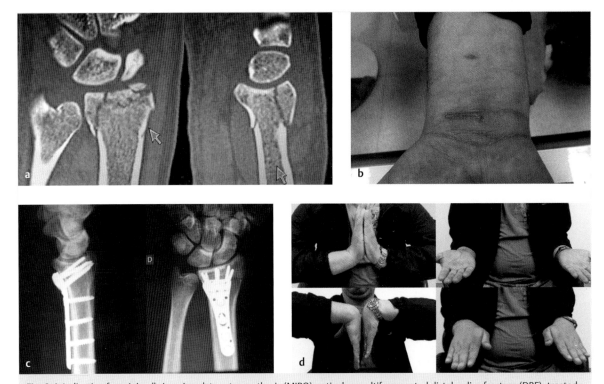

Fig. 9.4 Indication for minimally invasive plate osteosynthesis (MIPO): articular, multifragmented distal radius fracture (DRF), treated by MIPO technique and arthroscopic assistance for articular reduction. **(a)** Computed tomography (CT) scan of DRF. **(b)** Aspect of skin scar after 1 month. **(c)** Postoperative fixation. **(d)** Range of motion (ROM) after 1 month.

types C1 and C2). Lately, the combination of MIPO techniques with arthroscopic reduction assistance included more complex and displaced articular fractures (AO type C3) on the possible indications, making possible almost any fracture to be treated by this technique (▶Fig. 9.4).

The indication of mini approaches for complex articular fractures depends on surgeon's experience, using percutaneous reduction techniques and arthroscopic approach, having in mind that a MIPO technique can be easily and anytime converted to a traditional approach if a good reduction is not feasible to be obtained.

The great concern dealing with a complex fracture is to consider the fracture pattern and all the fragments present, when choosing the proper implant. Comminuted articular fractures may require anatomically designed distal radius plates with large distal rows of screws to provide wide subchondral support and fixation of many different articular fragments. Usually, those plates are wide and big and may be more difficult to be applied by MIPO technique. The new MIPO plates are smaller and simpler and may not provide the required stability for all the articular fragments on a complex DRF, as we show in our complications description below.

9.4 Surgical Technique

9.4.1 Single Longitudinal Incision

The group from Strasbourg, France, promoted this technique. The incision is marked on FCR line, with 15 to 20 mm, centered on the final position of the plate (we recommend the use of fluoroscope with the plate over the skin to determine the perfect position for the plate over the fracture and consequently the best position of skin incision).

Dissect the subcutaneous tissue along the FCR line distally and proximally to the skin incision and expose FCR sheath. Note that the skin incision is used during all the procedure as a "mobile window" to visualize the deeper layers of the approach. Using the natural skin elasticity and mobility, move the skin approach distally and proximally to access all the area usually necessary to be exposed on the conventional volar approach (▶ Fig. 9.5).

Incise the FCR sheath and expose the FCR tendon, proximally and distally to the skin incision. Retract FCR tendon medially (this allows to naturally protect median nerve and palmar cutaneous branch) and expose the floor of the FCR sheath. Incise the FCR sheath floor proximally and distally to the skin exposition, exposing the PQ muscle, while sustaining the FCR retracted medially.

Make a sharp incision on the transition between PQ muscle and volar capsule, transversely to skin incision. Using a periosteal elevator, clean the volar aspect of the distal radius on the distal fragment. With the periosteal elevator, create a space below the PQ muscle and prepare the place for the plate, exposing the fracture site for reduction. Usual reduction maneuvers and cleaning of fracture site can be easily done at this moment.

Insert the plate below the PQ and perform reduction/fixation according to the surgeon preferred method:
- First, fix the plate on the distal fragment and use the plate as a reduction device.
- First, fix the plate on the proximal fragment and perform a reduction maneuver for the distal fragment with traction and wrist flexion. Fix the distal screws with one hand, while holding the reduction with another hand.
- Alternatively, some surgeons prefer to perform a closed reduction and a temporary K-wires fixation before starting the mini approach and then fix the plate on a previously reduced fracture (▶ Fig. 9.7).

Plate positioning, reduction, and fixation are controlled by fluoroscopy. Proximal screws are fixed on the plate using small incisions on the PQ fibers, or simply dissect the fibers with a small forceps and fix the locking guide.

Once fixation is complete, close the skin incision, preferably with intradermal suture for cosmetic reasons. Usually, no immobilization is required as the soft tissue damage is not relevant, and expected postoperative pain is minimal.

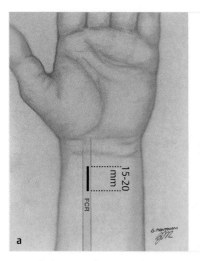
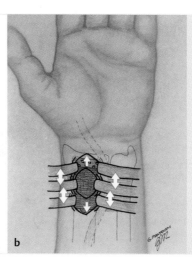

Fig. 9.5 Longitudinal incision technique for minimally invasive plate osteosynthesis (MIPO).

9.4.2 Transverse Incision

The first to describe this technique was a group from Japan[26] in 2011. In its paper, the transverse distal incision was illustrated on figures with 30 mm and another proximal incision around 20 mm. We propose that the same technique could be performed using a smaller skin incision.

Mark the transverse skin incision with 15 to 20 mm, depending on surgeon experience and size of implant (the width of the plate used is the limitation for the size of the distal incision). The skin incision is transverse to FCR, centered on the tendon line on the proximal wrist crease (usually 15 mm proximally to the distal wrist crease when there is no proximal crease visible).

Dissect the subcutaneous tissue proximally and distally over the FCR sheath. Open the FCR sheath and retract the tendon medially, so it protects the median nerve and palmar cutaneous branch. Incise the FCR sheath floor and expose the PQ muscle, keeping the FCR medially.

Incise the edge of PQ muscle, along the transition between muscle fibers and the volar capsule, transverse to the FCR. Expose the volar cortex on the distal fragment and create a space below the PQ using a periosteal elevator.

Insert the plate under the PQ muscle and align the distal part of the plate to the distal fragment, under fluoroscopic control (▶ Fig. 9.6).

Reduction and fixation of the fracture may be done using two different methods:

- First, do the distal fixation of the plate, under fluoroscopic control. Use a long cortical screw as the first distal screw in a central hole on the distal row of the plate, to promote the intimate contact of the plate to the distal fragment volar cortex. The plate must be anatomically aligned to the distal fragment, using fluoroscopic control and the other three or four screws on the distal row of the plate are fixed using locking screws. Lastly, the first cortical screw can be changed for another locking screw. Because the fracture is not perfectly reduced yet, the position of the plate at this moment will show the proximal part not perfectly aligned to the proximal fragment of the radius. It stays medially to the proximal fragment in the anteroposterior view of fluoroscopy and away from volar cortex in the lateral incidence of fluoroscopy. Secondary, using fluoroscopic control, mark the skin over the oblong proximal hole of the plate and make a punctual incision (size enough for the insertion of soft tissue protector guide) around 3 to 5 mm, over the FCR line. With a small forceps, do a blunt dissection until the plate, radially to the FCR. Insert the protector guide until to the oblong hole, check under fluoroscopy, and drill a hole. Then perform light traction to gain the radial shortening and partially reduce the fracture, and insert a long cortical screw (20 mm) on the oblong

hole. Sustain the traction to correct the radial length, while inserting the cortical screw, bringing the proximal part of the plate to the proximal fragment volar cortex, and reducing the dorsal tilt. With a satisfactory reduction achieved, fix the other proximal screws, using the same punctual incision, mobilizing the skin proximally, and distally using the natural skin mobility. Lastly, the first cortical long screw used on the oblong hole to reduce the fracture must be changed to another screw with the proper size of the bone (usually 12 or 14 mm). This method of reduction implies that the normal volar tilt of the radius is corrected by the plate, after it being fixed to the distal fragment, and then the proximal part of the plate stands initially around 1 cm away from the volar cortex of the proximal fragment. That is the reason for using the first cortical screw on the oblong hole long enough to reach the dorsal cortex of the proximal fragment before reach the plate, and thus have the screws threads fixed on both cortices (volar and dorsal) and enough torque to promote the approach of the plate to the bone and consequently reduce the fracture dorsal tilt.

- Perform a closed reduction and K-wires fixation before the mini approach and plate fixation, so the technique will not require the reduction maneuvers and tips above, being basically an "in situ" fixation according to the quality of the reduction obtained with the K-wires (▶ Fig. 9.7). We recommend always the use of the first cortical screw distally, to have the most intimate contact of the plate to the volar cortex of distal fragment, avoiding flexor tendons complications when the plate stands 2 to 3 mm away from the bone. Once the exposition is minimal, visualization of this contact may be tricky, and using initially a cortical screw on the distal fragment prevents this complication.

9.5 Evolution of Distal Radius Fractures Minimally Invasive Plate Osteosynthesis

9.5.1 Special Plates

The philosophy of minimally invasive surgery is becoming more popular and accepted globally. On the MIPO DRF techniques, this popularity is reflected by industry reaction, producing new plate designs adapted to the MIPO techniques.

The major restriction for the minimal size of the longitudinal technique skin incision is the size of the implant on its length (▶ Fig. 9.8b). Thus, a smaller plate in length could permit a surgeon to decrease the skin incision size from 15 to 10 mm. Some industries on the market already provide small implants for the longitudinal incision technique (▶ Fig. 9.8a).

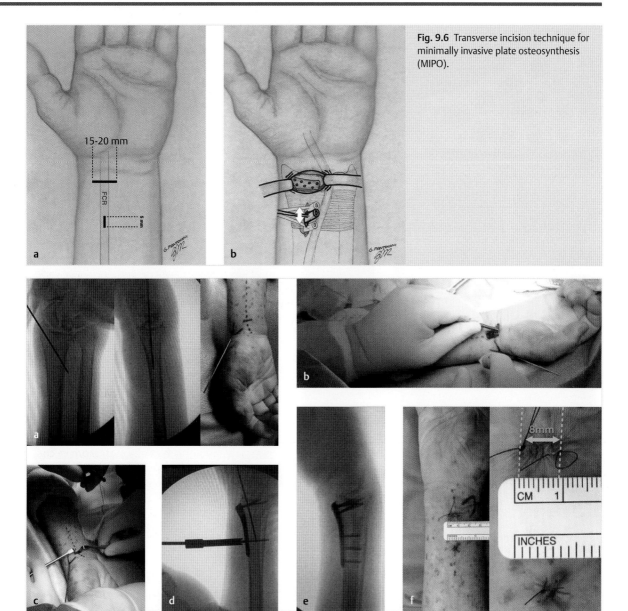

Fig. 9.6 Transverse incision technique for minimally invasive plate osteosynthesis (MIPO).

Fig. 9.7 Minimally invasive plate osteosynthesis (MIPO) transverse technique sequence with previous closed reduction and percutaneous temporary fixation with one K-wire. **(a)** Fluoroscopy after K-wire fixation. **(b)** Insertion of the plate by the mini approach. **(c, d)** Plate fixation. **(e)** Final fixation in lateral view. **(f)** Final skin aspect with less than 10-mm scar.

On the contrary, for the transverse technique, the major restriction for the minimal size skin incision is the size of the implant width (▶Fig. 9.8b). In this direction, new implants designed for this technique are narrower plates. Another tricky step on the transverse incision technique is the insertion of proximal screws, done almost percutaneous. In this way, the quality of soft tissue guides on the plates' instruments setup is relevant. In the same way is the grip of screwdriver to the screws; once during the insertion of the screws proximally, if it sets free from the screwdriver, it becomes lost inside soft tissues and it may be more difficult to find the screw and remove it than the whole programmed surgery. To prevent these difficulties, some special setups for MIPO techniques were made with larger soft tissues protector guides where the screws and screwdriver can be inserted, making easier to mark the screw hole position and avoid soft tissues to disconnect the screw from the screwdriver (▶Fig. 9.8c). Another innovative system to facilitate this step of the surgery is a targeting device, presented in a new Medartis (Basel, Switzerland) MIPO set, in a limited release process on the European market, when this chapter was written (▶Fig. 9.9).

Using those new implants, experienced surgeons can decrease the incision size to less than 10 mm, bringing the DRF MIPO techniques to a new stage.

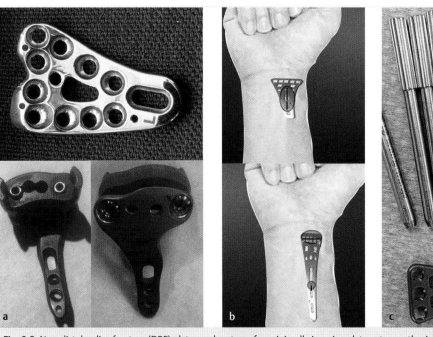

Fig. 9.8 New distal radius fracture (DRF) plates and systems for minimally invasive plate osteosynthesis (MIPO) technique.
(a) Examples of plates for longitudinal incision MIPO technique (silver plate—Osteomed, Addison, TX, USA; green plate—Newclip, Haute Goulaine, France). **(b)** Logics behind the new design for DRF plates for MIPO: short plates for longitudinal technique and narrow/long plates for transverse technique. **(c)** Example of plate for transverse incision MIPO technique: narrow plate with special guides to assist in proximal screws fixation (GMReis, Campinas, SP, Brazil).

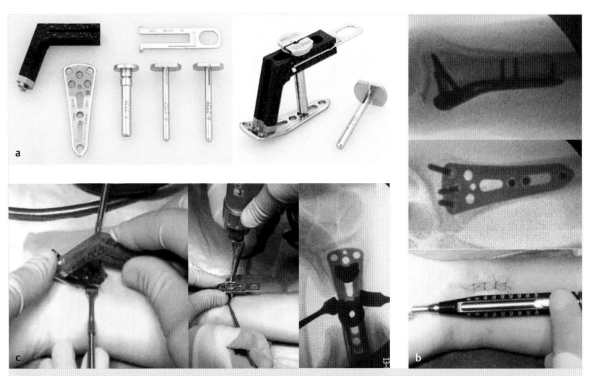

Fig. 9.9 (a-c) Special distal radius fracture (DRF) plate for minimally invasive plate osteosynthesis (MIPO) technique (all intellectual property owned by Medartis, Basel, Switzerland) with external targeting device, pictures of the first prototype limited release product, and one of the first clinical cases done on a limited release evaluation. (This case is provided courtesy of Dr. Pedro Delgado, Madrid, Spain).

9.6 Results, Clinical Examples, and Unusual Minimally Invasive Plate Osteosynthesis Cases

Literature is unanimous, showing equivalent results between MIPO techniques and conventional volar plates techniques. However, the cosmetic benefit is obvious, and some comparative studies and better outcomes on the earlier evaluations demonstrated a faster recovery.[14,26–28]

Coincidentally to the literature, in our clinical experience, using MIPO technique on the last 8 years, from 2010 to 2018, we perceived as the most impressive aspect on the clinical outcome the painless postoperative recovery on the first consultation after the surgery. It was very surprising for us, in the great majority of the cases, how independent the patients were and the good range of motion (ROM; more than 70% of normal ROM) right on the first consultation after surgery 3 to 5 days postoperatively, using normally the affected hand for DLA with almost no pain. This recovery for DLA since the first days after the surgery was quite different from the conventional technique, where patients usually achieved the same function around 2 to 3 weeks, after primary soft tissues healing. This fast recovery is considerably important to elder patients and moreover on bilateral fractures, to provide independence to DLA and self-care (▶Fig. 9.10).

Complications on both literature and our clinical experience are equivalent on MIPO and conventional volar plate techniques and are basically related to technique errors on the plate fixation or to the complexity of the fractures, but not correlated to the mini approaches. As mentioned before, one must not give priority to the mini approach instead of a perfect alignment of the fracture and the best plate position. If it becomes technically demanding to reach the optimal fracture reduction and plate fixation, the mini approach must be abandoned and converted to the traditional FCR approach.

Some special cases are worthy to be illustrated in this chapter, showing unusual indications for mini approaches. One is the combined DRF with a good indication for MIPO technique, but presenting a combined distal ulna fracture on the neck, requiring a combined fixation. It makes no sense to apply a stable fixation method to one bone and an unstable method to the other, obliging the patient to an immobilization postoperative protocol. Thus, we decided to fix the distal ulna as well using a fixed-angle mini plate and properly by a mini approach. That resulted in a very quick recovery and painless postoperative recovery to the patient as shown in ▶Fig. 9.11c. The technique for mini approach to the ulna is not the topic of the chapter but follows a short description. Basically, it consists on the distal ulna fixation by two locking screws of 2.5 mm in a mini T-shape plate and three screws on the proximal fragment, using two mini skin incision (15 mm) over the lateral aspect of the ulna head between flexor carpi ulnaris and extensor carpi ulnaris (▶Fig. 9.11). The major pitfall on this technique is the dorsal sensory branch of the ulnar nerve, during the distal mini approach on the ulna head.

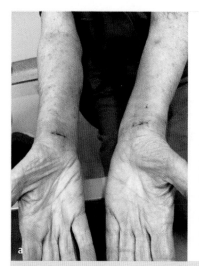
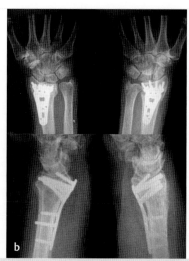
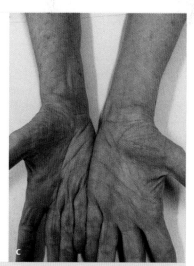

Fig. 9.10 Example of good indication for minimally invasive plate osteosynthesis (MIPO) technique on an 80 years old patient with bilateral distal radius fracture (DRF) due to the fast recovery for daily life activities (DLA). **(a)** Clinical aspect of the skin scars with 5 days after surgery with total independence for DLA. **(b)** X-rays with fractures fixed and healed. **(c)** Final aspect of the scar with 6 months after surgery showing a good cosmetic aspect.

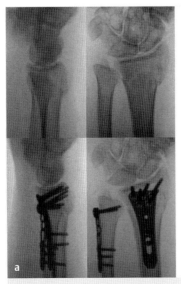
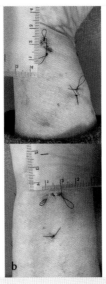
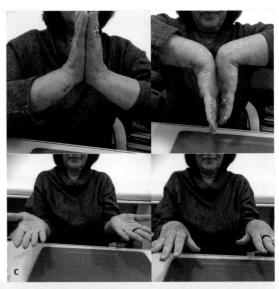

Fig. 9.11 Special case showing a combination of mini approaches for both distal radius fracture (DRF) and distal ulna fracture (DUF). **(a)** Intraoperative fluoroscopy before and after the fixation. **(b)** Clinical aspects of scars with less than 10-mm incisions 7 days after surgery. **(c)** ROM only 7 days after surgery, with total independence for DLA.

9.7 Pitfalls and Contraindications

When a surgical exposure is limited, the major difficulty is to visualize and avoid injury on the noble anatomic structures on the surgical exposition. In the MIPO techniques for DRF, the most at-risk structures are: median nerve, palmar cutaneous branch, and sensitive branch of radial nerve and radial artery. The main advice to avoid the damage to those structures is to stay on the line of FCR from the skin to the bone. When retracting the FCR, do it medially, so your retractor will hold the FCR between the surgical instruments and implants (plate, drill guides, drills, screws, etc.) and the nervous structures (palmar cutaneous branch and median nerve). The radial retractor protects the structures on the radial side (▶ Fig. 9.12).

During the fixation of proximal screws on the transverse incision technique, always use the soft tissue protector guide, and insert it radially to the FCR. Again, the FCR will stay between your working area and the nerve structures. It will be more risky for the radial artery; thus, never neglect the use of the guide to drill. In the worst scenario, a radial artery injury is not as tragic as the median nerve damage, and that is the main reason for choosing the radial side of the FCR tendon.

As described before, with evolution of surgeon experience, one can dare to use mini approaches to more complex cases. The usual indication is extra-articular, unstable DRF. The problem when using the MIPO technique to a comminuted articular fracture may be on the inappropriate fixation and stabilization of all the fragments, when using a special MIPO plate design, which is more simple and smaller. The new MIPO plates were designed to extra-articular fractures, having less distal screws in a simpler arrange, which may not cover all subchondral surface area of distal radius and may not stabilize properly all the articular fragments. Thus, the contraindication for complex multifragmented articular fractures is more about the MIPO implant than the MIPO approach. The surgeon may only treat those fractures if he/she masters the mini approach technique, arthroscopic assistance maneuvers, and adapts carefully the fixation method to the fracture needs. It follows a complication example from the author, using MIPO technique to a complex articular fracture (▶ Fig. 9.13a), with arthroscopic reduction assistance, combined percutaneous screws on the articular fragments, and a special MIPO plate (▶ Fig. 9.13b). The result obtained on the fluoroscopic control on the surgery was satisfactory (▶ Fig. 9.13c) and we judged that the stability was strong enough to allow a fast mobilization protocol, allowing the patient to move his wrist after 1 week. The fixation construction was not sufficient and the fracture collapsed after 3 weeks (▶ Fig. 9.13d). Revising this case, we can criticize the implant election. Maybe, we could avoid the failure using a more robust and wide plate, providing a more extended subchondral area support with more screws in a better position. Maybe, a more conservative immobilization protocol, using a cast for 4 weeks or associating an external fixator, could sustain the initial reduction with the same implants construction. This case illustrates very well the potential contraindications to the MIPO technique and their complication, leaded by "MIPO" implants limitations or the surgeon's audacity.

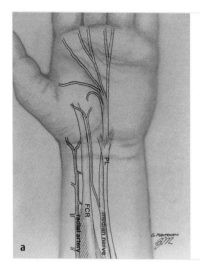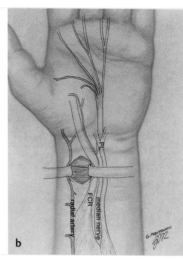

Fig. 9.12 Pitfalls: risky structures. **(a)** Relationship of the riskiest structures on the mini approach. **(b)** Retraction of the flexor carpi radialis (FCR) medially naturally protects the median nerve and palmar cutaneous branch.

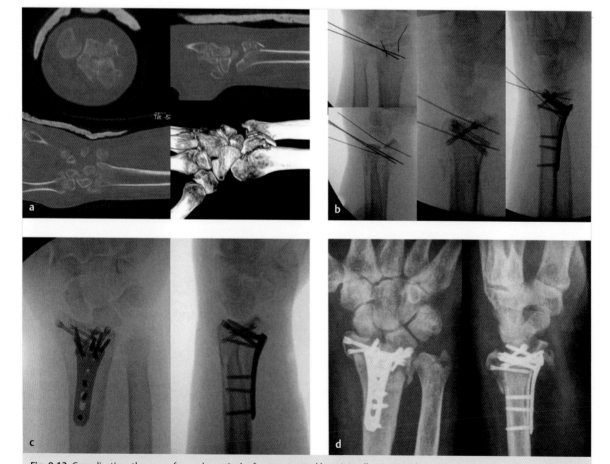

Fig. 9.13 Complication: the case of complex articular fracture treated by minimally invasive plate osteosynthesis (MIPO) technique combined to arthroscopy and percutaneous screws fixation for the articular fragments. **(a)** CT scan of the fracture. **(b)** Intraoperative fluoroscopy showing the articular reduction and fixation step by step. **(c)** Final fixation. **(d)** Late collapse of the fracture after 3 weeks.

Longitudinal technique:

- Start with a 20- to 30-mm incision and practice the principles of pronator-sparing technique and minimally soft tissue disruption during reduction and plate fixation. As your experience grows, start to decrease the size of the skin incision.
- If the case becomes difficult, remember that you can always enlarge your incision and convert the technique to your usual open approach. Do not expose your patient to a bad reduction and fixation to give priority to a small incision.
- Use the fluoroscope before starting to mark the best position of the plate and the skin incision, and be sure to center your skin incision on the plate position. The small skin incision must be centered exactly on the middle of the place where the plate will be fixed. Surgical skin marker is very useful.

Transverse incision:

- Very displaced fractures must be partially reduced before starting the approach. The volar cortex must be aligned, and dorsal tilt must not be very big. If the fracture is very dorsally displaced, the plate will stay too far away from the proximal fragment, in a distance that is impossible to stay below the PQ. Same way, if the volar cortex is not aligned, it becomes difficult to insert the plate below the PQ by the transverse distal incision. This is why most of surgeons, including the chapter's author, prefer to perform a previous closed reduction maneuver and K-wire temporary fixation before the MIPO approach, on those most displaced fractures.
- The first cortical screw, used on the distal row of the plate, must be long enough to cross the dorsal cortex, moreover on osteoporotic patient, to provide enough torque to bring the plate to touch the volar cortex. This screw (usually a 22–24 mm) will be changed for a locking screw with the correct size, to avoid damage to extensor tendons, just after the other locking screws on the distal row are fixed.
- The trickiest part on the transverse MIPO is to insert the proximal screw without loosening it from the screwdriver, inside the forearm. Test the screwdriver grip on the screw, by holding the screw connected to the screwdriver. If the screwdriver does not fall, disconnecting from the screw, it is ok. There will be less chance to loose the screw during the insertion. Another tip is to make a suture on the screw neck with a 3–0 Vicryl and hold this suture threads within the screwdriver, just in case it looses, to make the retrieval easier.
- To perform the transverse incision technique, a good quality setup of implants, a screwdriver with a strong grip on the screw head, and good soft tissue protector guides are mandatory. If the implant setup available does not provide those issues, choose the longitudinal MIPO technique.

9.8 Conclusion

Minimally invasive surgery is a worldwide tendency in every surgical specialty. Mini approach for volar locking plate on DRF is a feasible, safe, and technically reproducible method. It provides an immediate postoperative recovery with less pain, edema, and hematoma, consequently a faster recovery to DLA. This technique is indicated mainly to extra-articular, unstable, and reducible DRF fractures; however with a good learning curve, proper implants and instruments, most DRFs can be treated by this approach.

References

[1] Orbay JL, Badia A, Indriago IR, et al. The extended flexor carpi radialis approach: a new perspective for the distal radius fracture. Tech Hand Up Extrem Surg 2001;5(4):204–211

[2] Loisel F, Kielwasser H, Faivre G, et al. Treatment of distal radius fractures with locking plates: an update. Eur J Orthop Surg Traumatol 2018;28(8):1537–1542

[3] Forward DP, Lindau TR, Melsom DS. Intercarpal ligament injuries associated with fractures of the distal part of the radius. J Bone Joint Surg Am 2007;89(11):2334–2340

[4] Lindau T. Arthroscopic Evaluation of Associated Soft Tissue Injuries in Distal Radius Fractures. Hand Clin 2017;33(4):651–658

[5] Arora R, Lutz M, Hennerbichler A, Krappinger D, Espen D, Gabl M. Complications following internal fixation of unstable distal radius fracture with a palmar locking-plate. J Orthop Trauma 2007;21(5):316–322

[6] Thorninger R, Madsen ML, Wæver D, Borris LC, Rölfing JHD. Complications of volar locking plating of distal radius fractures in 576 patients with 3.2 years follow-up. Injury 2017;48(6):1104–1109

[7] Wilson J, Viner JJ, Johal KS, Woodruff MJ. Volar Locking Plate Fixations for Displaced Distal Radius Fractures: An Evaluation of Complications and Radiographic Outcomes. Hand (N Y) 2018;13(4):466–472

[8] Ruggiero GM. Saving Tendons on Distal Radius Fractures: A Simple Surgical Pearl to Prevent FPL Tendon Conflict with Volar Locking Plates. J Wrist Surg 2017;6(3):248–250

[9] Sen MK, Strauss N, Harvey EJ. Minimally invasive plate osteosynthesis of distal radius fractures using a pronator sparing approach. Tech Hand Up Extrem Surg 2008;12(1):2–6

[10] Cannon TA, Carlston CV, Stevanovic MV, Ghiassi AD. Pronator-sparing technique for volar plating of distal radius fractures. J Hand Surg Am 2014;39(12):2506–2511

[11] Chaudhry H, Kleinlugtenbelt YV, Mundi R, Ristevski B, Goslings JC, Bhandari M. Are Volar Locking Plates Superior to Percutaneous K-wires for Distal Radius Fractures? A Meta-analysis. Clin Orthop Relat Res 2015;473(9):3017–3027

[12] Peng F, Liu YX, Wan ZY. Percutaneous pinning versus volar locking plate internal fixation for unstable distal radius fractures: a meta-analysis. J Hand Surg Eur Vol 2018;43(2):158–167

[13] Dennison DG, Blanchard CL, Elhassan B, Moran SL, Shin AY. Early Versus Late Motion Following Volar Plating of Distal Radius Fractures. Hand (N Y) 2018:1558944718787880 doi:10.1177/1558944718787880.

[14] Aita MA, Vieira Ferreira CH, Schneider Ibanez D, et al. Randomized clinical trial on percutaneous minimally invasive osteosynthesis of fractures of the distal extremity of the radius. Rev Bras Ortop 2014;49(3):218–226

[15] Çalbıyık M, Ipek D. Use of Different Methods of Intramedullary Nailing for Fixation of Distal Radius Fractures: A Retrospective Analysis of Clinical and Radiological Outcomes. Med Sci Monit 2018;24:377–386

[16] Hardman J, Al-Hadithy N, Hester T, Anakwe R. Systematic review of outcomes following fixed angle intramedullary fixation of distal radius fractures. Int Orthop 2015;39(12):2381–2387

[17] Strassmair MK, Jonas M, Schäfer W, Palmer A. Distal Radial Fracture Management With an Intramedullary Cage and Fragment Fixation. J Hand Surg Am 2016;41(8):833–840

[18] Geissler WB, Fernandes D. Percutaneous and limited open reduction of intra-articular distal radial fractures. Hand Surg 2000;5(2):85–92

[19] Duncan SFM, Weiland AJ. Minimally invasive reduction and osteosynthesis of articular fractures of the distal radius. Injury 2001;32(Suppl 1):SA14–SA24

[20] Imatani J, Noda T, Morito Y, Sato T, Hashizume H, Inoue H. Minimally invasive plate osteosynthesis for comminuted fractures of the metaphysis of the radius. J Hand Surg [Br] 2005;30(2):220–225

[21] Lebailly F, Zemirline A, Facca S, Gouzou S, Liverneaux P. Distal radius fixation through a mini-invasive approach of 15 mm. PART 1: a series of 144 cases. Eur J Orthop Surg Traumatol 2013;24(6):877–890

[22] Liverneaux P, Ichihara S, Facca S, Hidalgo Diaz JJ. [Outcomes of minimally invasive plate osteosynthesis (MIPO) with volar locking plates in distal radius fractures: A review]. Hand Surg Rehabil 2016;35S:S80–S85

[23] Igeta Y, Vernet P, Facca S, Naroura I, Diaz JJH, Liverneaux PA. The minimally invasive flexor carpi radialis approach: a new perspective for distal radius fractures. Eur J Orthop Surg Traumatol 2018;28(8):1515–1522

[24] Liverneaux PA. The minimally invasive approach for distal radius fractures and malunions. J Hand Surg Eur Vol 2018;43(2):121–130

[25] Naito K, Zemirline A, Sugiyama Y, Obata H, Liverneaux P, Kaneko K. Possibility of Fixation of a Distal Radius Fracture With a Volar Locking Plate Through a 10 mm Approach. Tech Hand Up Extrem Surg 2016;20(2):71–76

[26] Zenke Y, Sakai A, Oshige T, et al. Clinical results of volar locking plate for distal radius fractures: conventional versus minimally invasive plate osteosynthesis. J Orthop Trauma 2011;25(7):425–431

[27] Pire E, Hidalgo Diaz JJ, Salazar Botero S, Facca S, Liverneaux PA. Long Volar Plating for Metadiaphyseal Fractures of Distal Radius: Study Comparing Minimally Invasive Plate Osteosynthesis versus Conventional Approach. J Wrist Surg 2017;6(3):227–234

[28] Zhang X, Huang X, Shao X, Zhu H, Sun J, Wang X. A comparison of minimally invasive approach vs conventional approach for volar plating of distal radial fractures. Acta Orthop Traumatol Turc 2017;51(2):110–117

10 Spanning Plates

Mitchell G. Eichhorn, Scott G. Edwards

Abstract

The dorsal spanning plate is a reasonable option in highly comminuted distal radius fractures. It allows adequate reduction of small fragments through traction ligamentotaxis and has a lower complication rate than external fixation. It is especially useful in intra-articular fractures that require offloading of the joint, and are too comminuted to allow dorsal or volar plate fixation. A dorsal spanning plate may be used alone or as an adjunct to other fixation methods, including K-wires and screws. The placement is simple and expedient with experience. It requires a second operation for removal several months later and most patients recover functional wrist motion. External fixation should still be applied in certain presentations, specifically in highly contaminated wounds; however, spanning plates are often a better alternative in cases that would traditionally require external fixation.

Keywords: distal radius fracture, comminuted distal radius fracture, spanning plate, external fixation, volar plate

10.1 Introduction

The treatment of distal radius fractures has evolved from nonoperative management to become one of the most commonly performed procedures in orthopaedic surgery.[1] Operative fixation of distal radius fractures was revolutionized by the advent of volar locking plates and fragment-specific fixation, which have become the primary methods of treatment in distal radius fractures requiring open reduction.[2] Since that time, the limitations of plates, specifically in the treatment of comminuted fractures, have become more clear.

Standard volar locking plates are not long enough to provide stability in fractures with extensive metaphyseal comminution. Longer locking plates have been designed to extend past metaphyseal comminution, but they cannot address intra-articular comminution or dorsal marginal impaction.[2] In these difficult fractures, external fixation can be utilized to hold the fracture out to length and to align the comminuted fragments with ligamentotaxis. External fixation neutralizes the force across the radiocarpal joint and prevents collapse of the distal radius in highly comminuted fractures.[3]

Although external fixation has excellent results and union rates, it is fraught with complications, mostly related to the external pins.[3,4,5,6] Complications of external pins include loosening, pin track infection, tendon injury, soft tissue scarring, osteomyelitis, and nerve injury.[4,7,8,9] Pin track infection is the most common problem, reported in up to half of external fixation cases.[10] Overall, the complication rate of external fixation is between 20 and 60%, and the risk of these complications increases with the duration of the fixation. Consequently, the external fixation construct often needs to be removed before the distal radius fracture is fully healed.[11]

The internal dorsal spanning plate was first introduced by Burke and Singer and Becton et al in 1998 as an alternative to external fixation in distal radius fractures.[12,13] The technique has been given many titles, including bridge plating, distraction plating, and spanning plate fixation. Spanning plates neutralize the load across the fracture and facilitate reduction by ligamentotaxis, similar to external fixation, but with many distinct advantages. Perhaps, the greatest of these advantages is the lack of external pins and their associated complications.

External fixation cannot fully correct volar tilt, as demonstrated in cadaveric and clinical studies.[2,4,14] Spanning plates buttress the dorsal cortex, allowing maintenance of volar tilt while the fracture is healing. A recent review of radiographic outcomes in distal radius fractures reported a volar tilt angle of 7.9 degrees with dorsal spanning plates compared to –5.5 degrees with external fixation.[2]

The rigidity of an external fixation construct is directly proportional to the pin length between the bone and the longitudinal bar.[15] A dorsal spanning plate essentially minimizes this length to the shortest possible distance. The plate sits directly on the bone and the bone-to-bar distance becomes zero. The advantages of zero bone-to-bar distance have been shown in ex vivo studies: spanning plates are much stiffer than external fixation in axial loading, wrist flexion, and wrist extension.[4,16] They provide a more stable and rigid fixation, allowing patients to bear weight on the wrist almost immediately. The stiffness of the construct is particularly important for bony union in comminuted fractures healing by secondary intention. The rigidity of spanning plates compared to external fixation may reduce the time required for fracture healing; however, additional clinical studies are needed.[17]

Spanning plates are also advantageous in patients with multiple injuries requiring a stable upper extremity to assist with transfers. In polytrauma, the ability to bear weight across the fracture, as soon as possible, is critical for rehabilitation. These patients often reside in the ICU where external fixation care is difficult and contamination can lead to infection.

The major disadvantage of a spanning plate is the secondary surgery required to remove it. There is also a risk of tendon impingement and nerve irritation, which is dependent on the surgical technique.[11,18] Plates left in place for an extended period of time can break at the level of the carpus and cause tendon injury.[19] There is also a concern for postoperative wrist stiffness, although this has been shown to improve within a year and may not be functionally significant after rehabilitation.[20]

The primary goal of treatment in any distal radius fracture is union of the bone with pain-free motion. Spanning plates restore radial length and congruency of the radiocarpal joint, allowing comminuted bone to heal in the most optimal position to preserve motion.[11,16] Dorsal spanning plates have become an integral part of distal radius fracture management and have largely superseded external fixation in certain situations. Upper extremity surgeons should be familiar with the application of both techniques.

10.2 Indications

Dorsal spanning plates are primarily used in distal radius fractures with severe comminution that precludes the placement of plates and screws. When the intra-articular fragments cannot be fixated or even buttressed by locking screws or fragment-specific fixation, the fracture must be reduced by ligamentotaxis. Proximally, metaphyseal bone loss with diaphyseal extension can prevent proximal screw placement.[21] The increased length of a spanning plate allows fixation into stable bone, proximal to the comminuted segment. Dorsal spanning plates are also suitable in comminuted fractures with dorsal marginal impaction. They buttress the dorsal cortex, reducing the dorsal lunate facet and restoring volar tilt.[2]

Spanning plates are an appropriate choice when a stable upper extremity is needed for early postoperative rehabilitation and mobility.[16,19,21] Patients with polytrauma and lower extremity injuries can bear weight across a dorsal spanning plate almost immediately, helping with transfers and gait assist devices. The same principle applies to patients with bilateral comminuted distal radius fractures who require their upper extremities for mobility.

Contraindications will be discussed below; please see ▸Table 10.1 for a full list of indications and contraindications. Case examples are provided in ▸Fig. 10.1, ▸Fig. 10.2, and ▸Fig. 10.3.

10.3 Surgical Technique

The first description of this technique by Burke and Singer placed the spanning plate in the floor of the fourth

Table 10.1 Indications and contraindications for dorsal spanning plates

Indications	Contraindications
Severe comminution	Volar plate or other fixation adequate
Metaphyseal bone loss	Volar comminution only
Diaphyseal fracture extension	Second and third metacarpal fractures
Polytrauma for rehabilitation	Unreliable follow-up
Bilateral for early mobility	Contaminated open wounds
Radiocarpal dislocations	Paucity of soft tissue coverage
Wrist and forearm amputations	

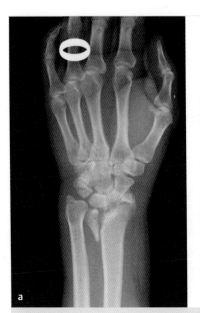
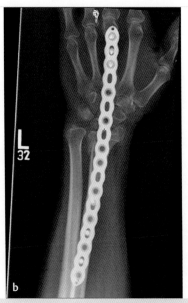
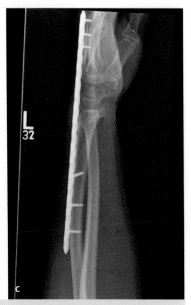

Fig. 10.1 (a) Anteroposterior view of an intra-articular distal radius fracture with severe comminution and near-complete loss of the lunate facet. **(b)** Six month postoperative radiographs after application of a curved 2.7-mm spanning plate to the third metacarpal position with restoration of length and radial inclination. **(c)** Lateral view 6 months postoperative with radiocarpal alignment and 0 degrees of dorsal angulation.

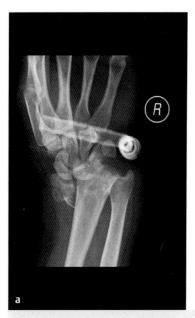
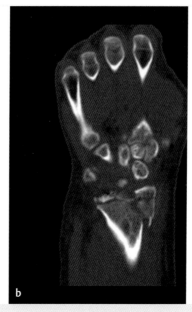
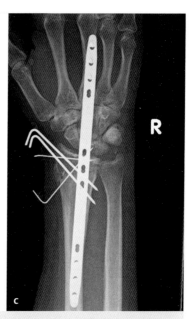

Fig. 10.2 (a) Intra-articular distal radius fracture with severe comminution and radiocarpal subluxation. **(b)** Computed tomography (CT) scan demonstrating intra-articular step off, comminution, and depression of the articular surface. **(c)** Dorsal spanning plate with neutralization of the radiocarpal joint, allowing pin placement and alignment of the articular bone fragments. (These images are provided courtesy of Gregory H. Rafijah.)

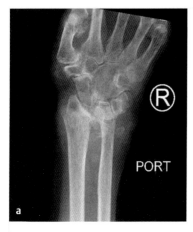
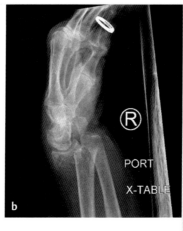

Fig. 10.3 (a) Distal radius fracture with comminution, loss of metaphyseal bone, and narrow distal fragment of subchondral bone. **(b)** Dorsal subluxation of the carpus and distal fragment. **(c)** Spanning plate application to the second metacarpal position with maintenance of length and radial inclination. **(d)** Lateral view with adequate alignment of the fracture. (These images are provided courtesy of Gregory H. Rafijah.)

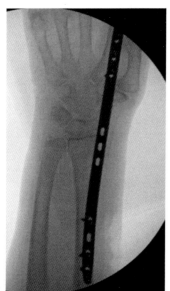
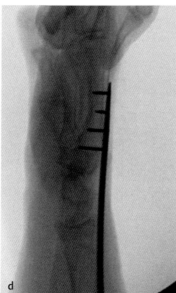

compartment, and the third metacarpal was chosen for distal fixation.[12] Hanel et al then introduced the "Harborview method," a more radially based approach utilizing the second dorsal compartment and the second metacarpal.[19] Biomechanical studies have shown little difference in plate position. Both have their advantages and can be used successfully in different situations.

The second metacarpal approach provides more traction across the radial side of the distal radius than the third metacarpal approach. This is ideal in comminuted fractures involving the radial column and it is the best method to restore both radial height and volar tilt.[2,22] Proponents of this approach also note increased grip strength due to ulnar deviation of the wrist.[22] The second metacarpal approach also has a theoretically lower rate of tendon entrapment and less tendon contact compared to third metacarpal placement; however, the plate is more prominent and may contact the superficial branches of the radial nerve.[11] When the second compartment is used, Lister tubercle and the extensor pollicis longus (EPL) tendon are avoided. This allows easier passage of the plate, and a third incision is not needed to release the EPL tendon.

The third metacarpal position is a stiffer construct, presumably due to better plate contact with the radius, although the clinical significance is debatable.[3] Perhaps, the greatest advantage of this approach is the ability to buttress the dorsal radius and directly off load the lunate facet.[21] It is important to note that the radius is not aligned with the third metacarpal. In order to make the transition across the wrist, the plate will override Lister tubercle.[11] This can impede passage of the plate and increases the risk of tendon entrapment.

The plate of choice has traditionally been a 3.5-mm dynamic compression plate, although a 2.4- or 2.7-mm plate can also be used.[16,23] A thicker plate is more rigid and less likely to break, but a larger screw size increases the risk of a metacarpal fracture.[10] The plate should be at least 12 to 16 holes in length to extend 4 cm proximal to metaphyseal comminution and proximal to the intersection of the first and second compartments. The plate is typically straight, although curved plates can be used as well. Specific plates have been designed for this application that have a tapered end for easier passage and smooth edges to facilitate removal.

10.3.1 Third Metacarpal Technique

Please refer to ▶ Fig. 10.4, ▶ Fig. 10.5, ▶ Fig. 10.6, ▶ Fig. 10.7, ▶ Fig. 10.8, ▶ Fig. 10.9, ▶ Fig. 10.10, ▶ Fig. 10.11, ▶ Fig. 10.12, and ▶ Fig. 10.13. A 5-cm dorsal longitudinal incision is made at the junction of the distal and middle thirds of the radius, proximal to the intersection of the first and second compartment tendons. Incision locations and plate length can be confirmed by placing the plate on the skin and marking its ideal location on FluoroScan. It should extend at least 4 cm proximal to comminuted segment.[24]

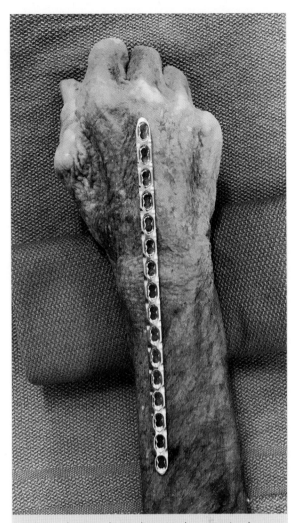

Fig. 10.4 This is a cadaveric dissection demonstrating the application of a third metacarpal position distal radius internal dorsal spanning plate. In this example, a 16-hole 2.7-mm locking dual compression plate was used (DePuy Synthes, Solothurn, Switzerland). Incision placement and plate size is determined radiographically and by placing the plate in the approximate position on the skin.

Dissection is continued down through skin and muscle until the radius is reached; the interval of this dissection is typically just ulnar to the brachioradialis.[11] A second longitudinal incision 2 to 4 cm in length is made over Lister tubercle and the dissection is carried down to the extensor retinaculum. Care should be taken not to injure dorsal sensory nerve branches over the forearm and hand. The third compartment is incised longitudinally and the EPL tendon is released and retracted radially. The plate is placed in the proximal incision and passed distally, along the periosteum of the fourth compartment and beneath the tendons, to a position over the third metacarpal. The plate will pass over Lister tubercle. If there is plate impingement on the tendons in the fourth compartment that prevents plate passage, the compartment can

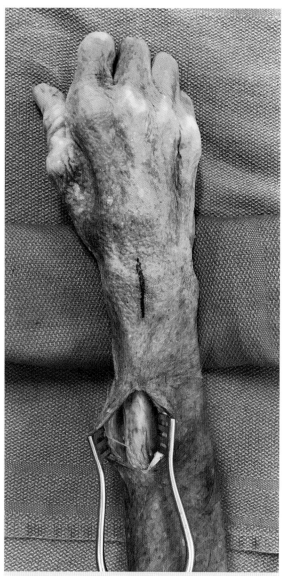

Fig. 10.5 A 5-cm incision is made proximally and carried down to the dorsal radius on the ulnar side of the brachioradialis tendon. The interval on the ulnar side of the second compartment tendons can be used as well.

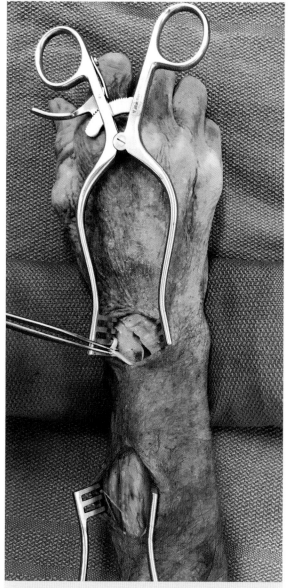

Fig. 10.6 A second 3-cm incision over the dorsal wrist is made and careful dissection is performed until the third compartment is visualized. The extensor pollicis longus (EPL) tendon is released from the compartment and retracted radially.

be elevated from radial to ulnar, off the distal radius. Also, Lister tubercle can be removed with a rongeur.

A third 5-cm longitudinal incision is made over the plate distally and the dissection is continued until the plate is reached. After confirming placement on fluoroscopy, fixation begins at the metacarpal level. A cortical screw is placed in the most distal or penultimate screw. Care should be taken to center the plate over the metacarpal. Traction is then applied across the fracture and it is reduced. Adding pronation to traction may facilitate reduction. We do not use external weight for traction, but others have reported the use of finger traps with

5 to 7 pounds of weight.[19,22] A locking drill guide provides a stable post to push the plate distally and create traction. To avoid overdistraction, the radiocarpal space should be less than 5 mm.[15,24] The plate is clamped proximally to the radius for provisional fixation, plate placement is checked on fluoroscopy, and then a cortical screw is placed proximally. At least three radial and three metacarpal locking or nonlocking screws are recommended.[25] Most authors prefer to place a single nonlocking screw in the metacarpal and one in the radius, then place the remaining screws after checking the plate position under fluoroscopy.[15,19,22]

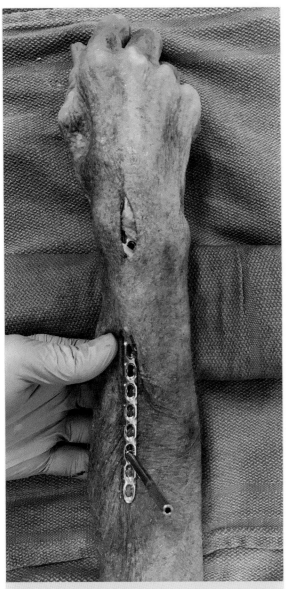

Fig. 10.7 A locking drill guide is placed in the plate to provide leverage during insertion. The plate is passed from proximal to distal, under the second and third compartment tendons. The floor of the fourth compartment may be elevated on the radial border to allow passage. Additionally, Lister tubercle may be removed with a rongeur.

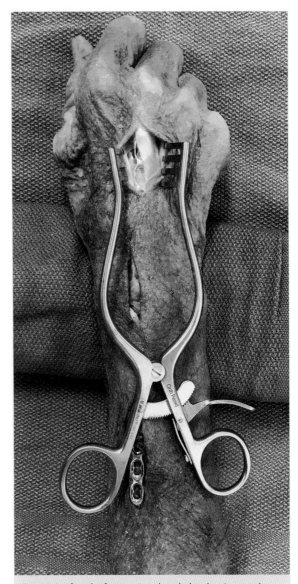

Fig. 10.8 After the fracture is reduced, the plate is passed distally, under the extensor tendons, until it is in line with the third metacarpal. A distal 5-cm incision is made over the plate and it is exposed with careful dissection. The extensor tendons are checked for entrapment and retracted.

At this point, small incisions can be made to reduce fragments and provide accessory fixation. K-wires, cannulated screws, and plates have been described. The third metacarpal position may not address the radial column and a radial styloid plate or pin is often a good adjunct. Depending on the fracture, a dorsal arthrotomy is used to visualize the intra-articular surface. Die punch fractures and intra-articular fragments are tamped into alignment and bolstered with hardware if needed. Demineralized bone matrix or bone graft may be utilized as well.

Before closure, ensure that there is no tendon impingement and no instability of the distal radioulnar joint (DRUJ). If the DRUJ is unstable, they should be treated accordingly and will require longer postoperative immobilization. The patient is placed in a short arm splint for comfort. They can start active and passive range of motion without a splint as soon as pain allows, typically 1 to 2 weeks. Digital range of motion should start the day after surgery. If early mobility is desired, they can bear weight up to 5 pounds immediately and can use crutches

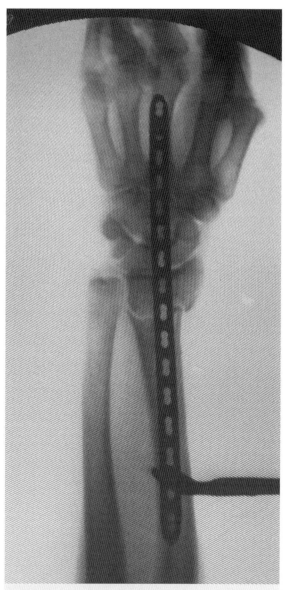

Fig. 10.9 Ensure the plate is in the correct position and centered, then place a cortical screw in the distal or penultimate screw hole. Traction is applied across the fracture with the plate; a locking drill guide can be used for leverage. Check the fracture on fluoroscopy and clamp the proximal plate to the bone when distraction is adequate. There should be no more than 5 mm of space at the radiocarpal joint. An artificial distal radius fracture was made for demonstration purposes.

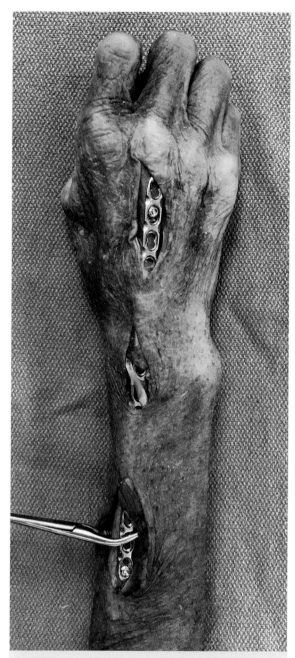

Fig. 10.10 A cortical screw is placed in the proximal plate; ensure that the plate is centered over the radius. Check alignment of fluoroscopy; small adjustments in plate position relative to the bone can still be made.

or a platform.[19,23] K-wires are typically removed at 6 weeks postoperatively and the plate is removed after 3 to 4 months if there is radiographic healing.

10.3.2 Second Metacarpal Technique

The same techniques are used for the second metacarpal position with a few modifications. Only two incisions are

needed since the third compartment is avoided. A proximal 5-cm longitudinal incision is made and the radius is exposed between the extensor carpi radialis longus (ECRL) and extensor carpi radialis brevis (ECRB) muscle bellies.[22] The superficial branch of the radial nerve is avoided if this interval is maintained. The plate is placed on the dorsal radial aspect of the radius and passed distally just above the periosteum, through the floor of

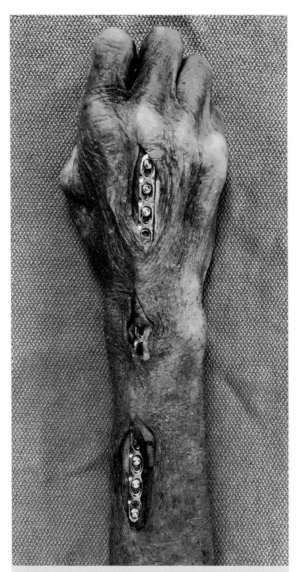

Fig. 10.11 Two additional locking screws are place in both the metacarpal and radius for a total of three on each side.

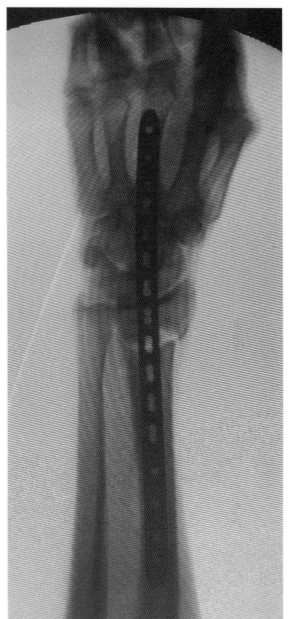

Fig. 10.12 Anteroposterior and lateral views of plate placement. Note restoration of volar tilt. At this point, further fixation could be performed with separate incisions.

the second compartment. It should pass under the first, second, and third compartment tendons. The plate is then exposed at the second metacarpal, with care to protect the radial nerve sensory branches.

Using the techniques described in the previous section, apply traction and fixate the plate first distally and then proximally. The wrist should be in slight ulnar deviation when the second metacarpal is collinear with the radius. Accessory fixation is performed as needed, the wounds are closed, and the patient is placed in a splint. The same postoperative course described above is followed.

10.4 Results

Multiple outcomes studies have been published on internal dorsal spanning plates; however, most studies are small and no prospective studies have directly compared spanning plates to external fixation.[10,15,19,21,22,26] External fixation has a high complication rate, ranging from 20 to 60%. The pin site infection rate alone with external fixation is up to 50%, compared to a 1.4% infection rate with spanning plates.[10] Although most of the pin site infections associated with external fixation are minor, there is no need for these complications if adequate functional and radiographic outcomes can be obtained with an internal spanning plate.[27]

A recent study by Lauder et al evaluated functional outcomes after spanning plate fixation and compared

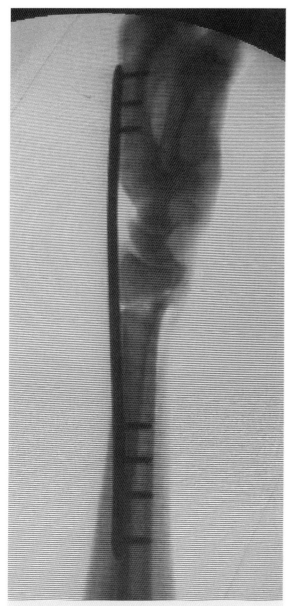

Fig. 10.13 Anteroposterior and lateral views of plate placement. Note restoration of volar tilt. At this point, further fixation could be performed with separate incisions.

within functional range. Functional range of wrist motion has been determined as 40 degrees of flexion and extension, with 50 degrees of pronation and supination.[15] Multiple studies have reported similar findings in postoperative wrist range of motion after internal spanning plates.[12,15,21,22]

The average volar tilt after spanning plate fixation ranges from 4.1 to 7.9 degrees and the average ulnar variance ranges from -0.3 to 0.18 mm.[2,21,22] The radiographic outcomes of dorsal spanning plates were compared to external fixation and volar plate fixation by Huish et al. The radial inclination was similar in all groups; however, the volar tilt of dorsal spanning plates was 7.9 degrees compared to –5.5 with external fixation and 6 degrees with volar plates.[2]

The union rates with a spanning plate range from 99 to 100%, compared to union rates of 96 to 98% with external fixation.[2,10,15,19,23,26,28,29] Reported complications of spanning plates include extensor tendon adhesions (1.4–76%), tendon ruptures (0–1.6%), and infection requiring plate removal (0–1.4%).[2,10,13,20,21,22,23] Dodds et al reported the highest rate of extensor tenolysis procedures at 76% (19/25); however, exploration of the extensor tendons was a routine part of their plate removal procedure.[22] Tendon entrapment is theoretical risk based on cadaveric studies, yet none were reported in the clinical literature.[11,18]

Other potential complications are plate failure (0–12%), metacarpal fracture (0–3%), and metacarpal screw failure (0–1.4%)[10,13,19,21,23] In the largest outcomes study, the rate of plate failure was 2% (3/144).[10] The average length of time before plate removal in patients with plate failure was 10 months, much longer than the typical 3 to 4 month interval. In the same study, the complication rate increased from 9 to 21% if the plate remained in place longer than 16 weeks. A similar trend was found by Dodd et al. Duration before plate removal was 13.5 months in the three (12%) patients with broken plates.[22]

10.5 Pitfalls and Contraindications

Dorsal spanning plates are not appropriate in noncomminuted distal radius fractures that can be easily fixated with a volar locking plate or other fixation method. They can, however, be considered as an adjunct to volar plating in patients with severely osteoporotic bone. They should not be used as the sole means of fixation if appropriate reduction is not achieved with ligamentotaxis. For example, a palmar lunate facet or volar shear fracture may require a separate incision, reduction, and fixation. Dorsal spanning plates are also contraindicated with concomitant second and third metacarpal fractures.

There are social factors to consider when choosing between an external fixation device and a dorsal spanning plate. Spanning plates can cause significant tendon

the function to the uninjured wrist.[20] At an average of 2.7-year follow-up in 18 patients, the injured wrist had 43 degrees of flexion, 46 degrees of extension, and 23 degrees of ulnar deviation compared to the uninjured hand with 58 degrees of flexion, 56 degrees of extension, and 29 degrees of ulnar deviation. Grip strength was 86% of the contralateral side. Pronation was 66 degrees and supination was 71 degrees in the injured wrist, while in the uninjured wrist pronation was 73 degrees and supination was 69 degrees.[20] Although range of motion was significantly less than the uninjured side, the absolute amount of reduction is minimal and well injuries if they are left in place too long and break. Every effort should be made to remove it in 3 to 4 months, after radiographic healing is confirmed. An alternative fixation method is a better choice in patients that may not return for plate removal.[22] Similarly, patients at risk for leaving against medical advice are less likely to do so with an external fixation device in place. Please see ▶ Table 10.1 for a full list of indications and contraindications.

Most of the complications associated with this procedure can be avoided with appropriate technique. Careful dissection is necessary to avoid branches of the superficial radial nerve. The plate should always be placed on the metacarpal first; otherwise, the metacarpal plate holes may not reach the metacarpal shaft after distraction, and the radius screws will need to be redrilled. At least three screws should be used on each side of the fracture, and ensure that the screws are placed in the center of the bone to prevent fractures.[10,16]

When using the third metacarpal approach, make a third incision to free the EPL and to confirm that tendons are not entrapped. To prevent plate failure, the plate should be at least 2.4 mm in thickness and it should be removed within 4 months. Complex regional pain syndrome is a possible consequence of overdistraction.[30] The fracture should not be distracted more than 5 mm and digital flexion should be checked after distraction.[24]

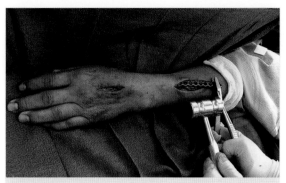

Fig. 10.14 Removal of a reconstruction plate with scalloped edges can be difficult. If "rolling" does not work, and the plate has some mobility but is not free, the plate can be hammered out of the posterior wound.

Tips and Tricks

- **Plate size and incision placement**: Place the plate on the skin and check length and incision placement on fluoroscopy before incision.
- **Plate passage**: If the plate will not easily pass, first try plate manipulation with different angles of attack. The extensor retinaculum can also be partially incised at it is most proximal extent.[19] Alternatively, a soft tissue plate track can be created from the distal incision to meet the soft tissue plate track created from the proximal incision.[22] A guide wire or suture retriever can be passed from distal to proximal, under the tendons. The wire or retriever is then attached to the plate and pulled through.[19]
- **Plate fixation**: The plate should always be fixated to the metacarpal first, and the most distal or penultimate screw should be used initially. This will provide good plate alignment along the shaft and will assure that metacarpal fixation is possible after distraction. If the radius is fixated first, the radial screws may need to be repositioned to allow metacarpal fixation.
- **Plate removal**: Mandibular plates and plates with scalloped edges can be difficult to remove. The plate can be "rolled" or rocked back and forth on its long axis until it is free from the soft tissue. If the plate is still is not completely free of soft tissue, grasp the proximal plate with pliers and gently hammer the plate out of the proximal incision (▶ Fig. 10.14). A locking drill guide can work for this purpose as well, although it may be damaged. A specifically designed spanning plate has smooth edges and is not as difficult to remove.

10.6 Conclusion

Dorsal spanning plates are a safe and effective option in highly comminuted distal radius fractures that require bridging fixation and neutralization of the radiocarpal joint. They have a lower complication rate than external fixation, they can be easily applied with the proper technique, and multiple studies have shown satisfactory clinical outcomes. In the properly selected patients, surgeons should consider their use in lieu of external fixation.

References

[1] Diaz-Garcia RJ, Chung KC. The evolution of distal radius fracture management: a historical treatise. Hand Clin 2012;28(2):105–111
[2] Huish EG Jr, Coury JG, Ibrahim MA, Trzeciak MA. Radiographic outcomes of dorsal distraction distal radius plating for fractures with dorsal marginal impaction. Hand 2018; 13(3)
[3] Alluri RK, Bougioukli S, Stevanovic M, Ghiassi A. A biomechanical comparison of distal fixation for bridge plating in a distal radius fracture model. J Hand Surg Am 2017;42(9):748.e1–748.e8
[4] Chhabra A, Hale JE, Milbrandt TA, Carmines DV, Degnan GG. Biomechanical efficacy of an internal fixator for treatment of distal radius fractures. Clin Orthop Relat Res 2001;(393):318–325
[5] Suso S, Combalía A, Segur JM, García-Ramiro S, Ramón R. Comminuted intra-articular fractures of the distal end of the radius treated with the Hoffmann external fixator. J Trauma 1993;35(1):61–66
[6] Bishay M, Aguilera X, Grant J, Dunkerley DR. The results of external fixation of the radius in the treatment of comminuted intraarticular fractures of the distal end. J Hand Surg [Br] 1994;19(3):378–383
[7] McKenna J, Harte M, Lunn J, O'Bierne J. External fixation of distal radial fractures. Injury 2000;31(8):613–616
[8] Klein W, Dée W, Rieger H, Neumann H, Joosten U. Results of transarticular fixator application in distal radius fractures. Injury 2000;31(Suppl 1):71–77
[9] Kapoor H, Agarwal A, Dhaon BK. Displaced intra-articular fractures of distal radius: a comparative evaluation of results following closed reduction, external fixation and open reduction with internal fixation. Injury 2000;31(2):75–79

[10] Hanel DP, Ruhlman SD, Katolik LI, Allan CH. Complications associated with distraction plate fixation of wrist fractures. Hand Clin 2010;26(2):237–243

[11] Dahl J, Lee DJ, Elfar JC. Anatomic relationships in distal radius bridge plating: a cadaveric study. Hand (N Y) 2015;10(4):657–662

[12] Burke EF, Singer RM. Treatment of comminuted distal radius with the use of an internal distraction plate. Tech Hand Up Extrem Surg 1998;2(4):248–252

[13] Becton JL, Colborn GL, Goodrich JA. Use of an internal fixator device to treat comminuted fractures of the distal radius: report of a technique. Am J Orthop 1998;27(9):619–623

[14] Bartosh RA, Saldana MJ. Intraarticular fractures of the distal radius: a cadaveric study to determine if ligamentotaxis restores radiopalmar tilt. J Hand Surg Am 1990;15(1):18–21

[15] Richard MJ, Katolik LI, Hanel DP, Wartinbee DA, Ruch DS. Distraction plating for the treatment of highly comminuted distal radius fractures in elderly patients. J Hand Surg Am 2012;37(5):948–956

[16] Wolf JC, Weil WM, Hanel DP, Trumble TE. A biomechanic comparison of an internal radiocarpal-spanning 2.4-mm locking plate and external fixation in a model of distal radius fractures. J Hand Surg Am 2006;31(10):1578–1586

[17] Wu JJ, Shyr HS, Chao EY, Kelly PJ. Comparison of osteotomy healing under external fixation devices with different stiffness characteristics. J Bone Joint Surg Am 1984;66(8):1258–1264

[18] Lewis S, Mostofi A, Stevanovic M, Ghiassi A. Risk of tendon entrapment under a dorsal bridge plate in a distal radius fracture model. J Hand Surg Am 2015;40(3):500–504

[19] Hanel DP, Lu TS, Weil WM. Bridge plating of distal radius fractures: the Harborview method. Clin Orthop Relat Res 2006;445(445):91–99

[20] Lauder A, Agnew S, Bakri K, Allan CH, Hanel DP, Huang JI. Functional outcomes following bridge plate fixation for distal radius fractures. J Hand Surg Am 2015;40(8):1554–1562

[21] Ruch DS, Ginn TA, Yang CC, Smith BP, Rushing J, Hanel DP. Use of a distraction plate for distal radial fractures with metaphyseal and diaphyseal comminution. J Bone Joint Surg Am 2005;87(5):945–954

[22] Dodds SD, Save AV, Yacob A. Dorsal spanning plate fixation for distal radius fractures. Tech Hand Up Extrem Surg 2013;17(4):192–198

[23] Jain MJ, Mavani KJ. A comprehensive study of internal distraction plating, an alternative method for distal radius fractures. J Clin Diagn Res 2016;10(12):RC14–RC17

[24] Ginn TA, Ruch DS, Yang CC, Hanel DP. Use of a distraction plate for distal radial fractures with metaphyseal and diaphyseal comminution. Surgical technique. J Bone Joint Surg Am 2006;88(Suppl 1 Pt 1):29–36

[25] Mann T, Lee DJ, Dahl J, Elfar JC. Can radiocarpal-spanning fixation be made more functional by placing the wrist in extension? A biomechanical study under physiologic loads. Geriatr Orthop Surg Rehabil 2016;7(1):23–29

[26] Mithani SK, Srinivasan RC, Kamal R, Richard MJ, Leversedge FJ, Ruch DS. Salvage of distal radius nonunion with a dorsal spanning distraction plate. J Hand Surg Am 2014;39(5):981–984

[27] Hayes AJ, Duffy PJ, McQueen MM. Bridging and non-bridging external fixation in the treatment of unstable fractures of the distal radius: a retrospective study of 588 patients. Acta Orthop 2008;79(4):540–547

[28] Anderson JT, Lucas GL, Buhr BR. Complications of treating distal radius fractures with external fixation: a community experience. Iowa Orthop J 2004;24:53–59

[29] Ma C, Deng Q, Pu H, et al. External fixation is more suitable for intra-articular fractures of the distal radius in elderly patients. Bone Res 2016;4:16017

[30] Chloros GD, Wiesler ER, Papadonikolakis A, Li Z, Smith BP, Koman LA. Complex regional pain syndrome after distal radius fractures. In: Slutsky DJ, Osterman AL, eds. Fractures and Injuries of the Distal Radius and Carpus: The Cutting Edge. Philadelphia, PA: Saunders; 2009:247

11 Arthroscopic Management

Yukio Abe

Abstract

Wrist arthroscopy is an efficient adjunct for intra-articular distal radius fracture fixation. However, performing wrist arthroscopy during the plate fixation is troublesome with the vertical traction applied and released. To facilitate the procedure, we developed a surgical technique, plate presetting arthroscopic reduction technique (PART), using a volar locking plate. Since July 2005, we have performed PART for 98 extra-articular and 358 intra-articular distal radius fractures with good and excellent results. The advantages of PART in the surgical treatment of distal radius fracture are: (1) accurate reduction of intra-articular fragments is possible compared with fluoroscopic reduction, (2) intra-articular fragments (free body) undetected with radiograph and CT can be recognized, (3) screw protrusion into joint surface can be monitored, (4) intra-articular soft tissue injury associated with fracture can be evaluated and treated, and (5) debridement of joint hematoma can be performed. Our results were superior to the results reported with using volar locking plate without arthroscopic intervention.

Keywords: wrist, distal radius fracture, intra-articular fracture, arthroscopy, volar locking plate, articular step-off

11.1 Introduction

The functional outcome of distal radius fracture (DRF) is affected by extra-articular alignment, anatomical reduction of the articular surface, intra-articular soft tissue injuries, and postoperative complications, similar with other peri- or intra-articular fracture.[1,2,3,4,5,6,7,8,9,10] From these aspects, wrist arthroscopy is recognized as an important adjunctive procedure in the management of DRF because precise reduction of the articular surface and the management of intra-articular soft tissue injuries can only be done by using wrist arthroscopy.[11,12,13,14] It would be easier if used in conjunction with percutaneous pinning and external fixation. However, volar locking plate (VLP) fixation markedly developed recently; performing wrist arthroscopy during plating becomes troublesome because vertical traction must be both applied and released during the surgery. Therefore, we have developed a plate presetting arthroscopic reduction technique (PART) using a VLP that can simplify the combination of plating and arthroscopy, and we have been using this technique since 2005.[15,16,17,18] This chapter describes the procedure of PART and its effectiveness for the treatment of DRF.

11.2 Indications

Intra-articular soft tissue injuries were found to have almost the same incidence in both extra-articular and intra-articular DRF from the author's experiences[16,17]; therefore, wrist arthroscopy may be indicated for any type of DRF. However, low-activity patients, extra-articular fractures in the elderly, open fractures, and DRF associated with other multiple fractures are considered to be contraindications for PART.

11.3 Surgical Technique

11.3.1 Preoperative Planning

Besides the standard posteroanterior and lateral radiographs, oblique radiographs at 45° of supination and pronation of the forearm, and computed tomography (CT), including three-dimensional (3D) reconstruction, are quite valuable in deciding a surgical strategy for the treatment of DRF. Especially the axial slice of 3D-CT including joint surface is useful for considering how to reduce and fix the intra-articular fracture fragments (▶Fig. 11.1).

11.3.2 Preparation and Patient Positioning

The monitors of arthroscopy and fluoroscopy, the fluoroscopy and the arthroscopic equipment, including a small diameter, 1.9- or 2.3-mm arthroscope with a 30° field of vision, a shaver, and a radiofrequency device must be positioned conveniently (▶Fig. 11.2). The patient, who has been placed under general or regional anesthesia, is placed in the supine position with the arm draped freely over a hand table. A tourniquet is wrapped around the upper arm and inflated. A palmar approach is used to apply the VLP before the arthroscopic procedure. Saline can flow away readily through the palmar incision, especially in an intra-articular fracture. Therefore, the surgeons are less concerned about swelling during the arthroscopy. We ordinarily use wet technique because blood clots and debris can be easily removed, and it can prevent the heat problem in using a radiofrequency device. However, in wet technique, bubbles sometimes disturb the surgeon's visualization. In that situation, the dry technique is useful.[19] The dry technique is also suitable to handle intra-articular fragments and pick up the free body because fragments do not move by water flow.

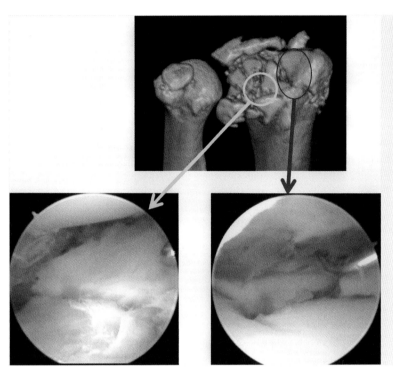

Fig. 11.1 Three-dimensional computed tomography (3D-CT) is quite useful to assess the condition of joint surface and make the strategy how to reduce the intra-articular fragments. *Arrows* indicate how the comminution of the joint surface was seen with arthroscopy.

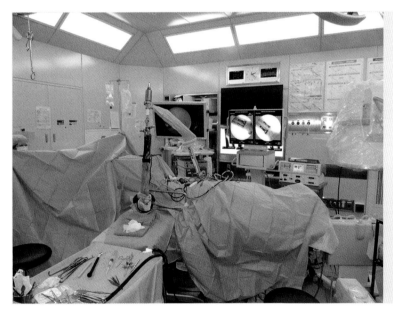

Fig. 11.2 The monitors, image intensifier, and surgical equipment have to be set conveniently.

11.3.3 Surgical Approach

Exposure

A longitudinal skin incision is made between the flexor carpi radialis (FCR) tendon and the radial artery (so-called Henry approach). The length of the incision can vary according to the severity of comminution at the palmar cortex. The shortest incision is about 2.5 cm for a simple metaphyseal fracture. The radial artery is retracted radially, and the FCR tendon is retracted ulnarly together with the median nerve. Retracting the flexor pollicis longus muscle ulnarly exposes the pronator quadratus muscle, which is split in its distal one-third for fracture site exposure and reduction.

Fracture Reduction

The fracture of the palmar site is reduced by manipulating the fragments using a periosteal elevator. As the palmar cortex of the radius is generally less comminuted, reduction of the palmar cortex is an indicator of anatomic reduction. If severe comminution of palmar

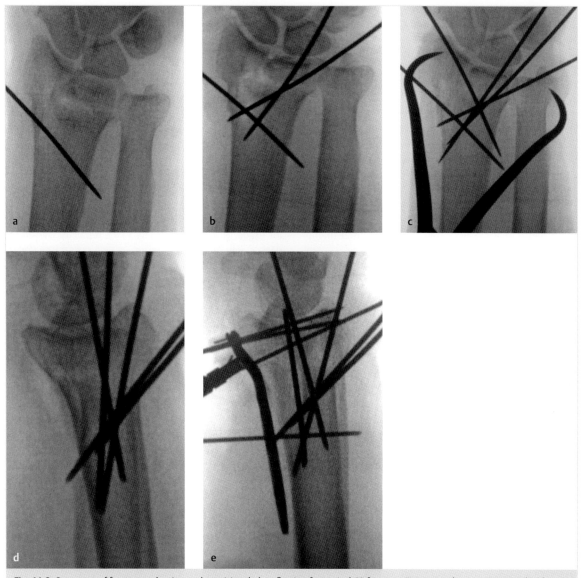

Fig. 11.3 Sequence of fracture reduction and provisional plate fixation for typical C3 fracture. Fracture reduction is acquired with manipulation and some intrafocal pinnings. **(a)** Intrafocal pinning from radial side and **(b)** from dorsal side; **(c, d)** interfragmental pinnings with tenaculum clamp; **(e)** a volar locking plate (VLP) is provisionally fixed.

cortex is recognized, the use of an external fixator with ligamentotaxis temporarily would be beneficial to maintain the reduction during surgery. Several intrafocal pins are inserted to reduce the alignment radially and dorsally (▶ Fig. 11.3). After anatomic reduction is achieved possibly including the articular surface, the fragments are subsequently fixed under fluoroscopy with several interfragmental pins percutaneously. Typically, for an intra-articular fracture, at least four to five Kirschner wires (K-wires), 1.5 mm in diameter, are inserted from the radial and dorsal aspects. Placement of the K-wires should not interfere with the placement of the VLP. The intrafocal pins are quite important to maintain the alignment if arthroscopic reduction of the intra-articular

fragments must be performed, because interfragmental pins must be removed to reduce the intra-articular fragments. After temporary fixation of the fracture by K-wires, the VLP is preset palmarly on the radius and temporarily fixed with pins inserted through the plate. Subchondral supporting wires are inserted into the distal fragment through the distal holes of the plate.

Wrist Arthroscopic Inspection

After the VLP has been preset, the wrist is suspended in a vertical traction tower, and wrist arthroscopy is carried out. The author generally uses two dorsal portals to evaluate and treat the intra-articular fragments and soft tissue injuries, the 3–4 portal (between the extensor pollicis longus tendon and the extensor digitorum communis tendons) and the 4–5 portal (between the extensor digitorum communis tendons and the extensor digiti minimi tendon). In addition, the author sometimes uses the palmar portal through the gliding floor of the FCR tendon to inspect the palmar segment tear of the scapholunate interosseous ligament (SLIL) and dorsal fracture fragment.[20,21] A 1.9- or 2.3-mm arthroscope with a 30° field of vision is introduced through the 3–4 portal, and a probe or a shaver is inserted through the 4–5 portal. The remaining hematoma in the joint should be removed for better visualization. The intra-articular condition, such as fracture fragments and soft tissue structures, is thoroughly inspected.

Fragments that are not reduced by the initial manipulation are now reduced under arthroscopic control. K-wires preventing reduction of the displaced intra-articular fragment must be removed or can be used as a joystick. Residual step-off of the fragment can be reduced by joystick maneuver using a K-wire inserted to the fragment (▶Fig. 11.4). Fragment just separated from each other are reduced by percutaneous tenaculum clamping (▶Fig. 11.5). Central depression is reduced by pushing up from the intramedullary canal using a probe inserted at the dorsal or palmar fracture site (▶Fig. 11.6). Free fragments, which are too small to fix, are removed.

After reduction of the fragments is achieved, temporary K-wire fixation is performed again. These K-wires are removed after inserting locking screws through the distal plate holes.

After reduction of the intra-articular fragments arthroscopically, associated soft tissue injuries should be evaluated and treated. The necessity of initial treatment of soft tissue injury is still controversial. The author's current principles are: if an SLIL injury is recognized, midcarpal arthroscopy is performed to evaluate scapholunate stability with a probe. Similarly, if distal radioulnar joint (DRUJ) instability is suspected, DRUJ arthroscopy should be performed to confirm a foveal tear of the triangular fibrocartilage complex (TFCC). Our strategy for the treatment of an SLIL injury is percutaneous pinning for grade III instability (▶Fig. 11.7), repair of the dorsal part of SLIL, and augmentation using a dorsal intercarpal ligament for grade IV instability according to the Geissler classification.[4] For foveal tear of TFCC,[22] the author performs the primary transosseous repair arthroscopically (▶Fig. 11.8). These procedures are basically indicated for younger and active patients. As soon as intra-articular fragments and soft tissue injuries are treated, vertical traction is removed, and the VLP is subsequently and securely fixed to the distal radius. The distal end of the VLP should be in contact with distal fragment of the radius to prevent flexor tendon attenuation. Since the introduction of the

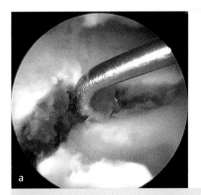 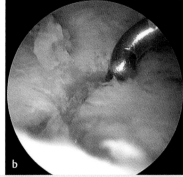 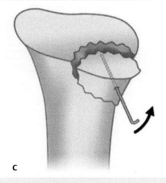

Fig. 11.4 The step-off is reduced by joystick maneuver: **(a)** prereduction, **(b)** postreduction, **(c)** joystick maneuver.

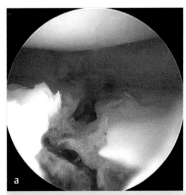 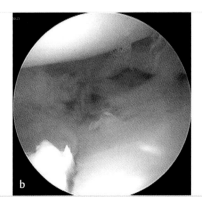 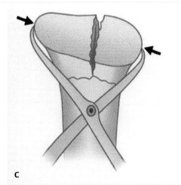

Fig. 11.5 Separation is reduced by tenaculum clamping. **(a)** Prereduction, **(b)** postreduction, **(c)** tenaculum clamping.

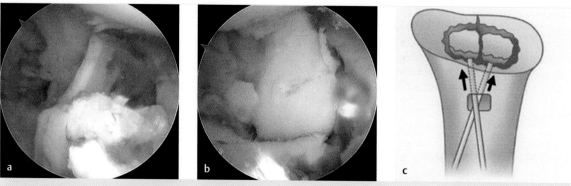

Fig. 11.6 Central fragment is reduced by pushing up from the intramedullary: **(a)** joint surface is severely comminuted, **(b)** postreduction, **(c)** push-up technique.

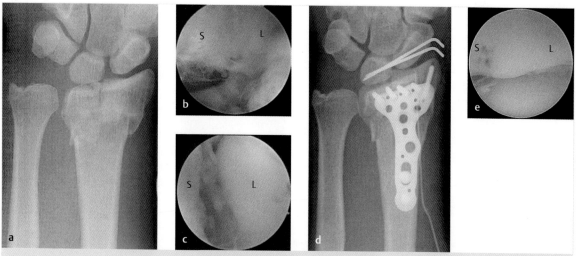

Fig. 11.7 A 47-year-old male had a C2 fracture **(a)** associated with grade III scapholunate interosseous ligament (SLIL) tear confirmed by radiocarpal **(b)** and midcarpal arthroscopy **(c)**. The fracture was fixed with a volar locking plate (VLP) **(d)**; the scapholunate joint was transfixed with two K-wires simultaneously. Six months after initial surgery at the plate removal, SLIL was confirmed to be completely healed **(e)**. L, lunate; S, scaphoid.

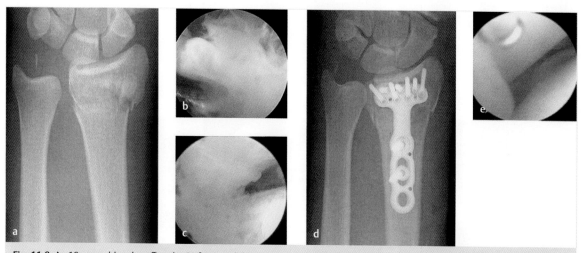

Fig. 11.8 An 18-year-old male suffered a C1 fracture **(a)** associated with complete triangular fibrocartilage complex (TFCC) foveal tear **(b)** as shown in distal radioulnar joint (DRUJ) arthroscopy. The fracture was fixed with a volar locking plate (VLP) **(d)** and TFCC foveal tear was fixed with arthroscopic transosseous repair **(c)**. TFCC fovea healing was confirmed with DRUJ arthroscopy **(e)** at the time of plate removal 6 months after the initial surgery.

VLP, the author rarely performed bone grafting for dorsal bone defects. However, artificial bone graft would facilitate to maintain the reduction of intra-articular fragment of central depression, and bone union in the severely comminuted fracture at the metaphysis, or severely osteoporotic bone. The wound is irrigated, a drain is inserted, and the overlying skin is closed with subcuticular absorbable suture.

11.3.4 Postoperative Care

Early rehabilitation can be allowed as VLP provides rigid fixation. A dorsal splint is applied just after surgery; the splint is removed and active wrist motion is started on the first day after surgery. Passive motion and grasping exercises are started from the second day with the therapist. Patients are encouraged to use the affected hand in daily living. Forearm rotation exercises are prohibited in patients who have ulnar side injuries, such as unfixed distal ulna fracture, ulnar styloid fracture, and TFCC repairs, until 3 weeks after surgery.

11.4 Results

11.4.1 The Advantages of Wrist Arthroscopy

From July 2005 to November 2017, PART was performed in 456 wrists of 449 consecutive DRF patients including both extra-articular and intra-articular fracture. The 110 men and 339 women ranged in age from 16 to 86 years (average age, 62 years). The authors classified all the fractures using the AO/ASIF (Association for Osteosynthesis/Association for the Study of Internal Fixation) classification system. The fractures consisted of 8 A2, 90 A3, 1 B2, 15 B3, 149 C1, 26 C2, and 167 C3 fractures. From these experiences, the author recognized several advantages of arthroscopic surgery for DRF.

First, during PART, anatomic reduction of the articular surface is initially achieved under fluoroscopy, and reduction is reconfirmed by arthroscopy. In this process, the author could recognize the difference of accuracy of reduction of articular surface between fluoroscopic and arthroscopic reduction (▶Fig. 11.9). The author hypothesized that after fluoroscopic reduction there will be no remaining gap and step-off of 2 mm or more in 302 intra-articular fractures. However, under arthroscopy, the author recognized more than 2-mm residual displacement in 67 wrists (22.2%). The residual displacement in the coronal plane was frequently observed.

Second, during arthroscopy, the author identified fracture fragments that could not be seen on preoperative radiographs and CT scan (▶Fig. 11.10). In 358 intra-articular fractures, the author arthroscopically could visualize free fracture fragments, including small cancellous bone chips in 30 wrists (8.4%). If these fragments were not removed, they might produce wrist pain because of impingement.

Third, a VLP produces maximal mechanical support when the distal screws are inserted into the subchondral

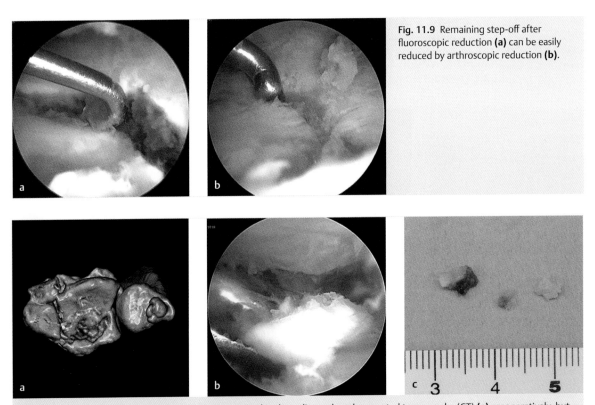

Fig. 11.9 Remaining step-off after fluoroscopic reduction **(a)** can be easily reduced by arthroscopic reduction **(b)**.

Fig. 11.10 Free fragments in the joint were not recognized in the radiograph and computed tomography (CT) **(a)** preoperatively, but were identified **(b)** and removed **(c)** arthroscopically.

zone of the distal radius. If the plate placement is too distal, screws may protrude into the joint surface (▶Fig. 11.11). Wrist arthroscopy can monitor any screw protrusion into the joint.

Finally, investigating the intra-articular soft tissue situation using wrist arthroscopy is one great advantage. In 456 DRFs, SLIL injury was recognized in 138 wrists (30.3%). Of these, grade III or IV instability according to the Geissler classification was recognized in 37 wrists (8.1%), and pinning or primarily repair was performed in 5 wrists (▶Fig. 11.12). Traumatic TFCC tear was recognized in 222 wrists (48.6%). Type of the injury was classified according to the Abe classification.[22] The slit tear of the disk was the most common. The TFCC foveal tear was repaired primarily in five out of six wrists (▶Fig. 11.13).

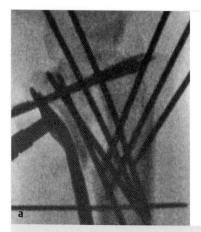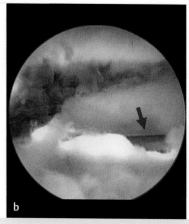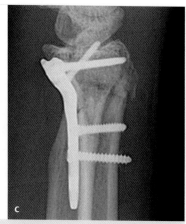

Fig. 11.11 A C3 distal radius fracture (DRF) was provisionally fixed with K-wires and a volar locking plate (VLP) **(a)**. A K-wire inserted to fix a VLP was protruded into the joint **(b)**. *Arrow* indicates K-wire for temporary fixation, which was protruded into the joint **(b)**. A VLP was set a little proximally **(c)**.

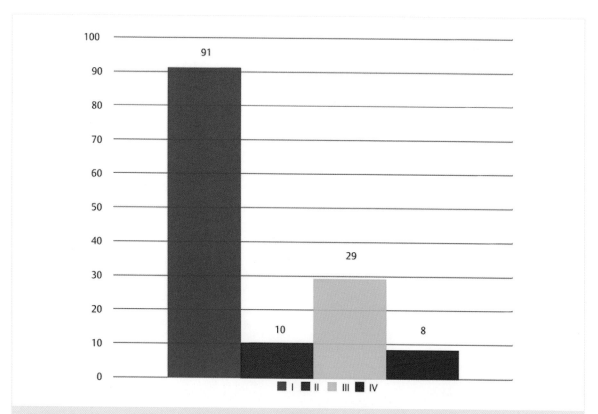

Fig. 11.12 The number of scapholunate interosseous ligament (SLIL)injury associated with distal radius fracture (DRF) classified according to the Geissler classification. In a total number of 456 DRF, SLIL injury was observed in 138 wrists (30.3%). Grade I central tears were the most common; however, grade III and IV tears showing severe instability were recognized in 37 wrists (8.1%).

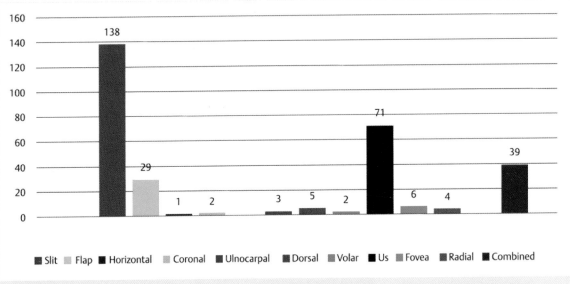

Fig. 11.13 The number of triangular fibrocartilage complex (TFCC) injury associated with distal radius fracture (DRF) classified according to the Abe classification. Traumatic tear was recognized in 222 wrists (48.6%).

In addition, wrist arthroscopy can remove the hematoma in the wrist joint. This could prevent the fibrous tissue formation in the joint that leads to wrist joint contracture.

11.4.2 Outcomes

A total of 282 wrists of 282 patients with intra-articular DRF treated with PART were followed up for more than 1 year. Those patients whose both wrists were affected were excluded. The follow-up period ranged from 12 to 72 months (average, 15 months). The age of the 73 men and 209 women ranged from 17 to 85 years (average age, 63 years). The fractures consisted of 10 B3, 132 C1, 18 C2, and 122 C3 fractures. The palmar tilt was 7.6° (range: −5° to 25°), radial inclination 26.1° (range: 18° to 33°), and ulnar variance 1.4 mm (range: −3 to 8.5 mm). The mean extension range of the wrist was 69° (range: 50° to 85°), and the mean flexion range was 64° (range: 35° to 85°), and the mean pronation range of the forearm was 83° (range: 70° to 90°), and the mean supination range was 89° (range: 75° to 95°). The mean grip strength was 91.3% (range: 38–133%) of the opposite side. The final results according to the Mayo Modified Wrist Score were 214 excellent (75.9%), 63 good (22.3%), 4 fair (1.4%), and 1 poor (0.4%). The mean Disabilities of the Arm, Shoulder and Hand score at final follow-up was 3.4 points (range: 0–33.0). There were few complications: five gross displacements of the distal fragment, two extensor pollicis longus tendon ruptures, and one complex regional pain syndrome. The final results of these eight cases were four good, three fair, and one poor.

11.5 Complications

The author has never experienced severe complications from arthroscopic reduction procedures, such as tendon rupture, major neurovascular injury, or compartment syndrome. There were several complaints of numbness at the dorsal wrist after surgery; however, the symptoms improved in 3 to 6 months.

11.6 Conclusion

Wrist arthroscopy is a feasible adjunct for the surgical treatment of DRF, especially as it can evaluate the reduction of intra-articular fragments and soft tissue injury. The VLP fixation and simultaneous arthroscopic intervention have become problematic because vertical traction must be applied and released during surgery. The author developed the original procedure, PART, to overcome these difficulties and achieved good final results.

References

[1] Catalano LW III, Barron OA, Glickel SZ. Assessment of articular displacement of distal radius fractures. Clin Orthop Relat Res 2004;(423):79–84

[2] Cheng HS, Hung LK, Ho PC, Wong J. An analysis of causes and treatment outcome of chronic wrist pain after distal radial fractures. Hand Surg 2008;13(1):1–10

[3] Fernandez DL, Geissler WB. Treatment of displaced articular fractures of the radius. J Hand Surg Am 1991;16(3):375–384

[4] Geissler WB, Freeland AE, Savoie FH, McIntyre LW, Whipple TL. Intracarpal soft-tissue lesions associated with an intra-articular fracture of the distal end of the radius. J Bone Joint Surg Am 1996;78(3):357–365

[5] Knirk JL, Jupiter JB. Intra-articular fractures of the distal end of the radius in young adults. J Bone Joint Surg Am 1986;68(5):647–659

[6] Lindau T, Arner M, Hagberg L. Intraarticular lesions in distal fractures of the radius in young adults. A descriptive arthroscopic study in 50 patients. J Hand Surg [Br] 1997;22(5):638–643

[7] Mehta JA, Bain GI, Heptinstall RJ. Anatomical reduction of intra-articular fractures of the distal radius. An arthroscopically-assisted approach. J Bone Joint Surg Br 2000;82(1):79–86

[8] Richards RS, Bennett JD, Roth JH, Milne K Jr. Arthroscopic diagnosis of intra-articular soft tissue injuries associated with distal radial fractures. J Hand Surg Am 1997;22(5):772–776

[9] Trumble TE, Schmitt SR, Vedder NB. Factors affecting functional outcome of displaced intra-articular distal radius fractures. J Hand Surg Am 1994;19(2):325–340

[10] Wadsten MA, Buttazzoni GG, Sjödén GO, Kadum B, Sayed-Noor AS, Sayed-Noor AS. Influence of cortical comminution and intra-articular involvement in distal radius fractures on clinical outcome: a prospective multicenter study. J Wrist Surg 2017;6(4):285–293

[11] Del Piñal F. Technical tips for (dry) arthroscopic reduction and internal fixation of distal radius fractures. J Hand Surg Am 2011;36(10):1694–1705

[12] Doi K, Hattori Y, Otsuka K, Abe Y, Yamamoto H. Intra-articular fractures of the distal aspect of the radius: arthroscopically assisted reduction compared with open reduction and internal fixation. J Bone Joint Surg Am 1999;81(8):1093–1110

[13] Lindau T. Arthroscopic evaluation of associated soft tissue injuries in distal radius fractures. Hand Clin 2017;33(4):651–658

[14] Ruch DS, Vallee J, Poehling GG, Smith BP, Kuzma GR. Arthroscopic reduction versus fluoroscopic reduction in the management of intra-articular distal radius fractures. Arthroscopy 2004;20(3):225–230

[15] Abe Y, Tsubone T, Tominaga Y. Plate presetting arthroscopic reduction technique for the distal radius fractures. Tech Hand Up Extrem Surg 2008;12(3):136–143

[16] Abe Y, Yoshida K, Tominaga Y. Less invasive surgery with wrist arthroscopy for distal radius fracture. J Orthop Sci 2013;18(3):398–404

[17] Abe Y. Plate presetting and arthroscopic reduction technique (PART) for treatment of distal radius fractures. Handchir Mikrochir Plast Chir 2014;46(5):278–285

[18] Abe Y, Fujii K. Arthroscopic-assisted reduction of intra-articular distal radius fracture. Hand Clin 2017;33(4):659–668

[19] del Piñal F, García-Bernal FJ, Pisani D, Regalado J, Ayala H, Studer A. Dry arthroscopy of the wrist: surgical technique. J Hand Surg Am 2007;32(1):119–123

[20] Abe Y, Doi K, Hattori Y, Ikeda K, Dhawan V. A benefit of the volar approach for wrist arthroscopy. Arthroscopy 2003;19(4):440–445

[21] Abe Y, Doi K, Hattori Y, Ikeda K, Dhawan V. Arthroscopic assessment of the volar region of the scapholunate interosseous ligament through a volar portal. J Hand Surg Am 2003;28(1):69–73

[22] Abe Y, Tominaga Y, Yoshida K. Various patterns of traumatic triangular fibrocartilage complex tear. Hand Surg 2012;17(2):191–198

12 Anterior Rim Fractures

Jorge L. Orbay, Gabriel Pertierra

Abstract

The volar marginal fragment (VMF) originates from the volar rim of the radius's lunate fossa. Though recorded incidence is low, the VMF is often missed during radiographic evaluation, leading to a lack of surgical planning. However, the VMF is essential to restoration of wrist function. Failed reduction of the small, avascular, and sometimes displaced fragment can yield catastrophic results (e.g., fragment resorption and carpal subluxation) that lead to wrist arthrodesis. Current surgical techniques that supplement volar plating for VMF management may include Kirschner wires (K-wire) or screw fixation, tension band wiring, fragment-specific plating, and modular plate extensions. In any case, the most important factor in VMF management is timeliness—identification and effective management upon index treatment. In order to effectively treat the VMF, the authors of this chapter recommend use of the extended FCR (flexor carpi radialis) approach for optimal operative visualization, and use of a volar hook plate extension.

Keywords: distal radius volar (anterior, palmar) rim fracture, volar marginal fragment, volar plating, volar locking plate, watershed line, lunate fossa, extended FCR approach, hook plate extension, wedge osteotomy

12.1 Introduction

12.1.1 Background

An anterior rim fragment, also known as a palmar rim, or volar marginal fragment (VMF), is a small fragment occurring at the volar rim of the lunate fossa, which complicates the management of distal radius fractures. They are difficult to fix because of their small size and distal location. They are uncommon, and their true incidence is unknown, but estimated to occur in 1 to 5% of distal radius fractures.[1,2] Despite its small size, the volar rim of the lunate fossa is a key part of the radiocarpal articulation and is essential in maintaining joint stability. Failure to properly address a VMF can lead to complications, particularly wrist subluxation (▶Fig. 12.1a, b).[2,3,4] After the advent of volar plating, it soon became apparent that volar fixed angle plates often failed to stabilize volar rim fragments.[3,4] The last few years have led to an increased awareness and understanding of this problem and have seen the development of new techniques for treatment.

12.1.2 Classification

VMFs are classified according to the primary distal radius fracture type and the timing of presentation. They can

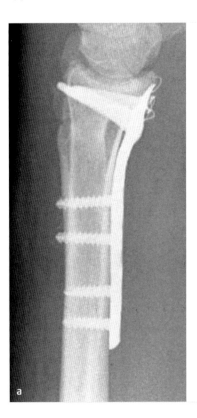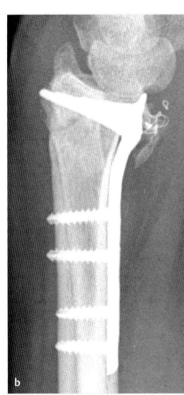

Fig. 12.1 Carpal subluxation resulting from failure to manage the volar marginal fragment (VMF) successfully. **(a)** Postoperative fixation with volar plating. **(b)** Failure of VMF fixation results in resorption, collapse, and palmar subluxation.

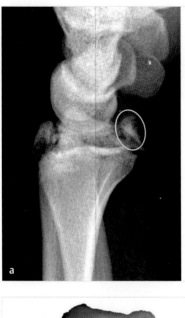
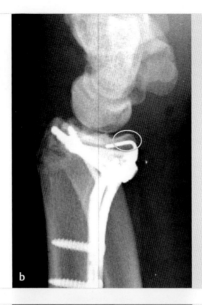

Fig. 12.2 Dorsal fracture-dislocation with a rotated volar marginal fragment (VMF). (a) Preoperative. (b) After volar plating and hook plate extension fixation. The *red line* represents the volar surface.

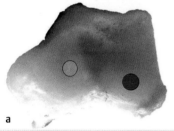
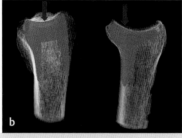
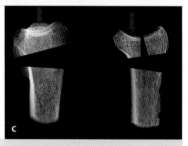

Fig. 12.3 (a) Centroids of joint reaction force. (b) Trabecular columns of subchondral plate support result in (c) different load and fracture patterns for the radius scaphoid fossa (left) and lunate fossa (right).

be present in dorsal- or palmar-directed fractures as extensions of articular comminution and in dorsal fracture-dislocations as avulsion injuries (▶Fig. 12.2a, b).[2,5,6,7] The presence of a VMF potentiates the instability of a palmar-directed fracture. This combination is particularly difficult to stabilize and may require extended buttressing support and/or direct fragment purchase. In dorsal-directed fractures or in dorsal fracture-dislocations, the pull of the short radiolunate ligament rotates the VMF into extension, requiring effective fragment purchase for reduction.[2,5,6,7] Often, volar marginal fractures are missed during initial presentation and treatment, only to be recognized when carpal subluxation is apparent (▶Fig. 12.1a, b). Fractures picked up more than 4 weeks after the index fracture are considered to have a late presentation; those diagnosed and treated early have a better prognosis than fractures diagnosed late or after failure of initial treatment.[3,8,9]

12.1.3 Anatomy and Biomechanics

The scaphoid and lunate fossae function differently. The geometric center of the scaphoid fossa is in line with the centerline of the radial shaft in the sagittal plane, and has two well-developed columns of trabecular bone transmitting articular loads to both the dorsal and palmar radial cortices.[10] The centroid of force application by the scaphoid coincides with the geometrical center of the fossa.[11] This renders an articular fracture fragment consisting mostly of the scaphoid fossa relatively stable and easy to fix with internal fixation. On the other hand, the geometric center of the lunate fossa is offset in the sagittal plane with respect to the radial centerline and has only one well-developed column of trabecular bone that transmits all articular loads to the palmar cortex. The centroid of lunate force application is located toward the palmar aspect of its articular surface and does not coincide with the geometric center. This arrangement renders lunate fossa palmar fragments relatively unstable, particularly in the case of palmar rim fragments. These have limited bony support. Therefore, articular loading results in shearing forces at the fracture surface[5,7,10] (▶Fig. 12.3a–c).

The scaphoid fossa concavity is directed in a more palmar direction (palmar tilt) than the lunate fossa, making the latter a more important restraint to palmar translation.[5] Also, because of the palmar location of the centroid of lunate force application, fracture of the palmar rim of the lunate fossa often results in palmar carpal dislocation.[5,7]

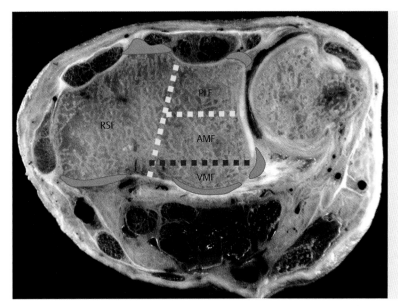

Fig. 12.4 *Blue zones* indicate the presence of ligaments. *Yellow dashed lines* indicate typical fracture lines that divide the radial scaphoid fragment (RSF), posterior lunate fragment (PLF), and anterior medial fragment (AMF). The *red dashed line* represents the zone from which volar marginal fragments (VMFs) may originate.

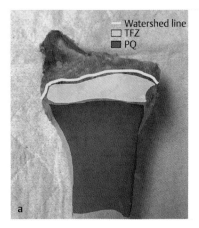
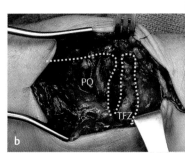

Fig. 12.5 (a) The watershed line (WL), transitional fibrous zone (TFZ), and pronator quadratus (PQ) are labeled on a cadaveric specimen. **(b)** Intraoperative view of dorsally displaced fracture with rupture between both structures.

When visualizing the radius from its distal end (▶ Fig. 12.4), the lunate fossa extends palmarly relative to the scaphoid fossa. The interfossa sulcus is a longitudinal groove on the palmar surface of the radius located between the scaphoid and lunate fossae. It limits the lateral or radial edge of the lunate fossa, narrowing its base and making it prone to fracture. Fracture lines that create a volar marginal fracture extend from the interfossa sulcus in a medial or ulnar direction, separating the palmar rim from the distal radius.

The palmar surface of the distal radius presents a transverse ridge called the watershed line (▶ Fig. 12.5a).[9] During wrist extension, it acts as a pulley for the digital flexors and extends in a generally transverse direction from the volar radial tubercle to the volar rim of the lunate fossa.[12] This ridge runs close to the joint line (2–3 mm proximal) over the palmar rim of the lunate fossa, and is incorporated in palmar rim fragments.

Blood supply to the volar rim of the lunate fossa depends on intraosseous vessels in the radius. The palmar rim fragment is small, covered distally by hyaline cartilage and palmarly by the volar wrist capsule and the origin of the short radiolunate ligament. The fractured volar rim fragment is often avascular, as often there is no retrograde vessel traversing proximally through its remaining soft tissue attachments. When not stabilized, the lack of blood supply to the fragment makes it prone to nonunion and resorption. When adequately stabilized, revascularization by primary bone healing or creeping substitution can allow it to heal.

After volar locked plating, rigidity of main fragment fixation by locking screws or pegs focuses stress at the volar rim fracture. Buttressing support by the plate surface is sufficient to stabilize some volar fragments of moderate or large size but insufficient to stabilize small fragments. The presence of the watershed line limits plate placement as more distal placement endangers flexor tendons.[13] Plates must be located at least 2 to 3 mm proximal to the watershed line in order to prevent flexor tendon injury.[9] Therefore, other fixation strategies besides buttressing support are used when managing small palmar rim fragments. Surgeons have used K-wires, individual screws, tension band fixation, extended buttressing, and hook plate extensions for this purpose. Hook plate extensions are different from fragment-specific hook plates; these are stand-alone implants intended for larger volar ulnar fragments.

Fixation of the VMF must be stable and rigid enough to allow healing, and be of low profile in order to prevent flexor tendon injury. K-wires and screws are not rigid enough unless they rest against the distal edge of the volar plate to increase stability, and they are prone to back out and irritate tendons. Tension banding of small VMFs to the volar plate is difficult due to fragment size. This technique also lacks rigidity, as purchase is often into capsular tissue or ligament, and the line of pull does not provide support against axial loads (▶Fig. 12.1a, b). Extending the plate's buttressing surface distal to the watershed line increases the risk of tendon injury, does not resist axial loads, and does not provide the rigidity needed for small or comminuted volar rim fragments. Direct purchase on the fragment is possible with a hook plate extension (Skeletal Dynamics, LLC; Miami, Florida, United States). This device is a modular extension of the volar plate that provides stability by skewering the VMF with two rigid tines, and allows effective resistance to axial loads (▶Fig. 12.6a–d). It is attached to the volar plate by an adjustable mechanism and a setscrew.

Unfortunately, it must cross the watershed line to reach and fix the volar rim. The risk of flexor tendon injury is ever-present and these cases must be followed closely to detect flexor tendon irritation early, and remove the hardware after fracture healing, if necessary.

12.2 Indications

Any distal radius fracture with a VMF is extremely unstable and should be considered for operative treatment. Commonly, VMFs are nondisplaced and difficult to visualize preoperatively. They are often identified during surgical treatment of an unstable distal radius fracture. Because they are nondisplaced and the surgeon is able to reduce the widely displaced major radial fragments, the volar rim fracture line may seem innocent and of no consequence. However, the surgeon must recognize the danger and address it properly. A VMF always occurs on the lunate fossa. It is defined by being too small to be supported by the volar plate's buttressing surface (▶Fig. 12.6a–d), and therefore, is variably identified according to the design of the volar plate used. Not all volar lunate fragments should be called VMFs, just those that are not stabilized by buttressing alone. A fragment considered a VMF could be of

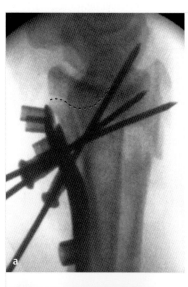
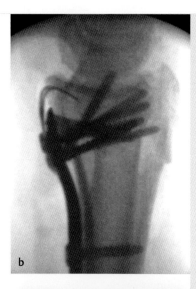
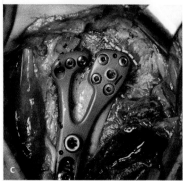
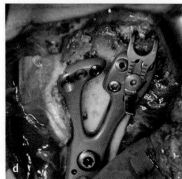

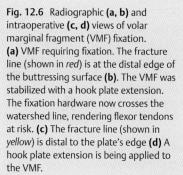

Fig. 12.6 Radiographic (a, b) and intraoperative (c, d) views of volar marginal fragment (VMF) fixation. (a) VMF requiring fixation. The fracture line (shown in *red*) is at the distal edge of the buttressing surface (b). The VMF was stabilized with a hook plate extension. The fixation hardware now crosses the watershed line, rendering flexor tendons at risk. (c) The fracture line (shown in *yellow*) is distal to the plate's edge (d) A hook plate extension is being applied to the VMF.

larger size when using a plate with a less effective buttressing surface. A plate with more effective distal support of the volar rim of the lunate fossa will adequately stabilize many volar lunate fragments and, therefore, only smaller fragments are considered VMFs.

After plate placement, the surgeon must check for adequate buttress stabilization of volar lunate fragments. If a fracture line is present close to or distal to the distal edge of the plate, it must be addressed with proper fixation.

12.3 Surgical Technique

Management of VMFs begins with proper surgical exposure. It is imperative to visualize and access the more lateral aspects of the volar radius while simultaneously being able to manage all the other components of the injury. Approaches between the flexor tendons and the ulnar neurovascular bundle do not allow treatment of the main fragments of the distal radial fracture. The ideal approach to the distal radius is the extended FCR (flexor carpi radialis) approach, as it provides global exposure to this area.[14] This distally extended Henry approach allows ulnar retraction of the flexor tendons and median nerve without undue tension.[15] This is accomplished by releasing the FCR tendon sheath distally over the scaphoid tubercle and the trapezial ridge. This surgical approach provides easy access to the volar rim of the lunate fossa, and therefore, to VMFs. In order to visualize these fragments, it is necessary to lift all soft tissues off the volar radius, proximal to the watershed line. To achieve this, a transverse incision is made sharply along the watershed line on the thick periosteum that covers the radius (transitional fibrous zone [TFZ]) (▶ Fig. 12.5a, b).[12] This incision is then continued proximally along the radial border of the pronator quadratus muscle. The pronator quadratus and the TFZ is lifted as an ulnar-based soft tissue flap. This provides exposure to the volar radius, while maintaining the origin of the volar carpal ligaments intact. In addition, by releasing the brachioradialis tendon, and pronating the proximal radial fragment, the extended FCR approach allows volar management of most complex dorsally displaced distal radius fractures.

Once the radius has been exposed and reduced, and the locking plate has been applied, the surgeon must check for the presence of a volar marginal fracture. Fracture lines that are distal enough to suggest that buttressing support will not suffice should be considered volar marginal fractures and treated accordingly. Ideally, fixation of a VMF is the last step in the procedure as it is difficult to assess volar ulnar fragment stability before the plate is applied. The surgeon must now decide the fixation method to use. All fixation hardware should be as low profile as possible. Because the watershed line must be crossed, implants should also be as narrow as possible and not present sharp edges. When using a hook plate extension, the surgeon must use careful technique.

The limbs of the hook plate extension must transfix the fragment and the base of the implant must be placed correctly in order to allow its attachment to the plate with a setscrew. A reduction instrument and a drill guide facilitate this step. Finally, the TFZ is sutured back distally at the watershed line, creating a soft tissue layer over the applied fixation hardware, therefore minimizing the possibility of tendon irritation.[16,17]

12.3.1 Salvage of a Collapsed VMF

When the VMF is not properly addressed, fragment collapse and resorption can yield catastrophic results such as articular instability and carpal subluxation.[8,18] When this occurs, simple repeat fixation with a hook plate extension and bone grafting is seldom effective. Therefore, salvage procedures are often necessary, including partial or total wrist arthrodesis. Alternatively, we prefer to utilize a volar opening wedge osteotomy. This procedure salvages the wrist by redirecting the remaining articular surface in a dorsal direction, therefore providing volar stability, and redistribution of the joint loads to the remaining articular surface (dorsal aspect). Use of an opening wedge technique also restores radial length, and requires the use of cancellous bone autograft. The opening wedge osteotomy decreases load on the volar lunate facet. Repeat fixation and bone grafting of the volar rim may succeed if the biomechanical environment is improved with the osteotomy procedure.

An extended FCR approach is used and a K-wire is inserted parallel to the articular surface in the lateral view, serving as a guide for a sagittal plane correction. A small sagittal saw is then used to cut the distal radius transversely and parallel to the k-wire, leaving a dorsal cortical hinge to rotate the distal fragment into extension. In this sagittal plane, the goal of the correction is to achieve at least neutral volar tilt of the residual lunate fossa concavity (slight dorsal is best). Radial inclination may be addressed simultaneously, and restoration of radial length is prioritized. A volar plate is then shaped to reduce its volar tilt, allowing the plate to sit flush on the now deformed volar radial bone surface. After plate application, cancellous autograft is inserted into the opening wedge defect.[9]

12.4 Results

A study conducted in 2016 showed that 19/21 patients with unilateral distal radius fracture and a VMF who were treated with volar plating and hook plate extension had successful outcome and maintained reduction through final follow-up.[9] Of these 21 cases, 17 were primary interventions in which the surgeon judged that hook plate extension treatment of a concomitant VMF to a distal radius fracture was indicated. All 17 of these primary cases healed uneventfully. Of the 21 cases, 4 were treated with volar plate and hook plate extension as a secondary or revision surgery of a previously surgically treated distal radius fracture in which a VMF had been missed and subsequently displaced. Of these four revision cases, two failed to heal (50% failure rate). In this study, there were no flexor tendon complications, despite crossing the watershed line. Indeed, such occurrences would have led to removal of the hook plate. Hook plate fixation seems to be best indicated in the primary concomitant VMF; salvage of failed VMFs is not reliably achieved by the use of the hook plate extension.

12.5 Pitfalls and Contraindications

Any case in which volar fixed angle plating is contraindicated is also a contraindication for a hook plate extension. Fractures that present significant resorption of the VMF are also contraindicated.

> **Tips and Tricks**
>
> - Use extended FCR approach.
> - Identify VMF intraoperatively after plate application.
> - VMF fixation method should be as low profile as possible to avoid tendon irritation.
> - Follow-up closely with patient and remove hardware if there are signs of flexor tendon irritation.

12.6 Conclusion

The VMF has proven a formidable problem that was brought to the attention of the surgical community by the use of volar locking plates. Understanding the biomechanics, blood supply, and anatomy of the radiocarpal joint is key to its proper management. The extended FCR approach allows access to the most ulnar aspect of the distal radius without tension on the median nerve, and management of the rest of the fracture fragments.[9,16,17] It is imperative that the presence of a VMF is recognized, but radiography often fails to identify its presence. Intraoperative inspection of the fracture lines is what often identifies the problem. There are multiple methods of fixing the VMF and the hook plate extension has many advantages. The decision to use it can be made intraoperatively, fixation is very reliable, and tendon irritation and hardware removal has not been common.[9]

References

[1] Pattee GA, Thompson GH. Anterior and posterior marginal fracture-dislocations of the distal radius. An analysis of the results of treatment. Clin Orthop Relat Res 1988(231):183–195

[2] Marcano A, Taormina DP, Karia R, Paksima N, Posner M, Egol KA. Displaced intra-articular fractures involving the volar rim of the distal radius. J Hand Surg Am 2015;40(1):42–48

[3] Beck JD, Harness NG, Spencer HT. Volar plate fixation failure for volar shearing distal radius fractures with small lunate facet fragments. J Hand Surg Am 2014;39(4):670–678

[4] O'Shaughnessy MA, Shin AY, Kakar S. Volar marginal rim fracture fixation with volar fragment-specific hook plate fixation. J Hand Surg Am 2015;40(8):1563–1570

[5] Teunis T, Bosma NH, Lubberts B, Ter Meulen DP, Ring D. Melone's concept revisited: 3D quantification of fragment displacement. J Hand Microsurg 2016;8(1):27–33

[6] Medoff RJ. Essential radiographic evaluation for distal radius fractures. Hand Clin 2005;21(3):279–288

[7] Melone CP Jr. Open treatment for displaced articular fractures of the distal radius. Clin Orthop Relat Res 1986;(202):103–111

[8] Berglund LM, Messer TM. Complications of volar plate fixation for managing distal radius fractures. J Am Acad Orthop Surg 2009;17(6):369–377

[9] Orbay JL, Rubio F, Vernon LL. Prevent collapse and salvage failures of the volar rim of the distal radius. J Wrist Surg 2016;5(1):17–21

[10] Mandziak DG, Watts AC, Bain GI. Ligament contribution to patterns of articular fractures of the distal radius. J Hand Surg Am 2011;36(10):1621–1625

[11] Majima M, Horii E, Matsuki H, Hirata H, Genda E. Load transmission through the wrist in the extended position. J Hand Surg Am 2008;33(2):182–188

[12] Clement H, Pichler W, Nelson D, Hausleitner L, Tesch NP, Grechenig W. Morphometric analysis of lister's tubercle and its consequences on volar plate fixation of distal radius fractures. J Hand Surg Am 2008;33(10):1716–1719

[13] Soong M, Earp BE, Bishop G, Leung A, Blazar P, Blazar P. Volar locking plate implant prominence and flexor tendon rupture. J Bone Joint Surg Am 2011;93(4):328–335

[14] Orbay JL, Gray R, Vernon LL, Sandilands SM, Martin AR, Vignolo SM. The EFCR approach and the radial septum-understanding the anatomy and improving volar exposure for distal radius fractures: imagine what you could do with an extra inch. Tech Hand Up Extrem Surg 2016;20(4):155–160

[15] Henry MH. Distal radius fractures: current concepts. J Hand Surg Am 2008;33(7):1215–1227

[16] Orbay JL, Mijares MR. History and complications of volar locking plate fixation for distal radius fractures. J Minim Invasive Orthop Surg 2015;75:S1–S8. ISSN: 13423991

[17] Orbay J, Shah A, White BD, Patel A, Vernon L. Volar plating as a treatment for distal radius fractures. Plast Reconstr Surg Glob Open 2016;4(9):e1041

[18] Harness NG, Jupiter JB, Orbay JL, Raskin KB, Fernandez DL. Loss of fixation of the volar lunate facet fragment in fractures of the distal part of the radius. J Bone Joint Surg Am 2004;86-A(9):1900–1908

13 Dorsal Rim Distal Radius Fractures with Radiocarpal Fracture-Dislocation

Rohit Garg, Jesse Jupiter

Abstract

Dorsal rim distal radius fractures involving either the shear injuries or fractures associated with radiocarpal fracture-dislocations are unstable injuries and operative fixation is recommended. Dorsal approach is preferred for these fracture patterns. This chapter outlines many case examples of such injuries and surgical technique for their operative repair.

Keywords: distal radius fracture, radiocarpal fracture-dislocation, dorsal approach, fragment-specific fixation

13.1 Introduction

Radiocarpal fracture-dislocations are complex injuries characterized by dislocation of the radiocarpal joint (▶Fig. 13.1). It is important to differentiate these from a Barton or reverse Barton (dorsal) fracture (▶Fig. 13.2). Barton fracture involves a shear fracture of the articular surface of distal radius with the fractured fragment attached to the carpus. In addition, the displaced fragment forms a substantial part of the distal radius articular surface. In contrast, radiocarpal fracture-dislocation is a high-energy injury with disruption of the radiocarpal ligaments. It is typically associated with a small cortical rim and/or radial styloid fracture (▶Fig. 13.1). According to the Association for Osteosynthesis (AO) classification, partial articular distal radius fractures are classified as type B. B2.1 fractures involve the dorsal rim of the distal radius. In B2.2, fracture of the dorsal rim is associated with fracture of the radial styloid as

well. In B2.3 fractures, the fracture of the dorsal rim is associated with a radial styloid fracture as well, with greater instability than in B2.2 fractures and radiocarpal dislocation.

Radiocarpal fracture-dislocations are rare injuries and their real prevalence is disputed, ranging from 0.2 to 20%.[1,2] This wide variation in prevalence is likely because of lack of strict definition and grouping radiocarpal dislocations with other injuries including a reverse Barton fracture. In addition, a very distal, severely displaced intra-articular distal radius fracture may resemble a radiocarpal dislocation (▶Fig. 13.3). Dislocation can be dorsal or volar; however, dorsal injuries are more common.[3] These are high-energy injuries primarily seen in younger males in early 30s.[3,4,5] Associated fractures and dislocations, open injuries, tendon ruptures, and neurovascular injuries have all been reported.[3,6,7] The exact mechanism of injury is unclear. It has been postulated to involve a rotational force that is consistent with the high incidence of associated distal radioulnar joint (DRUJ) injuries.[3,5]

Dumontier et al[3] proposed a classification system dividing these injuries into two groups. Type 1 radiocarpal dislocations are primarily ligamentous injuries. They have a small (less than one-third of width of scaphoid fossa) or absent radial styloid fragment. These dislocations are very rare and accounted for 7/27 cases described in this series. The authors suggested that in this group all volar radiocarpal ligaments are torn and posteriorly the ligamentous injury most often presented as a capsuloperiosteal avulsion. Ligamentous injuries make type 1 injuries globally unstable. Type 2 radiocarpal dislocations are associated with fractures of the radial styloid that

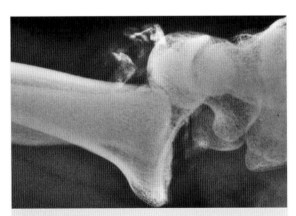

Fig. 13.1 Radiocarpal dislocation with dorsal dislocation of carpus relative to the radius and small cortical rim and radial styloid fractures.

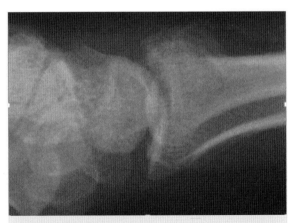

Fig. 13.2 Dorsal shear fracture of articular surface of distal radius (reverse Barton).

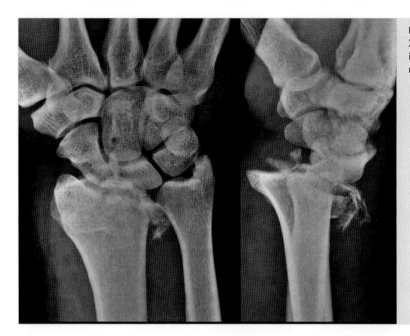

Fig. 13.3 Posteroanterior (PA) and lateral X-rays of a very distal, severely displaced intra-articular distal radius fracture resembling radiocarpal dislocation.

involves more than one-third of the width of scaphoid fossa. This fracture usually includes all of the scaphoid fossa and may continue to the dorsal margin of distal radius. The volar radiocarpal ligaments are believed to be attached to the radial styloid fragment and posteriorly there is capsuloperiosteal avulsion. The authors recommended repair of the volar ligamentous structures for type 1 injuries and a dorsal approach with fixation of the radial styloid fragment for type 2 injuries.

A dorsal approach is also recommended for dorsal shear fractures (reverse Barton) and articular surface reconstruction (▶ Fig. 13.2). Lozano-Calderón et al[8] described 20 patients with dorsal shear fractures associated with radiocarpal subluxation or dislocation. The authors found that these fractures involved dorsal shear fragments associated with: (1) central impaction; (2) impaction of majority of distal radius articular surface; (3) radiocarpal dislocations with rupture of the radiolunate ligaments or fracture of the volar portion of the lunate facet where radiolunate ligaments originate. The authors recommended dorsal approach to buttress the dorsal shear fractures and reconstruct the articular surface for associated central impaction. A combined volar approach was recommended for volar ligamentous repair or fixation of small volar avulsion fracture in radiocarpal dislocations with dorsal shear fractures.

13.2 Indications

Operative management is recommended because of the high energy and unstable nature of these injuries. A thorough history and physical examination should be performed to identify any associated neurovascular injuries. Since most of the radiocarpal dislocations are

dorsal with a fracture of the radial styloid and fracture of dorsal cortical rim, a dorsal approach is preferred. Similarly, a dorsal approach is utilized for dorsal shear fractures (reverse Barton) and articular surface reconstruction. These fractures may be accompanied by avulsion of the ulnar styloid and/or disruption of the DRUJ. If there is gross instability after fixation of the radial fracture, it is recommended that the ulnar styloid and/or triangular fibrocartilage complex (TFCC) is reattached. If there is any sign of median nerve injury, it should be decompressed using an additional palmar approach. Every patient should also be assessed for associated carpal injuries.

13.3 Surgical Technique

13.3.1 Case 1

A 30-year-old male sustained a fall from a height and presented with right distal radius fracture. Posteroanterior (PA) and lateral radiographs reveal a complex radiocarpal fracture dislocation of his right wrist (▶ Fig. 13.4). Sagittal two-dimensional computed tomography (2D-CT) views demonstrate the very small shearing fracture of the dorsal aspect of the distal radius with dislocation of the carpus (▶ Fig. 13.4). 3D-CT reconstructions show the volar rim of the radius to be intact with the dorsal small shearing fracture fragments (▶ Fig. 13.4). Also seen in all the preoperative images is the radial styloid fracture. Note the horizontal fracture line involving the entire scaphoid fossa and continuing to the dorsal cortical rim. Operative fixation was recommended. A standard dorsal approach to the wrist was used with a longitudinal incision over distal radius and radiocarpal joint

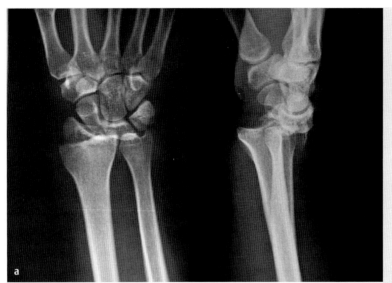

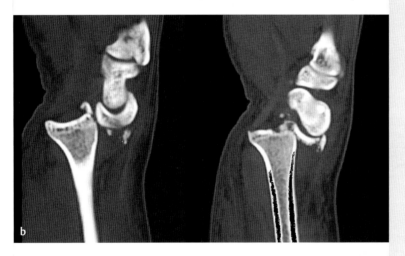

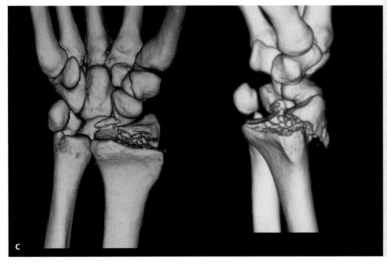

Fig. 13.4 (a-c) X-rays, two-dimensional computed tomography (2D-CT) sagittal views, and three-dimensional computed tomography (3D-CT) reconstruction showing dorsal radiocarpal dislocation with radial styloid and dorsal cortical rim fracture.

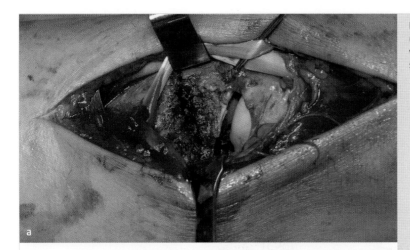

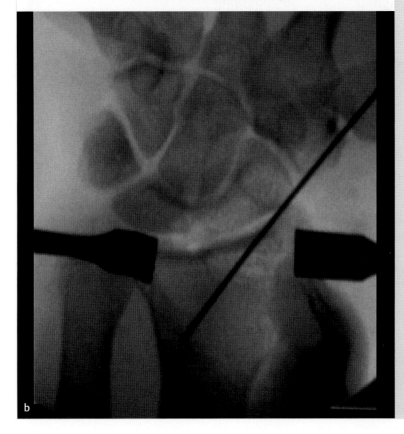

Fig. 13.5 (a, b) Standard dorsal approach (hand to the right of the clinical image) with provisional fixation of the radial styloid fragment using 0.062 K-wire.

in line with the third metacarpal. The extensor pollicis longus tendon was mobilized from the third dorsal compartment and the tendons of the second and fourth dorsal compartment were retraced to gain exposure (▶Fig. 13.5). The dorsal small rim and the radial styloid fractures are clearly visualized. Usually, the capsule is torn (▶Fig. 13.5), but if it is intact, a dorsal arthrotomy is made parallel to the dorsal rim to inspect the articular surface and look for any associated carpal injury. At this point, carpus is reduced and fixation is started with the less comminuted fracture fragment. In this case, a 0.062 smooth K-wire was used for provisional fixation

of the radial styloid fracture and articular reduction was also confirmed using intraoperative fluoroscopy (▶Fig. 13.5). If dorsal rim fragments are large enough, provisional fixation can be obtained with K-wires. If they are too small, they can be held with suture anchors or transosseous sutures. Low-profile dorsal distal radius plates were then used for fragment-specific fixation (▶Fig. 13.6). Radial column plate and 2.4-mm dorsal plate were used. Capsule was repaired using resorbable suture (▶Fig. 13.6). Follow-up at 8 months shows excellent function with some loss of wrist extension and flexion (▶Fig. 13.7). Many plates are available for these

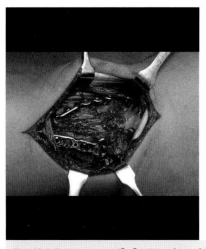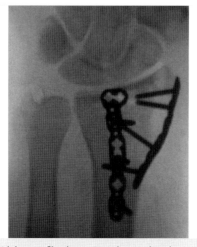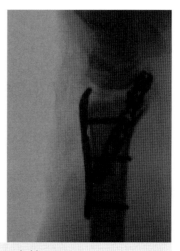

Fig. 13.6 Fragment-specific fixation achieved with low profile plates. Capsule was closed using resorbable sutures.

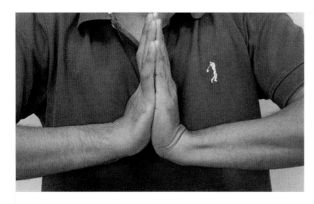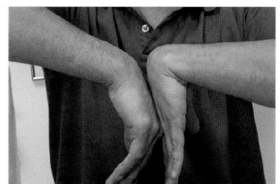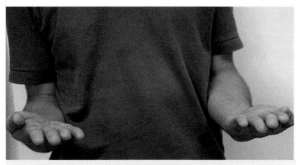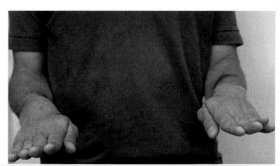

Fig. 13.7 Clinical result at 8-month follow-up for case 1.

fractures. The most recently designed plates have variable angle locking screws. The dorsal plate should be applied as distally as possible. These plates might need some contouring to fit the distal radius metaphysis and the radial styloid.

13.3.2 Case 2

A 34-year-old male laborer sustained a fall from scaffolding and presented with a radiocarpal dislocation with fractures of the radial styloid, dorsal cortical rim of distal radius, and ulnar styloid (▶ Fig. 13.8). A standard dorsal approach as described above was used and the radial styloid was fixed using a 3.0-mm cannulated screw and dorsal distal radius plate was used to buttress the dorsal cortical rim (▶ Fig. 13.9). DRUJ stability was checked after fixing the radial fracture and it was unstable. Separate ulnar-sided incision was made to use a cannulated screw with washer for the ulnar styloid (▶ Fig. 13.9). Excellent range of motion was obtained postoperatively (▶ Fig. 13.10).

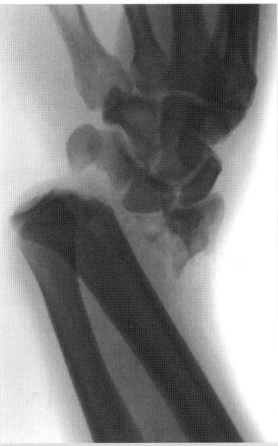

Fig. 13.8 Radiocarpal dislocation with fractures of the radial styloid, dorsal cortical rim of distal radius, and ulnar styloid.

13.3.3 Case 3

This is another example of dorsal radiocarpal fracture dislocation with fractures of the radial styloid involving the entire scaphoid fossa, dorsal cortical rim, and distal ulna (►Fig. 13.11). A standard dorsal approach was used to achieve fragment-specific fixation of the distal radius. A radial column buttress plate and a 2.4-mm **L**-shaped dorsal plate were used (►Fig. 13.12a). A nonlocking, standard screw long enough to engage the opposite cortex was first placed through the oblong hole but not fully tightened. The reduction and plate position was confirmed using intraoperative fluoroscopy. If necessary, plate position can be adjusted until it is as distal and central as possible, and then the screw can be tightened. Once the plate position is satisfactory, it should be secured with a screw (locking) in the proximal screw hole. Screws are then inserted through the distal plate holes (L part of the plate). Variable angle locking plate was applied to the radial column (►Fig. 13.12). Locking head screws were inserted into the distal locking hole of the plate. The position of these screws should be just under the subchondral bone (►Fig. 13.12). The tip of these screws should not penetrate the sigmoid notch. It is safer to leave these screws a little short and should not be drilled into the opposite cortex (►Fig. 13.12). Screws were also placed in the proximal screw holes of this plate (►Fig. 13.12). A true joint view using intraoperative fluoroscopy should be obtained to confirm that there are no screws penetrating into the joint. DRUJ stability was checked at this point. A separate ulnar side incision along the subcutaneous border of distal ulna was utilized to fix the distal ulna with a hook plate (►Fig. 13.12).

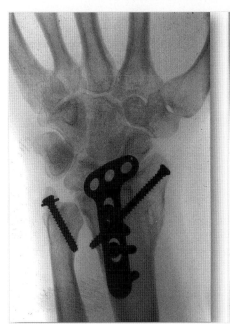

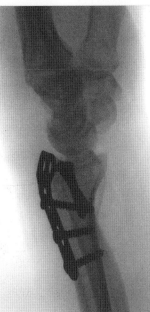

Fig. 13.9 Fixation using 3.0-mm cannulated screw for radial styloid and a cannulated screw with washer for ulnar styloid. A dorsal distal radius plate was used to buttress the cortical rim.

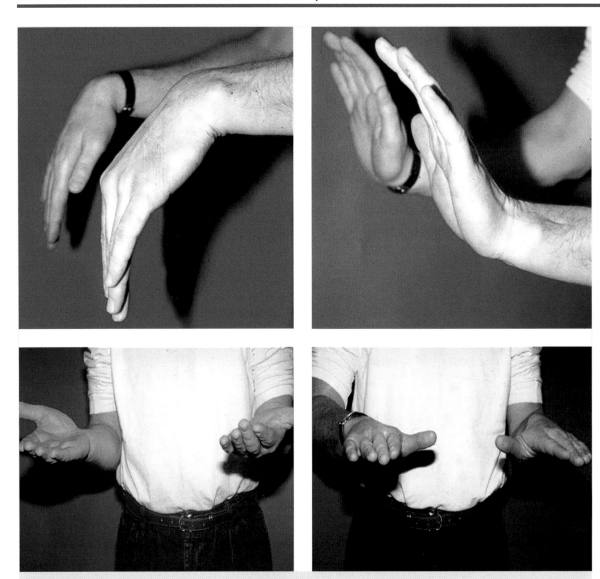

Fig. 13.10 Range of motion (ROM) at follow-up for case 2.

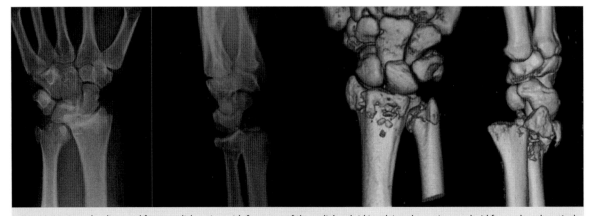

Fig. 13.11 Dorsal radiocarpal fracture dislocation with fractures of the radial styloid involving the entire scaphoid fossa, dorsal cortical rim, and distal ulna.

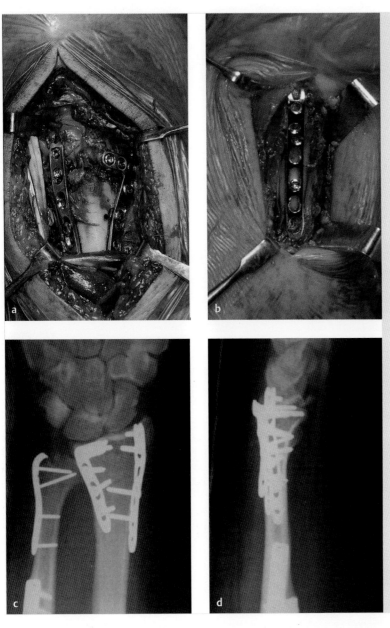

Fig. 13.12 (a–d) Fragment-specific fixation of distal radius and a separate ulnar side incision along the subcutaneous border of distal ulna was utilized to fix the distal ulna with a hook plate.

13.3.4 Case 4

A 42-year-old male involved in a bicycle accident sustained a dorsal shear fracture associated with central impaction and radial styloid fracture (▶Fig. 13.13). A dorsal approach was utilized to reconstruct the articular surface and achieve fragment-specific fixation (▶Fig. 13.14).

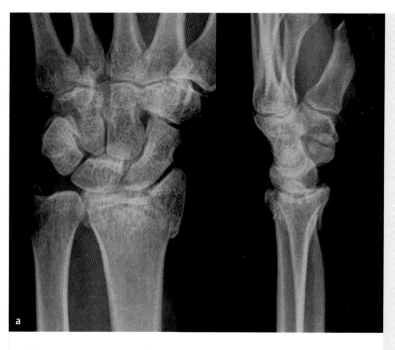

Fig. 13.13 **(a, b)** Dorsal shear fracture associated with central impaction and radial styloid fracture.

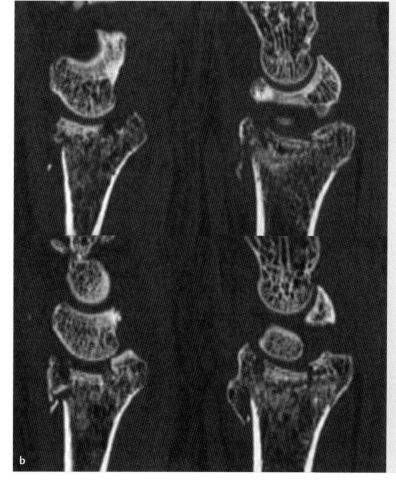

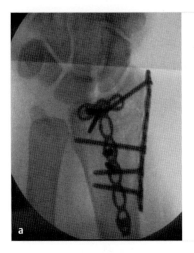 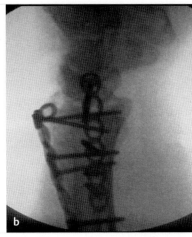

Fig. 13.14 (a, b) Dorsal approach used to reconstruct the articular surface and achieve fragment-specific fixation.

13.4 Results

Loss of about 30 to 40% of total wrist flexion/extension arc has been reported in literature with radiocarpal fracture dislocations.[3,4] Worse outcomes are associated with persistent articular incongruity, persistent neurological deficit, associated carpal fractures and residual ulnar translocation of the carpus.[3,4,9] Chronic radiocarpal and distal radioulnar instability or ulnar translation of the carpus are more common with type 1 radiocarpal fracture dislocations.[3,9] Good to excellent short-term outcomes have been reported in literature.[3,4,8] Posttraumatic arthritis is commonly seen in these patient and is likely related to persistent articular incongruity. Posttraumatic arthritis does not necessarily result in a painful wrist at short-term follow-up. With the design of new lower profile systems, rate of hardware removal is not higher for dorsal plates in our experience.

Tips and Tricks

- Preoperative CT scan including 3D reconstruction is often helpful in making treatment decisions and operative planning.
- Identify median nerve compromise that will require an additional palmar approach.
- Look out for any intercarpal ligament injuries.
- Carpal stability needs to be assessed after fracture fixation. As additional palmar approach might be needed to repair volar capsule and ligaments.
- Ulnar styloid and/or TFCC might need to be reattached for DRUJ instability.

13.5 Conclusion

Distal radius dorsal rim shear fractures or fractures associated with radiocarpal dislocation are unstable injuries and operative treatment is recommended. Dorsal approach to the distal radius is preferred and allows for fixation of dorsal radiocarpal fracture-dislocations, dorsal shearing fractures, articular surface reconstruction, associated scaphoid fractures and other carpal injuries, and displaced dorsal ulnar fragment of the distal radius. DRUJ stability needs to be assessed and often a separate ulnar-sided incision is needed to reattach the ulnar styloid and/or TFCC. Carpal instability after fixation and/or median nerve injury necessitates a separate volar incision to repair the volar capsule and ligaments and decompress the median nerve.

References

[1] Dunn AW. Fractures and dislocations of the carpus. Surg Clin North Am 1972;52(6):1513–1538

[2] Moneim MS, Bolger JT, Omer GE. Radiocarpal dislocation--classification and rationale for management. Clin Orthop Relat Res 1985;(192):199–209

[3] Dumontier C, Meyer zu Reckendorf G, Sautet A, Lenoble E, Saffar P, Allieu Y. Radiocarpal dislocations: classification and proposal for treatment. A review of twenty-seven cases. J Bone Joint Surg Am 2001;83-A(2):212–218

[4] Mudgal CS, Psenica J, Jupiter JB. Radiocarpal fracture-dislocation. J Hand Surg [Br] 1999;24(1):92–98

[5] Ilyas AM, Mudgal CS. Radiocarpal fracture-dislocations. J Am Acad Orthop Surg 2008;16(11):647–655

[6] Nyquist SR, Stern PJ. Open radiocarpal fracture-dislocations. J Hand Surg Am 1984;9(5):707–710

[7] Fernandez DL. Irreducible radiocarpal fracture-dislocation and radioulnar dissociation with entrapment of the ulnar nerve, artery and flexor profundus II-V-case report. J Hand Surg Am 1981;6(5):456–461

[8] Lozano-Calderón SA, Doornberg J, Ring D. Fractures of the dorsal articular margin of the distal part of the radius with dorsal radiocarpal subluxation. J Bone Joint Surg Am 2006;88(7):1486–1493

[9] Penny WH III, Green TL. Volar radiocarpal dislocation with ulnar translocation. J Orthop Trauma 1988;2(4):322–326

14 Multiplanar Fixation in Severe Articular Fractures

Peter C. Rhee, Alexander Y. Shin

Abstract

Severely comminuted distal radius fractures can pose tremendous challenges in restoring articular congruity and achieving anatomic alignment. Successful management of these fractures requires a thorough understanding of the osteoligamentous fracture fragments and the deforming forces that must be mitigated. Although volar locking plates (VLPs) can be used in the management of most distal radius fractures, their use should be limited in complex, multi-fragmentary fractures. In these situations, the surgeon must be facile with various surgical approaches and be ready to provide alternative methods to stabilize unstable fragments.

Keywords: comminuted distal radius, combined approach, articular fragment, dorsal-ulnar fragment, volar rim

14.1 Introduction

Volar locking plate (VLP) fixation can be utilized in the surgical management of most distal radius fractures to effectively stabilize sizable fracture fragments. The fixed-angle construct of a VLP provides stable fixation, even in the setting of metadiaphyseal comminution, by transferring forces from the distal fragments to the volar cortex of the intact radial shaft.[1,2] However, there are limitations to these implants when used in isolation to reconstruct multifragmentary distal radius fractures, especially in the setting of marked articular comminution with small fracture fragments. Successful surgical management of complex distal radius fractures requires versatility in surgical approaches and techniques, in addition to a familiarity with a variety of fixation methods including multiplanar fragment-specific (F-S) fixation.[2]

14.1.1 Understanding the Fracture Characteristics

Multifragmentary distal radius fractures result in characteristic fracture fragments.[3,4,5] Melone noted that intra-articular fractures of the distal radius often results in a coronal plane fracture line that separates the dorsal and volar surfaces of the lunate facet.[6] Teunis et al reviewed computed tomography (CT) scans of 41 intra-articular distal radius fractures (Association for Osteosynthesis [AO] type C3) and noted that 93% ($n = 38$) fit the Melone distribution of fracture fragments.[4] Rikli and Regazzoni initially described the distal end of the radius as two columns, radial and intermediate, which contain bony and ligamentous structures that provide stability to the radiocarpal and distal radioulnar joints (DRUJs).[2,7] Medoff further classified the common fracture fragments that reside within these columns (▶Fig. 14.1).[2,3] The intermediate column is composed of the volar rim, dorsal ulnar corner, dorsal wall, and a free intra-articular fragment, while the radial column consists of the radial styloid fragment alone (▶Fig. 14.2).

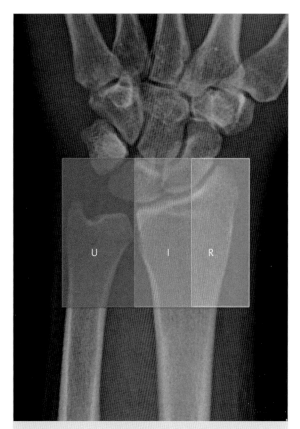

Fig. 14.1 Column model for distal radius fractures. Intermediate (I), radial (R), and ulnar (U) columns.

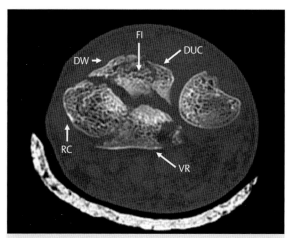

Fig. 14.2 Common fracture fragments in comminuted, intra-articular distal radius fractures. An axial computed tomography scan of the articular surface of a multifragmentary distal radius fracture illustrates the volar rim (VR), dorsal ulnar corner (DUC), free intra-articular (FI), dorsal wall (DW), and radial column (RC) fragments.

Articular fractures at the distal radius occur at inherent areas of weakness between sites of ligamentous attachments.[4,5,8,9] Mandziak et al reviewed CT scans of 100 intra-articular distal radius fractures to identify common patterns and locations of fracture lines.[8] They noted that fractures sites commonly occurred between ligament attachments. Similarly, Bain et al utilized CT scans of 42 intra-articular distal radius fractures and observed cortical breaches in an interligamentous zone in 85% of cases (71 of 84 fracture lines), thus resulting in three characteristic fracture fragments involving the radial styloid and the dorsal or volar articular surfaces of the lunate facet, each with their own subtypes.[9] Given the fact that ligamentous origins were relatively preserved despite marked comminution, the authors suggested that the fracture fragments should be conceptualized as osteoligamentous units that should be taken into consideration during reconstruction.

Understanding the fracture fragments and their role in providing stability to the radiocarpal and distal radioulnar joints is paramount to successful reconstruction of complex distal radius fractures. Teunis et al utilized quantitative CT to evaluate the articular surface area of the radial styloid (radial column), volar lunate facet (volar rim), and dorsal lunate facet (dorsal ulnar corner and dorsal wall) fragments in 41 intra-articular distal radius fractures.[4] They noted decreasing mean articular surface area from the volar lunate facet (39%) and radial styloid (37%) to the dorsal lunate facet (24%) fragments. The authors concluded that anatomic reconstruction of the radial styloid and volar rim fragments may be the key elements to imparting a stable foundation for the radiocarpal joint. However, the volar rim and dorsal ulnar corner fragments create the sigmoid notch as well as the lunate facet; thus, both fragments are indispensable to providing stability at both the radiocarpal and distal radioulnar joints.[2,3,4] Unfortunately, the volar rim and dorsal ulnar corner fragments can often malrotate and may be irreducible with ligamentotaxis and manipulation alone.[3,4,5]

14.1.2 Limitations of Volar Locking Plate Fixation

Although versatile, the VLP may not provide stability to all critical fracture fragments in many multifragmentary distal radius fractures.[10,11,12] Harness et al initially described the inability of a VLP, appropriately placed proximal to the so-called watershed line at the junction of the pronator fossa and the volar rim of the lunate, to stabilize a small volar rim fragment, thus resulting in loss of fixation and radiocarpal instability in seven patients.[12] Beck et al further noted that volar shear fractures with separate radial styloid and lunate facet fragments (AO type B3.3) with less than 15 mm of lunate facet volar cortical length available for VLP fixation or greater than 5 mm of initial lunate facet subsidence were at risk for failure with a properly positioned VLP alone.[11] In these instances, additional fixation methods should be implemented in addition to the VLP to stabilize the unstable volar rim fragment or to utilize alternative forms of fixation and techniques such as F-S fixation, external fixation, or distraction bridge plate fixation.[2,10]

14.1.3 Rationale for Fragment-Specific Fixation

Due to the inability of a single implant or technique to reconstruct all unstable distal radius fractures, the concept of F-S fixation was introduced.[13,14] F-S fixation involves the application of individualized, low-profile implants and the use of corresponding surgical exposures to stabilize all unstable fracture fragments with only a minimal footprint within the fragment itself.[2] These implants create a multiplanar, load-sharing construct that anatomically restores the articular surface while providing enough stability to allow immediate motion after surgery.[2,13,14]

Although small and low profile, F-S implants can provide tremendous stability to comminuted distal radius fractures, particularly the dorsal ulnar corner fragment.[15,16] Dodds et al performed a cadaveric biomechanic study comparing the stability of three- and four-part distal radius fractures reconstructed with dedicated F-S implants to external fixation with 0.062-inch Kirschner wires (K-wires) in each fracture fragment.[15] Although both forms of fixation provided equal stability in a simulated three-part fracture, F-S fixation alone resulted in greater stability in all six axes of motion compared to external fixation with supplemental pin fixation in four-part fractures of the distal radius. Taylor et al compared the stability of a fixed-angle VLP to F-S implants in a cadaveric, biomechanic study with a simulated AO type C2 fracture.[16] The authors noted that although there were no significant differences in load to failure between groups, the F-S group resulted in significantly stiffer fixation of the dorsal ulnar corner fragment in cyclic-loading compared to the VLP group.

14.2 Indications

The indications for operative management of distal radius fractures include postreduction radial shortening > 3 mm, dorsal tilt > 10°, and intra-articular displacement or step-off > 2 mm. Distal radius reconstruction with F-S fixation is indicated when fracture fragments are too small for screw fixation through a VLP or when the fracture line courses distal to the watershed line.[10,11,12] In many instances, supplemental F-S fixation can be utilized in addition to a VLP if reduction and stabilization of a free intra-articular fragment is necessary or if the dorsal ulnar corner, dorsal wall, or radial column fragments remain unstable after initial VLP fixation.[2]

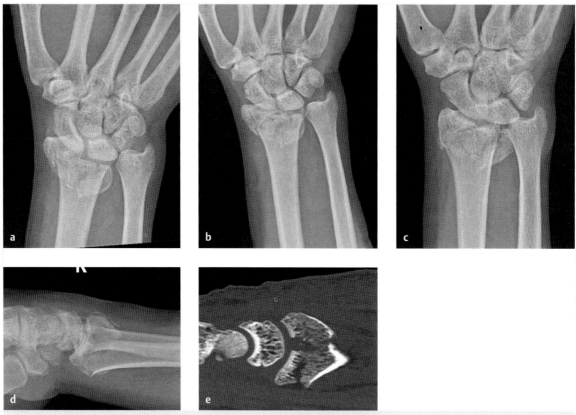

Fig. 14.3 Radiographs and CT scan of a multifragmentary, intra-articular distal radius fracture. Posteroanterior (PA) radiographs upon presentation **(a)**, traction view **(b)**, oblique **(c)**, and lateral **(d)** can identify most fracture fragments. The sagittal reformat of the volar rim fragment **(e)** clearly identifies the small fragment with a very distal fracture line that may not be amenable to standard volar locking plate fixation.

14.3 Surgical Technique (Authors' Preferred)

14.3.1 Preoperative Planning

Traction or reduction radiographs (posteroanterior, lateral, and oblique views) are and can be used to visualize the fracture fragments more clearly than the nonreduced injury images. More complex fractures may require CT images with sagittal and coronal reformats to clearly delineate the fracture patterns (▶Fig. 14.3). As one gain more experience in correlating CT findings with radiographic findings, the need for CT diminishes. However, CT scan should be obtained for fractures where the fragments are not clearly identified or is unusual, or if there is concern for concomitant carpal injuries.

14.3.2 Sequence of Reconstruction

The sequence of reconstruction starts with the volar rim fragment and progresses in a step-wise fashion addressing all of the unstable fracture fragments (▶Fig. 14.4). The volar rim fragment is the cornerstone of the other fragments within the intermediate column. With its

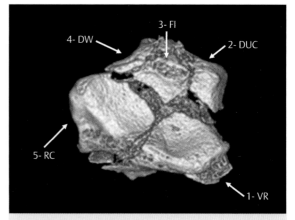

Fig. 14.4 Sequence of reconstructing the comminuted distal radius fracture. Step-wise reconstruction of the volar rim (VR), dorsal ulnar corner (DUC), free intra-articular (FI), dorsal wall (DW), and radial column (RC) fragments.

attachment to the short radiolunate ligament, it also has the ability to reduce the displaced carpus that often follows the volar rim fragment. The next fragment to address is the dorsal ulnar corner fragment. Note that reduction of the volar rim and dorsal ulnar corner fragments permit

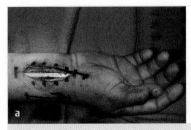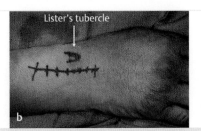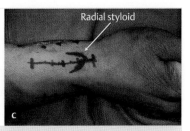

Fig. 14.5 Incisions utilized to approach multifragmentary distal radius fractures. Volar flexor carpi radialis–based approach **(a)**, dorsal approach **(b)**, and direct radial approach **(c)**.

restoration of the lunate facet and sigmoid notch articular surfaces. Reduction of any depressed free intra-articular fragments is then performed followed by reduction and fixation of the dorsal wall fragments. At this point, the intermediate column is fully reconstructed and the radial column (styloid) fragment can then be reduced and buttressed to the intermediate column, thus completing the reconstruction of the distal radius. Lastly, fractures and soft tissue injuries involving the distal ulna or the triangular fibrocartilage complex (ulnar column) are addressed if the DRUJ remains unstable. However, this will be further discussed in Chapter 19.

Examination of the normal, uninjured wrist is extremely helpful prior to surgery. It will allow for comparison of motion and stability of the DRUJ. When planning for F-S fixation, understanding the angiosomes of the wrist as well as incision placement is essential.[17,18] As multiple incisions may be needed to approach the various fragments, they should be longitudinal while preserving the angiosomes demarcated by the radial and ulnar arteries. Up to four longitudinal incisions can be placed on the wrist without skin necrosis or wound issues in the authors' experience. These incisions include a volar incision, dorsal midline incision, radial incision, and, when necessary, an ulnar incision (▶ Fig. 14.5). The specific approaches will be detailed with each fragment.

14.3.3 Management of the Volar Rim Fragment

The surgical approach for the volar radius, in particular the volar rim fragment, can be accomplished either with a flexor carpi radialis (FCR) approach or a volar-ulnar approach.[19] When part of a multi-incision approach, the longitudinal skin incision of the FCR approach can be made slightly ulnar to the FCR tendon, with caution to not injure the palmar cutaneous branch of the median nerve, to allow for a greater skin bridge between the volar and radial approaches. The skin incision is made from the distal wrist crease and extended proximally as dictated by the proximal extent of the fracture. The skin flap is elevated radially to visualize the FCR tendon sheath that is then incised as distal as possible to allow for adequate radial or ulnar retraction of the FCR tendon.

The pronator quadratus is reflected from the volar cortex of the radius taking care to not divide the volar radiocarpal ligaments. The brachioradialis is divided as needed to permit reduction of a proximally displaced radial column fragment.

An alternative approach to the volar rim fragment is the volar-ulnar approach with the incision made 1 cm radial to the FCU tendon. In this approach, the flexor tendons and median nerve are reflected radially and the ulnar neurovascular bundle is reflected ulnarward. The pronator quadratus is split longitudinally over the ulnar border of the radius and reflected radially to expose the volar rim fragment. In the authors' experience, this approach is useful for small volar rim fragments in patients with a wide distal radius where the tradition FCR approach may inhibit adequate exposure.

The volar rim fragment is often impacted, malrotated, and flexed or extended based on the injury pattern. Reduction starts with longitudinal traction and realignment of the volar cortex. Disimpaction of this fragment can be aided with a dental pick. Once accomplished, a K-wire can be temporarily placed across the radial styloid, if not comminuted, into the proximal radius to provisionally hold the reduction. Not infrequently, the volar rim fragment remains unstable and requires the use of a dental pick to hold it in place while flexing the wrist to prevent extension of the fragment. The apposition site of the volar rim fragment to the distal radius metaphysis, on the volar-ulnar surface of the distal radius, is evaluated to confirm that adequate reduction has been achieved and that coronal shift of the volar rim fragment relative to the proximal radius has not occurred.

Once the fragment is reduced, fixation of the volar rim fragment can be accomplished with a VLP if the fragment is large enough. When using a VLP as part of a multi-incision F-S approach, the surgeon must consider space available for other screws/pins that may need to be placed from supplemental F-S implants. For example, the VLP may block screws and pins placed from the dorsum of the radius. Additionally, if a dorsal ulnar corner fragment requires F-S fixation, the ulnar-sided screws through the VLP should be initially inserted short and only into the volar fragment so the dorsal ulnar corner fragment can be reduced without hindrance from long screws (▶ Fig. 14.6).

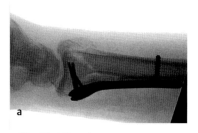
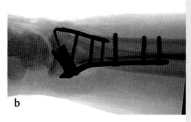

Fig. 14.6 Volar locking plate fixation with subsequent fragment-specific fixation for an unstable dorsal ulnar corner fragment. A volar locking plate is first inserted to stabilize a sizable volar rim fragment with forethought to place short distal row screws **(a)** as to not impede reduction of the dorsal ulnar corner fragment that requires supplemental fragment-specific fixation **(b)**.

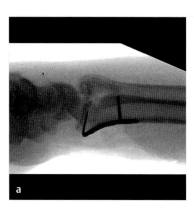
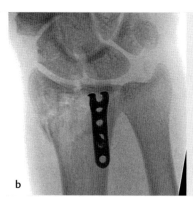

Fig. 14.7 Fragment-specific fixation of the volar rim fragment. Lateral **(a)** and posteroanterior **(b)** radiographs of a volar hook plate (TriMed Inc, Valencia, California, United States).

For very distal volar rim fragments, several options exist: combination of K-wires and VLP,[20] volar wireforms,[2,21] and volar hook plate (▶Fig. 14.7).[22,23] The surgical techniques of each of these techniques has been previously described and a full description is beyond the scope of this chapter.[2,13,14,23,24] The key points for fixation of the volar rim are that it needs to be anatomic, as it is the cornerstone on which all other fragments are reduced to, and it needs to be low profile to prevent injury to the flexor pollicis longus or flexor digitorum profundus tendons. Start with the simplest technique and advance to more difficult techniques when required. Be cognizant of hardware needs from dorsal and radial approaches before placing a VLP to secure the volar rim fragment.

14.3.4 Management of the Dorsal Ulnar Corner Fragment

The dorsal ulnar corner fragment is the second fragment to be addressed after the volar rim fragment. The dorsal ulnar corner fragment is approached through a dorsal, midline longitudinal incision centered over the carpus and slightly ulnar to Lister tubercle. While there remains controversy on the necessity of an arthrotomy to evaluate the adequacy of reduction versus use of indirect means such as fluoroscopy, it has been our practice to directly visualize the articular reduction via a dorsal arthrotomy at the radiocarpal articulation.[25] Although arthroscopy can be performed to evaluate for articular

congruity and even assist in reduction efforts, severely comminuted distal radius fractures that require multiplanar fixation must utilize a dorsal approach. Therefore, direct visualization through an arthrotomy is preferred.

After the skin incision is made, skin flaps are carefully elevated with preservation of perforators from the radial and ulnar arteries supplying their respective angiosomes. The third extensor compartment is opened and an ulnarly based retinacular flap is created by dividing the septation between the 3–4 and 4–5 extensor compartments (▶Fig. 14.8). It is essential to expose the extensor digiti minimi as the dorsal ulnar corner fragment is at the floor of the fifth extensor compartment. A posterior interosseous nerve neurectomy is performed, not only for potential pain relief, but to prevent traumatic neuroma from occurring from the arthrotomy or with placement of dorsal hardware. The proximal limb of a ligament-sparing capsulotomy as described by Berger et al is performed to expose the radiocarpal joint.[26] If carpal work is necessary, the distal limb of the ligament-sparing capsulotomy can be made, by splitting the dorsal intercarpal ligament, and the entire carpus can be exposed.

Traction on the digits and a freer-elevator can be used to visualize and palpate the articular surface of the radius to assess the intra-articular fragments and step-off (▶Fig. 14.9). There is a paradox to visualization of the articular surface: the more articular surface that can be seen implies that there are dorsal fragments that are unreduced, and when the dorsal fragments are reduced,

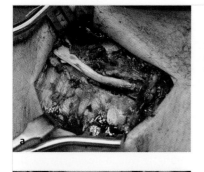
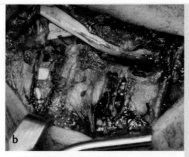
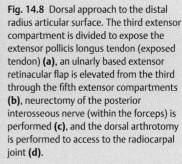
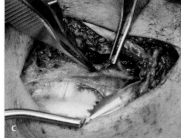
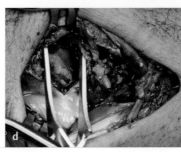

Fig. 14.8 Dorsal approach to the distal radius articular surface. The third extensor compartment is divided to expose the extensor pollicis longus tendon (exposed tendon) **(a)**, an ulnarly based extensor retinacular flap is elevated from the third through the fifth extensor compartments **(b)**, neurectomy of the posterior interosseous nerve (within the forceps) is performed **(c)**, and the dorsal arthrotomy is performed to access to the radiocarpal joint **(d)**.

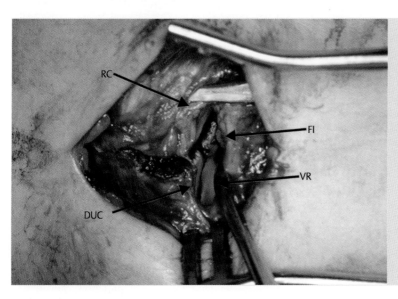

Fig. 14.9 Visualization of the articular fracture fragments. Through the dorsal radiocarpal arthrotomy, the volar rim (VR), dorsal ulnar corner (DUC), free intra-articular (FI), and radial column (RC) fragments can be visualized to assess for displacement and to perform a direct open reduction.

it is more difficult to visualize the distal radius articular surface.

The dorsal radioulnar ligament attaches the dorsal ulnar corner fragment to the distal ulna, yet the dorsal ulnar corner fragment has no ligament attachments to the carpus. As such, no amount of longitudinal traction will reduce the impacted and malrotated dorsal ulnar corner fragment by closed means. A freer-elevator is placed into the transverse component of the fracture over the radius and is used to elevate the fragment and rotate it back into a reduced position. A dental pick is helpful to hold the fragment in place and determine the location of placing a K-wire into the fragment. If markedly impacted, allograft bone graft can be inserted to backfill the defect to aid in maintaining reduction. The adequacy of

reduction is visualized directly and also can be palpated with the freer-elevator. If the lunate facet is reconstructed anatomically, the sigmoid notch has been reduced indirectly. Much like the concept of a broken tea cup handle, if one portion of the handle is accurately reduced the other break is reduced as well. Once the dorsal ulnar corner fragment is reduced, fixation can be afforded by K-wires or an F-S implant can be inserted (▶ Fig. 14.10).

14.3.5 Management of Free Intra-articular Fragments

Oftentimes, there are concomitant free intra-articular fragments that require reduction and stabilization. These

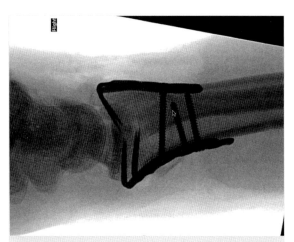

Fig. 14.10 Fragment-specific fixation of the dorsal ulnar corner fragment. An unstable dorsal ulnar corner fragment is stabilized with a fragment-specific implant (Dorsal hook plate, TriMed Inc., Valencia, California, United States).

are all visualized via the dorsal arthrotomy. Reduction of these fragments can be very challenging since they are frequently impacted and rotated. Very small fragments should be debrided and discarded to prevent the occurrence of symptomatic loose bodies. The larger fragments should be reduced and stabilized. In cases where there is tremendous impaction, longitudinal traction and placement of allograft bone into the impacted defect proximal to the impacted fragment through dorsal wall defect allows for accurate reduction of the intra-articular fragments. It is important to make sure enough allograft bone is used to buttress the now disimpacted free intra-articular fragment. Fixation of the intra-articular fragments can be with subchondral K-wires, screws through the VLP, or F-S implants. Typically, the fixation is in combination with the dorsal wall fragment. When these elements are securely fixed, the intra-articular fragments lock into place.

14.3.6 Management of the Dorsal Wall Fragment

The dorsal wall fragment size can vary from a thin shell to a sizable fragment. The need to adjust the technique for fixation is imperative. For thin shell fragments, pull-through sutures, K-wires, dorsal buttress plates, or F-S implants can be used. For larger fragments, F-S implants such as dorsal hook plates, K-wires, or dorsal buttress plates can be used.

14.3.7 Management of the Radial Column Fragment

The final step in reconstructing the radius is to reduce and secure the radial column fragment. The surgical approach to the radial column can be through an extension of the volar approach (a combined volar and radial column approach) or a direct radial approach. The combined volar and radial column approach requires a curvilinear incision that crosses the radial artery, and it can be challenging to place the radial column plate accurately due to the limited exposure. It is the authors' preference to utilize a direct radial approach for the benefits of easier plate/pin placement. However, the direct radial approach potentially places the superficial branch of the radial nerve (SBRN) at risk and adds a third incision with potential wound issues. To mitigate wound-healing issues, the soft tissues beneath the skin flap and radial artery are not to be disturbed. The decision for a third incision versus a combined volar-radial approach is made by the surgeon and is often dictated by surgeon experience and preference, and radius fracture characteristics. Anecdotally, in over 400 multi-incision cases performed by the authors of this chapter, there have been no significant wound issues noted.

A direct radial incision is made and meticulous skin flaps are raised. The SBRN is identified and protected with direction of retraction of the SBRN selected based on its course through the surgical field. Occasionally, the SBRN bifurcates within the exposure and an internal neurolysis can be performed to increase its split proximally to ensure its safety while retracting. The first and second extensor compartments are identified and the radial styloid tip is palpated between these extensor compartments. The retinaculum of the first compartment is preserved distally for 1 to 1.5 cm, while the proximal extent of the first extensor compartment is divided (▶ Fig. 14.11). The abductor pollicis longus and the extensor pollicis brevis are retracted dorsally exposing the brachioradialis tendon. If this tendon has not been previously divided, its insertion onto the radial styloid is elevated at this point.

Utilizing a dental pick, K-wire, or ulnar deviation of the wrist, the radial styloid is reduced and a temporary K-wire can be placed from the distal aspect of the radial styloid, between the first and second extensor compartments, across the fracture engaging on the ulnar side of the intact radial metadiaphysis. The adequacy of articular reduction can be visualized directly from the dorsal arthrotomy, indirectly by evaluating the reduction of the radial and intermediate columns via the volar approach, or with fluoroscopy. Once the adequacy of reduction has been confirmed, the radial column can be definitively stabilized with an additional antirotation K-wire or an F-S implant (▶ Fig. 14.12).

14.3.8 Finishing Steps

Once all fragments are reduced and fixated, and the stability of the ulnar column has been confirmed, the wounds are then copiously irrigated with sterile saline. With the tourniquet still inflated, the dorsal capsule from the arthrotomy is closed with nonabsorbable

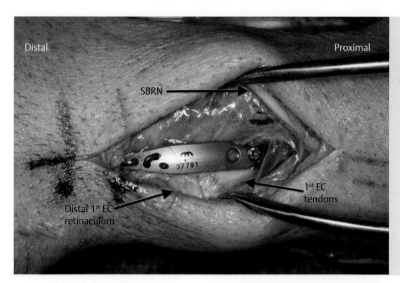

Fig. 14.11 Direct radial approach to the radial column fragment. The distal one-half of the first extensor compartment (EC) retinaculum is left intact, while the proximal one-half is divided to accommodate plate passage onto the radius. Note the superficial branch of the radial nerve (SBRN) which is in the surgical field.

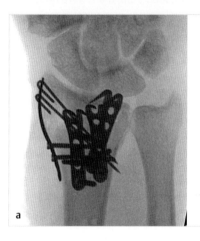
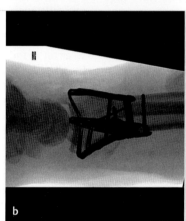

Fig. 14.12 Radial column stabilization with a fragment-specific implant. Posteroanterior **(a)** and lateral **(b)** fluoroscopic images after fragment-specific fixation of the radial column fragment to the reconstructed intermediate column.

2–0 sutures followed by repair of the extensor retinaculum with the extensor pollicis longus (EPL) left transposed dorsal to the retinaculum to assist with retinacular closure and to prevent attritional injury with in the extensor compartment.

Prior to deflation of the tourniquet, temporary sutures/ staples holding the dorsal and volar skin incision are placed if preoperative swelling and edema was a concern. The tourniquet is deflated and hemostasis obtained followed by closure of the radial incision with interrupted horizontal mattress sutures with a 4–0 nonabsorbable, monofilament suture. The dorsal incision is addressed next. A dorsal drain is placed if necessary. Finally the volar wound is closed. A well-padded, sugar tong splint is applied in neutral forearm rotation to immobilize the wrist and DRUJ. If laxity was noted in the DRUJ, the forearm can be splinted to 45° of supination. Elevation of the operative extremity commences as soon as possible with initiation of hand range of motion immediately postoperative.

14.4 Results for Multiplanar Plate Fixation with Fragment-Specific Implants

14.4.1 Functional Outcomes

Satisfactory wrist range of motion and patient reported functional outcome can be attained after F-S fixation for complex distal radius fractures.[13,24,27] Konrath and Bahler noted mean wrist palmar flexion of 54°, dorsiflexion of 61°, radial deviation of 18°, ulnar deviation of 25°, and mean grip strength of 83% of the uninjured contralateral side after F-S fixation for AO type A (n = 4), type B (n = 4), and type C (n = 19) fractures.[13] At a mean follow-up of 29 months (range: 24–36 months), the mean Disabilities of the Arm, Shoulder, and Hand (DASH) was 17 and the mean Patient-Rated Wrist Evaluation (PRWE) score was 19. Similarly, Benson et al reported on 85 intra-articular distal radius fractures, AO type B (n = 9) and type C

(n = 76), which were reconstructed with a dedicated F-S fixation system (TriMed Inc., Valencia, California, United States).[24] At a mean clinical follow-up of 32 months, the mean DASH score was 9 with wrist flexion, wrist extension, and grip strength at 85, 91, and 92% compared to the uninjured wrist, respectively. In addition, Saw et al observed a mean PRWE score of 20 (range: 2–68) in 21 intra-articular fractures, AO type C2 (n = 10) and type C3 (n = 12), at a mean follow-up of 10 months (range: 6–25 months).[27]

14.4.2 Radiographic Outcomes

Multiplanar, F-S fixation of multifragmentary distal radius fractures results in satisfactory radiographic outcomes despite early rehabilitation.[13,14,28] Konrath and Bahler initially reported their results in 27 distal radius fractures, 23 intra-articular and 4 extra-articular, that were reconstructed with an F-S fixation system.[13] All fractures were noted to achieve radiographic union by 6 weeks with 96% of fractures (24 of 25) maintaining 0° or greater of volar tilt without evidence of loss of reduction between initial postoperative and final follow-up radiographs. Similarly, Gavaskar et al performed a prospective study in 105 distal radius fractures, consisting of AO type C1 (n = 41), type C2 (n = 31), and type C3 (n = 33) fractures, reconstructed with an F-S fixation system (2.4-mm locking distal radius system, Synthes, India).[28] They noted radiographic union in all patients without interval fracture displacement between immediate to final postoperative radiographs at 1 year. Anatomic reconstruction of the articular surface was achieved in 74 patients (71%).

14.4.3 Complications

The use of F-S fixation in the management of complex distal radius fractures can result in some minor and major complications.[13,27,29,30] Galle et al reported on 61 patients who underwent VLP with radial column plating (RCP, n = 55), dorsal locking plate fixation and RCP (n = 3), or RCP alone (n = 3) for AO type A (5, 8%), type B (13, 21%), and type C (43, 71%) fractures.[29] Although the authors noted no cases of tendon attritional wear or rupture, 28% (n = 17) of patients required RCP removal secondary to symptomatic hardware. Konrath and Bahler noted numbness in the distribution of the SBRN in 8 of 27 wrists after F-S fixation that completely resolved by 3 months in seven patients and persisted in one patient.[13] Symptomatic hardware removal was necessary in three patients; two of these were due to the F-S implant being placed too close to the DRUJ. In parallel, Saw et al reported transient median nerve paresthesias in four patients that resolved within 1 week and two patients that required symptomatic hardware removal.[27] Lastly, Landgren et al noted more complications with F-S (n = 13) compared to VLP (n = 5),

which included transient SBRN neuritis (n = 6), median nerve neuropathy (n = 2), complex regional pain syndrome, radial-sided implant loosening, tendinitis, skin adherence, and EPL rupture requiring tendon transfer (n = 1 each).[30]

14.4.4 Comparison of Fragment-Specific to Volar Locking Plate Fixation

The benefits of F-S fixation are best appreciated in the reconstruction of complex, multifragmentary distal radius fractures not amenable to VLP fixation. Landgren et al compared the patient-reported, clinical, and radiographic outcomes of 49 distal radius fractures, with equal distribution of AO type A and type C fractures, that were randomized to VLP (n = 24) or F-S fixation (n = 25).[30] At 12-month follow-up, there were no significant differences in grip strength, wrist range of motion, or quick DASH scores between the two groups. Conversely, Sammer et al noted significantly worse correction of volar tilt in the F-S fixation (n = 14) group compared to the VLP (n = 85) group with a mean value of –10° versus 10°, respectively.[31] Additionally, grip strength, lateral pinch, ulnar deviation, and wrist flexion–extension arc were significantly better in the VLP group at 6-month postoperative, which continued to be significantly different at 12 months for wrist flexion–extension, forearm pronation, and supination. However, the authors stated that F-S fixation was preferentially performed to treat comminuted intra-articular AO type C fractures (n = 11 or 79% for F-S vs. n = 39 or 46% for VLP).

14.5 Pitfalls and Contraindications

Although F-S fixation is a powerful tool that can be utilized to reconstruct highly comminuted distal radius fractures, there are pitfalls associated with this technique. Due to the fact that F-S fixation is utilized to stabilize small fracture fragments, these fragments can further displace during implant insertion or even fracture. Thus, fragments should be at least 7 mm wide, 5 mm long, and 4 mm in the dorsal to volar dimension to avoid iatrogenic comminution or fragmentation with subsequent loss of fixation (▶ Fig. 14.13).[23] Additionally, there is a steep learning curve in understanding the functional anatomy of the distal radius and considerable experience is needed to apply F-S implants into the reconstructive efforts of complex distal radius fractures.[27] Contraindications to F-S fixation include fractures associated with severe osteoporosis, segmental bone loss in the metadiaphyseal region, or in cases of marked comminution not amenable to any form of direct fixation.[2]

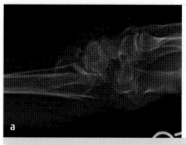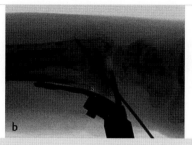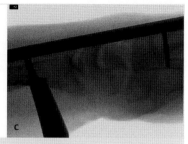

Fig. 14.13 Iatrogenic fragmentation of a small volar rim fragment with fragment-specific fixation. Injury posteroanterior radiographs of a highly comminuted distal radius fracture **(a)**. Fragment-specific fixation of a small volar rim fragment was attempted that resulted in comminution of the fragment **(b)**, thus requiring salvage to a dorsal spanning plate fixation **(c)**.

Tips and Tricks

- Prior to the first case, know the implants and the surgical techniques.
- Start with easier cases to get experience with various approaches and implants.
- Know all surgical approaches and pertinent surgical anatomy.
- Understand the sequence of column and fragment reconstruction:
  - Intermediate column:
    - Volar rim.
    - Dorsal ulnar corner.
    - Free intra-articular.
    - Dorsal wall.
  - Radial column/styloid.
  - Ulnar column.
- Plan surgical exposures prior to first incision.
- Use bone graft to maintain reduction after disimpaction of free intra-articular fragments.
- Judiciously place multiple plates with careful forethought of final implant positioning and construct.
- Keep tourniquet time under 2 hours.
- Meticulous dissection and elevation of skin flaps to minimize wound healing issues with multiple incision approaches.
- Some complex intra-articular fractures are not amenable to VLP or F-S fixation; thus, be prepared to perform distraction bridge plate or external fixation if required.

14.6 Conclusion

Surgical management of multifragmentary distal radius fractures can present many challenges, particularly when all unstable fracture fragments cannot be effectively stabilized with one implant, technique, or approach. Understanding the functional anatomy of common fracture fragments that compose the intermediate and radial columns in distal radius fractures can be beneficial in preoperative planning and intraoperative decision making to reconstruct highly comminuted distal radius fractures in a step-wise approach. Successful surgical management of complex distal radius fractures requires versatility in surgical approaches and techniques, particularly the implementation of multiplanar fixation with F-S implants alone or as adjuncts to VLP fixation.

References

[1] Schneppendahl J, Windolf J, Kaufmann RA. Distal radius fractures: current concepts. J Hand Surg Am 2012;37(8):1718–1725

[2] Rhee PC, Medoff RJ, Shin AY. Complex distal radius fractures: an anatomic algorithm for surgical management. J Am Acad Orthop Surg 2017;25(2):77–88

[3] Medoff RJ. Essential radiographic evaluation for distal radius fractures. Hand Clin 2005;21(3):279–288

[4] Teunis T, Bosma NH, Lubberts B, Ter Meulen DP, Ring D. Melone's concept revisited: 3D quantification of fragment displacement. J Hand Microsurg 2016;8(1):27–33

[5] Zumstein MA, Hasan AP, McGuire DT, Eng K, Bain GI. Distal radius attachments of the radiocarpal ligaments: an anatomical study. J Wrist Surg 2013;2(4):346–350

[6] Melone CP Jr. Articular fractures of the distal radius. Orthop Clin North Am 1984;15(2):217–236

[7] Rikli DA, Regazzoni P. Fractures of the distal end of the radius treated by internal fixation and early function. A preliminary report of 20 cases. J Bone Joint Surg Br 1996;78(4):588–592

[8] Mandziak DG, Watts AC, Bain GI. Ligament contribution to patterns of articular fractures of the distal radius. J Hand Surg Am 2011;36(10):1621–1625

[9] Bain GI, Alexander JJ, Eng K, Durrant A, Zumstein MA. Ligament origins are preserved in distal radial intraarticular two-part fractures: a computed tomography-based study. J Wrist Surg 2013;2(3):255–262

[10] Harness NG. Fixation options for the volar lunate facet fracture: thinking outside the box. J Wrist Surg 2016;5(1):9–16

[11] Beck JD, Harness NG, Spencer HT. Volar plate fixation failure for volar shearing distal radius fractures with small lunate facet fragments. J Hand Surg Am 2014;39(4):670–678

[12] Harness NG, Jupiter JB, Orbay JL, Raskin KB, Fernandez DL. Loss of fixation of the volar lunate facet fragment in fractures of the distal part of the radius. J Bone Joint Surg Am 2004;86-A(9):1900–1908

[13] Konrath GA, Bahler S. Open reduction and internal fixation of unstable distal radius fractures: results using the trimed fixation system. J Orthop Trauma 2002;16(8):578–585

[14] Gerostathopoulos N, Kalliakmanis A, Fandridis E, Georgoulis S. Trimed fixation system for displaced fractures of the distal radius. J Trauma 2007;62(4):913–918

[15] Dodds SD, Cornelissen S, Jossan S, Wolfe SW. A biomechanical comparison of fragment-specific fixation and augmented external fixation for intra-articular distal radius fractures. J Hand Surg Am 2002;27(6):953–964

[16] Taylor KF, Parks BG, Segalman KA. Biomechanical stability of a fixed-angle volar plate versus fragment-specific fixation system: cyclic testing in a C2-type distal radius cadaver fracture model. J Hand Surg Am 2006;31(3):373–381

[17] Taylor GI. The angiosomes of the body and their supply to perforator flaps. Clin Plast Surg 2003;30(3):331–342

[18] Inoue Y, Taylor GI. The angiosomes of the forearm: anatomic study and clinical implications. Plast Reconstr Surg 1996;98(2):195–210

[19] Tordjman D, Hinds RM, Ayalon O, Yang SS, Capo JT. Volar-ulnar approach for fixation of the volar lunate facet fragment in distal radius fractures: a technical tip. J Hand Surg Am 2016;41(12):e491–e500

[20] Moore AM, Dennison DG. Distal radius fractures and the volar lunate facet fragment: Kirschner wire fixation in addition to volar-locked plating. Hand (N Y) 2014;9(2):230–236

[21] Rhee PC, Shin AY. Management of complex distal radius fractures: review of treatment principles and select surgical techniques. J Hand Surg Asian Pac Vol 2016;21(2):140–154

[22] O'Shaughnessy MA, Shin AY, Kakar S. Volar marginal rim fracture fixation with volar fragment-specific hook plate fixation. J Hand Surg Am 2015;40(8):1563–1570

[23] O'Shaughnessy MA, Shin AY, Kakar S. Stabilization of volar ulnar rim fractures of the distal radius: current techniques and review of the literature. J Wrist Surg 2016;5(2):113–119

[24] Benson LS, Minihane KP, Stern LD, Eller E, Seshadri R. The outcome of intra-articular distal radius fractures treated with fragment-specific fixation. J Hand Surg Am 2006;31(8):1333–1339

[25] Thiart M, Ikram A, Lamberts RP. How well can step-off and gap distances be reduced when treating intra-articular distal radius fractures with fragment specific fixation when using fluoroscopy. Orthop Traumatol Surg Res 2016;102(8):1001–1004

[26] Berger RA, Bishop AT, Bettinger PC. New dorsal capsulotomy for the surgical exposure of the wrist. Ann Plast Surg 1995;35(1):54–59

[27] Saw N, Roberts C, Cutbush K, Hodder M, Couzens G, Ross M. Early experience with the TriMed fragment-specific fracture fixation system in intraarticular distal radius fractures. J Hand Surg Eur Vol 2008;33(1):53–58

[28] Gavaskar AS, Muthukumar S, Chowdary N. Fragment-specific fixation for complex intra-articular fractures of the distal radius: results of a prospective single-centre trial. J Hand Surg Eur Vol 2012;37(8):765–771

[29] Galle SE, Harness NG, Hacquebord JH, Burchette RJ, Peterson B. Complications of radial column plating of the distal radius. Hand (N Y) 2018

[30] Landgren M, Abramo A, Geijer M, Kopylov P, Tägil M. Fragment-specific fixation versus volar locking plates in primarily nonreducible or secondarily redisplaced distal radius fractures: a randomized controlled study. J Hand Surg Am 2017;42(3):156–165.e1

[31] Sammer DM, Fuller DS, Kim HM, Chung KC. A comparative study of fragment-specific versus volar plate fixation of distal radius fractures. Plast Reconstr Surg 2008;122(5):1441–1450

15 Management of Wrist Open Fractures and Bone Defects

Rames Mattar Junior, Emygdio Jose Leomil de Paula, Luciano Ruiz Torres, Tiago Guedes da Motta Mattar, Gustavo Bersani Silva

Abstract

Open fractures remain challenging due to the combination of bone and soft tissue injuries as the result of high energy trauma. Contamination and tissue damage predispose to a higher risk of infection. Principles of treatment include prompt diagnosis, debridement, skeletal stabilization with reduction and fixation of fractures, soft tissue repair or reconstruction, and frequent treatment of segmental bone loss. Damage control using an external fixation device is usually indicated in more complex settings. Early treatment of soft tissue (muscles, tendons, peripheral nerves) and bone lesions provides the best functional results. The treatment of osteoarticular injuries involves fracture reduction and stabilization, ligament repair, and treatment of segmental bone loss, either by conventional or vascularized bone grafts. Injuries of tendons, muscles, and peripheral nerves should be treated primarily or as early as possible. If necessary, arteries and veins should be mended. Soft tissue repair or reconstruction is essential for satisfactory outcome. Local, pedicle, or free flaps should be performed to promote coverage as early as possible, and preferably within the first 72 hours posttrauma. Gustilo and Anderson classified open fractures in three types: I, II, and III. Antibiotic prophylaxis should be recommended for Gustilo type III open fractures of the hand and wrist (first-generation cephalosporins). Situations that contraindicate reconstructive procedures are rare and usually related to the patient's clinical condition. Early specialized treatment carried out by skilled hand surgeons significantly improves outcomes, with decreased infection rates, shorter hospitalization time, and better functional and aesthetic results.

Keywords: wrist open fractures, skeletal stabilization, tendon repair, nerve repair, bone reconstruction, local flaps, free flaps

15.1 Introduction

Management of open fractures remains a challenge due to the combination of bone and soft tissue injuries in different magnitudes. Contamination and tissue damage predispose to a higher risk of infection. About 25% of polytrauma patients have injuries to the wrist and hand.[1] According to Schädel-Höpfner and Siebert,[1] and Ciclamini et al,[2] uncomplicated hand or wrist fractures are the most common form of injury (2–16%), followed by soft tissue lesions (2–11%). Severe combined lesions and amputations are rare (0.2–3%). These lesions have a large incidence in young individuals (between 20 and 40 years of age), with increased incidence of hand trauma due to motorcycle accidents.[2] In polytraumatized patients, it is frequent that injuries to the wrist or hand go unnoticed or are underdiagnosed.[2]

Orthopaedic approach must be based on the advanced trauma life support protocol,[3] with immediate attention to restore airway, breathing, and circulation. Similarly, orthopaedic, trauma, and hand surgeons should consider each patient and his/her clinical situation as unique and plan treatment based on individualized evaluation. High-energy injury induces local and systemic release of proinflammatory cytokines, which often results in a systemic inflammatory response syndrome.[4,5]

Procedures for damage control are based on minimizing surgical trauma in a critical period for the patient, reducing surgical time, blood loss, and tissue damage. For damage control in more severe patients, fractures should be stabilized with external fixators.[6] In open fractures, the mechanism and energy of trauma must always be considered. Meticulous clinical examination is critical and challenging in the unconscious patient. Image exams should be performed in the emergency room. Life-threatening injuries should be a priority, and the multidisciplinary care team should define the timing and approach of open fractures according to the following principles: preserve life, preserve tissue, and preserve and restore function.[7]

The principles of local treatment include irrigation, debridement, soft tissue repair or reconstruction, skeletal stabilization with reduction and fixation of fractures, and treatment of segmental bone loss. Early and adequate debridement decreases contamination and risk of infection. Very few structures in the hand and wrist can be debrided and sacrificed without predictable functional impairment; therefore, the surgeon must decide between how much to debride and preserve according to each situation.

Primary and early repair or reconstruction of soft tissue (muscles, tendons, peripheral nerves) provides the best functional results. Small bone segmental loss (less than 6 cm) in well-vascularized recipient beds can be treated with conventional bone graft. Large segmental losses (more than 10 cm) and hypovascular recipient areas are best treated with vascularized bone graft.

There is no consensus on how to define and classify open fractures of the hand and wrist. From the clinical point of view, it is possible to consider that open fractures of the wrist or hand have similar behaviors because of the similar anatomy. Gustilo and Anderson[8] published the most commonly used classification for open fractures. This classification is based mainly on the size and contamination of the wound:

- Type I: wound less than 1 cm, little soft tissue damage with no crushing. Type I fractures usually occur by mechanism from the inside to outside, when a misaligned bone fragment pierces the skin.
- Type II: wound more than 1 cm in length, slight or moderate crushing injury, moderate fracture

fragmentation and moderate contamination. There is no extensive soft tissue damage.

- Type III: wound with extensive soft tissue damage with a high degree of contamination and caused by high-energy trauma. There is a severe bone fragmentation and instability. There are three subtypes:
  - III-A: soft tissue preserved despite extensive laceration.
  - III-B: loss of soft tissue. After surgical irrigation and debridement, there is an exposed bony segment, which imposes the need for a flap (cutaneous, muscular, or muscle-cutaneous).
  - III-C: open fracture associated with arterial laceration. Arterial repair is necessary regardless of the degree of soft tissue injury.

Swanson et al[9] classified open fractures of the hand based on wound size, degree of contamination, and host factors. The authors recommended fracture stabilization based on fracture classification or instability, and primary wound closure for type I and delayed for type II:

- Type I: clean wound and no systemic factors.
- Type II: contaminated wound, delay in treatment greater than 24 hours, or significant systemic illness.

McLain et al[10] and Duncan et al[11] modified the classification by Gustilo and Anderson[8] for open hand fractures. McLain et al[10] classification:

- Type I: laceration less than 1 cm, no signs of contamination, crush or fracture fragmentation.
- Type II: laceration greater than 1 cm, no contamination, crush or fracture fragmentation.
- Type III: laceration greater than 10 cm, contamination, crush, comminuted/segmental fractures, blast injuries, and all farm injuries.

Duncan et al[11] classification: the philosophy of this classification was to downscale the wound size of Gustilo–Anderson classification to apply to the open fractures of the hand:

- Type I: clean laceration less than 1 cm (puncture wound), no crush or tissue loss.
- Type II: clean laceration from outside less than 2 cm, no crush or tissue loss.
- Type III-A: laceration greater than 2 cm, soiled wound, and penetrating or puncturing projectile wound.
- Type III-B: III-A with periosteal elevation or stripping.
- Type III-C: III-B with neurovascular injury.

Duncan et al[11] showed an infection rate of 3.5% in Gustilo–Anderson type III hand open fractures. Capo et al[12] showed a 1.4% infection rate, even in a series with a high proportion (91 out of 145) of Gustilo–Anderson type III open fractures of the hand. Saint-Cyr and Gupta[13] found a 0% infection rate with the use of bone grafting to treat more severe open fractures of the hand. A retrospective review from Bannasch et al[14] found no significant difference in infection rates between the open (133 fractures) and closed (299 fractures) hand fractures. Ketonis et al,[15] in a systematic review, found that the infection rate after open hand fracture remains relatively low. Timing of debridement has not been shown to alter infection rates and the majority of infections can be treated with antibiotics alone. We believe that open fractures of the wrist behave similarly to those of the hand.

On the other hand, in many countries, over 50% of open fractures of the wrist are caused by motorcycle or motor vehicle accidents with high level of dissipated energy resulting in severe injury to bone and soft tissues.[16] There is a loss of periosteal and intramedullary blood supply to the fractured bone. That could result in tissue necrosis, both from direct trauma and from secondary ischemia. The association of avascular bone, soft tissue damage, and contamination makes some open fractures of the wrist region a challenging treatment. Open fractures imply that wrist bones and soft tissue have been exposed to a nonsterile environment. Injuries with large skin defects or soft tissue losses can have gross wound contamination with high pathogen titers and foreign bodies. In the initial treatment of these skeletal injuries, aggressive infection control and wound management often take precedence over definitive fracture fixation. Local or systemic damage control using an external fixation device is usually indicated in more complex and severe situations.

Following a violent injury, soft tissue necrosis and contamination cause an inflammatory response composed of immune cells along with a host of molecular mediators which collectively increase soft tissue permeability and promote phagocytosis. Contaminated hematomas dissect along affected tissue, resulting in dead spaces, becoming an ideal culture medium for bacterial growth.[16]

Gram-positive bacteria *Staphylococcus* and *Streptococcus* are the most frequent infectious agents in the hand and wrist open fractures.[17] Infections acquired at the hospital often involve *Staphylococcus* and gram-negative bacteria (*Pseudomonas*, *Klebsiella*, *Acinetobacter*).[17] Wounds contaminated by soil are usually infected with gram-negative and anaerobic bacterias.[17] Infections acquired in the aquatic environment often involve *Aeromonas*, *Pseudomonas*, and *Mycobacterium*.[18] Wounds contaminated with saliva (human bites) can be infected by *Eikenella corrodens* and anaerobic bacteria.[19] Animal bites can cause mixed infections, with both aerobic and anaerobic bacterias.[20,21] Cat and dog bites can cause infections associated with *Pasteurella multocida*.[20,21,22] The presence of devitalized and necrotic tissue is related to the development of clostridial gas gangrene.[23]

Empirical antibiotic therapy should be initiated as soon as possible based on the probable infectious agent and according to the nature of wound contamination until the final culture and sensitivity tests are conclusive. Intravenous antibiotics should be given before, during, and for at least 5 days after surgery. Antibiotic coverage must remaining while the wound is still open (primary closure types I and II, delayed type III).[23]

Nylén and Carlsson correlate the delay in treatment with increased risk for infection.[24] Swanson et al[9] relate a higher incidence of infection in open fractures of the hand to the presence of wound contamination, systemic illness (malnutrition, diabetes, renal or hepatic failure, malignancy, immune deficiency, drug, alcohol, or tobacco abuse) and delay in treatment greater than 24 hours.

We do not have specific data on the importance of using antibiotics in wrist open fractures. Therefore, we use the same principles of open fracture management, but add some specific concepts for hand open fractures. Some publications report the importance of antibiotic therapy in hand injuries. Sloan et al[25] indicated prophylactic antibiotic therapy to reduce the risk of infection in open fractures of the distal phalanx. However, Peacock et al[26] considered that antibiotic prophylaxis is not necessary in open wounds of the hand with moderate contamination and adequate debridement. Similarly, Suprock et al[27] showed no benefit of prophylactic antibiotic therapy in open fractures of fingers after irrigation and debridement. Other authors emphasize the need for debridement in the management of an open fracture and that antibiotics are not a substitute for surgical debridement.[28,29] Antibiotic prophylaxis should be recommended for Gustilo type III open fractures of the hand and wrist.[30] It is our opinion that wounds with minimal contamination can be treated with first-generation cephalosporins. Aminoglycosides should be used in more contaminated wounds.[5] In anaerobic infections, penicillin is the drug of choice. Prophylactic antibiotics should be used for no longer than 48 to 72 hours.[25] In the management of complex open hand and wrist trauma, there seems to be little benefit in extending antibiotic treatment beyond 5 days if there is no clinical sign of infection.[23,25]

15.2 Indications

Wrist open fractures usually occur from high-energy trauma. The primary or early treatment of all lesions provides the best functional results. The treatment of these lesions is an emergency and should be carried out mainly in reference centers with trained staff. Irrigation and debridement should be carried out properly and as early as possible. The treatment of osteoarticular injuries involves fracture reduction and stabilization, ligament repair, and treatment of segmental bone loss, either by conventional or vascularized bone grafts. Injuries of tendons, muscles, and peripheral nerves should be treated primarily or as early as possible. If necessary, arteries and veins should be mended. Soft tissue repair and reconstruction of the bone envelope are essential for satisfactory outcome. Local, pedicle, or free flaps should be performed to promote coverage as early as possible, and preferably within the first 72 hours posttrauma.

15.3 Surgical Technique

15.3.1 Fracture Management

Anatomical reduction with rigid fixation of fractures promotes bony union and allows early mobilization and the best functional result.

Gustilo type I injuries have a very low infection rate comparable with closed fractures.[8,16] The choice of fixation method and tactic depends on the fracture pattern. Most often, class I open fractures with little fragmentation, clean wound, and well-vascularized soft tissues are treated by reduction and definitive fixation with plates and screws.

Gustilo type II open fractures have a higher rate of infection with an increased degree of bony fragmentation and soft tissue injury (►Fig. 15.1a–h). For patients who present dirtier wounds and greater compromise of tissue viability,

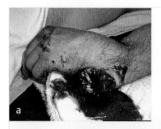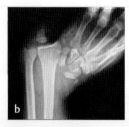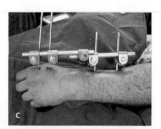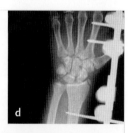
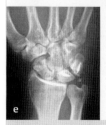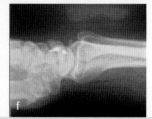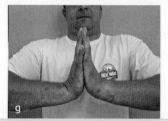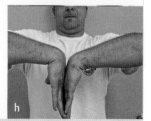

Fig. 15.1 Open dorsal transstyloid perilunate fracture dislocation of left wrist. **(a, b)** Clinical and radiographic appearance. **(c, d)** After debridement, reduction, and temporary stabilization. **(e–h)** Radiographic and clinical aspect after 6 years of follow-up.

the treatment should be based on immediate irrigation and debridement with stabilization with an external fixation or spanning plate, followed by wound closure and definitive internal fixation some days after injury depending on the clinical evolution of the wound. If it is considered clean, it is possible to perform internal fixation of the fracture and even use bone graft if necessary.[12,14,31,32] In polytraumatized patients with systemic impairment, a damage control protocol must be adopted, and fractures should be stabilized with an external fixator.[6]

In type III fractures, treatment principles are roughly the same as type II fractures. Of note is the necessity to repair associated arterial lesions in type IIIC, step that should be undertaken right after debridement and judicious osseous stabilization. Fasciotomy can also be employed in selected cases in which vascular repair was somewhat delayed. Also depending on the extension of the soft tissue lesion, coverage should be performed at the same time of the vascular reconstruction.

15.3.2 Soft Tissue Repair

Soft tissue lesions represent a very complex challenge for the hand surgeon. Soft tissue repair should follow the ladder of complexity, including wound suture (after debridement), skin grafting (appropriate receptor bed), local flaps (preserved local anatomy), and free flaps. The complexity of soft tissue reconstruction after a devastating trauma often requires major surgical procedures that cannot be performed early in a polytraumatized unstable or borderline patient. The first step in any major reconstructive effort is initial adequate debridement and skeletal reduction. The complete removal of all necrotic tissue and wound irrigation to remove debris and reduce bacterial colonization prevents infection. All other major reconstructive procedures should be postponed and performed as early as possible, depending on the patient's clinical course and local wound conditions.[33] In such cases, after an adequate debridement the vacuum-assisted closure therapy system has become an important temporary tool that offers a "bridge" until definitive surgery can be performed safely.[34]

In more complex cases with loss of skin and bone exposure, the choice of flap will depend on the preservation of the local anatomy, the possibility of local flaps (minor cutaneous losses), and the viability of the vascular pedicles for microanastomoses (free flaps) (▶ Fig. 15.2a–e). These choices depend on the patient's condition and the experience of the surgical team. We prefer to use pedicled or free cutaneous flaps since in most cases there is no dead space in this region and these flaps allow secondary procedures to be performed more adequately. It is our opinion that muscular or musculocutaneous flaps leave the region bulkier and create less

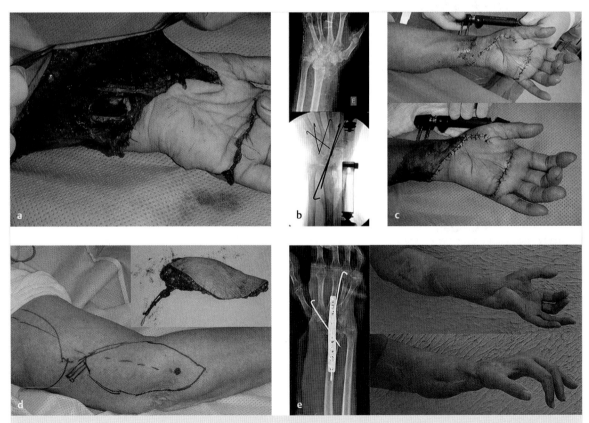

Fig. 15.2 Open fracture of the distal extremity of the radius and ulna. (a, b) Clinical and radiographic appearance. (c) Immediate postoperative result after debridement, reduction, and temporary stabilization (above). Skin necrosis at day 7 (below). (d) Lateral arm flap planned to cover the soft tissue defect. (e) Radiographic and clinical appearance at 8 years of follow-up.

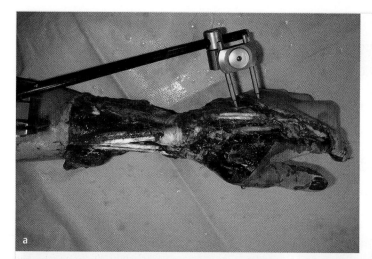
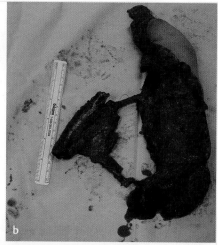
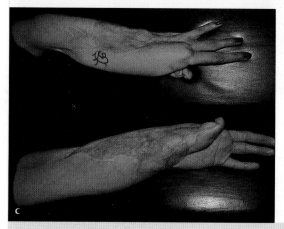
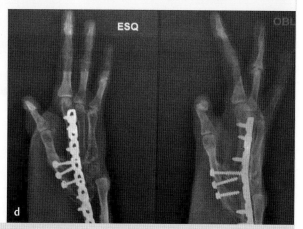

Fig. 15.3 A 20-year-old female presented with mangling lesion to her left upper extremity. **(a)** Gustilo IIIB open fracture of the distal radius with carpal and metacarpal bone loss. **(b)** Chimeric osteomyocutaneous flap (free latissimus dorsi myocutaneous flap connected at the back table to rib osseous flap, both harvested from the same donor site, which was closed primarily). **(c)** Patient at late follow-up. **(d)** Final radiographic appearance. Wrist and thumb arthrodesis were possible following microsurgical bone reconstruction.

adequate sliding planes than cutaneous flaps. Regarding the pedicled flaps, the most commonly used options are the radial forearm flap (using the main vessels or perforating branches), the dorsoulnar flap, and the posterior interosseous artery flap. As for the free flaps, there are many options, but we prefer the lateral arm flap for minor cutaneous losses and the anterolateral thigh flap for greater defects. When there are composite losses (e.g., bone and soft tissue), chimeric flaps can be used. In these conditions, osteocutaneous or osteomyocutaneous flaps may be indicated (e.g., osteocutaneous flaps from fibula, iliac, rib, lateral humerus, medial femoral condyle) (▶ Fig. 15.3a–d).

15.3.3 Nerve Injuries

General principles for repairing or reconstructing peripheral nerves should be adopted in the treatment of open fractures with severe upper limb injuries. Definitive treatment may be hindered due to systemic conditions, multiple compromised regions, and difficulties to determine limits of nerve tissue viability. Primary or delayed primary suture under appropriate conditions has proven to be superior to secondary repairs or grafts in animal models and in clinical series.[35] According to damage control principles, stable patients can undergo delayed surgery a few days after the trauma but nerve repair surgery should be performed as fast as possible, preferably within up to 4 days (delayed primary procedure). In some rare situations, due to lesion's severity or poor local conditions, nerve repair should be delayed. However, even in these cases, the earlier the procedure is performed, the better for the patient.

15.3.4 Tendons

Tendon injuries vary in severity and location (tendon, muscle–tendon transition, laceration, avulsion, combined lesions) on the volar and/or dorsal aspect of the forearm, wrist, or hand.[2] Simple inspection of posture of the fingers and clinical tests (tendon tension,

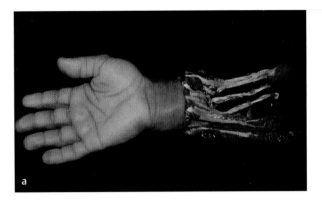
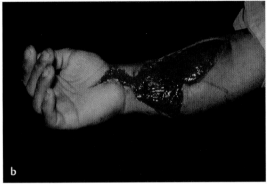
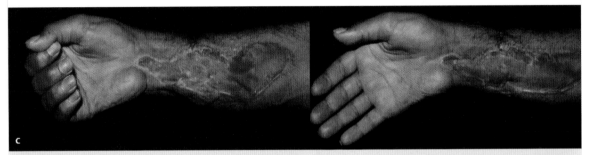

Fig. 15.4 Young male presented with amputation of his dominant hand. **(a)** Avulsion type amputation at midforearm level. **(b)** Early outcome of replantation surgery. Bone, vessels, tendons, and nerves primarily repaired. **(c)** Late follow-up with good functional and aesthetic result. The remaining soft tissue defect was skin-grafted after a few days. Hardware was not exposed; it could be covered with healthy muscle after skeletal shortening. The metal seen in **(b)** is a microvascular clamp.

forearm compression test) are useful for a correct diagnosis.[2,36] Treatment options may include primary repair, delayed primary repair, or secondary repair, depending on associated injuries and the patient's general condition.[37] One-stage reconstruction, when possible, with early primary repair or reconstruction promotes better functional outcomes. A two-stage approach using initial placement of a silicone rod followed by a free tendon graft is the treatment of choice in more complex cases with loss of substance, according to damage control protocol principles.[38,39]

15.3.5 Amputations and Devascularizations

Trauma can result in complete amputation or devascularization at forearm, wrist, hand, or fingers level. At the initial clinical examination, the state of the perfusion of the extremities should be carefully analyzed. Finger color, turgor, and temperature are usually sufficient to determine the perfusion status. In patients with hypotension or hypovolemic shock, Doppler may better access vascular integrity. The ideal candidates for replantation or revascularization are hemodynamically stable patients who sustained a sharp lesion with only minimal contamination. Classically, reimplantation or revascularization may be indicated within 6 hours of

warm ischemia or within 12 hours of cold ischemia. For finger reimplantation, a longer period of ischemia can be tolerated.[40] Immediate replantation should be attempted if the clinical condition of the patient is stable (▶ Fig. 15.4a–c). In some special situations, the limb salvage should be emphasized as in patients with bilateral lesions in the upper limbs, severe lesions in the lower limbs, or at risk of paraplegia. In these situations, all efforts should be made for preservation of the upper limb. In some cases, when possible, two teams of surgeons treating separate injury sites may decrease surgical time. Advances in polytraumatized patient clinical care and in anesthesia procedures have enabled earlier and effective clinical stabilization, allowing for a greater number of reconstructive surgeries in the early phase of the treatment to be performed.[41] In amputations or devascularizations, the primary repair of all damaged structures promotes the best functional results.

15.4 Results

Patients with open fractures of the wrist region with different degrees of local and systemic involvement are better treated in tertiary reference trauma centers.

Since 2010, with the establishment in São Paulo (Brazil) of a trauma unit formed by hand surgeons skilled in microsurgical techniques managing high-complexity lesions, we witnessed significant improvement in outcomes, with decreased infection rates, shorter hospitalization time, and better functional and aesthetic results. Our experience emphasizes the importance of adequate treatment in the acute period of trauma, made possible by the existence of a reference center with multidisciplinary care including hand surgeons trained in reconstructive microsurgery.

15.5 Pitfalls

Open fractures in the wrist region should be treated as an emergency and may require sophisticated reconstructive techniques. Multidisciplinary support team and the hand surgeons must be trained to allow the earliest possible treatment obeying damage control protocols. Such requirements reinforce the importance of creating tertiary reference trauma centers strategically distributed to attend the entire population.

Situations that contraindicate reconstructive procedures are rare and usually related to the patient's clinical condition. The decision to abort a replantation or reconstruction surgical plan is always a multidisciplinary decision. Likewise, in the unfavorable outcome after the treatment of an open fracture generating poor functional results, with stiffness, loss of sensation, presence of pain, and/or infection (osteomyelitis), the decision to amputate or indicate other invasive surgical treatments is not always simple and should involve several specialists (hand surgeon, infectious disease specialist, rehabilitation, psychologist).

Tips and Tricks

- After thorough debridement, irrigate the wound profusely.
- Ensure good perfusion of distal segment.
- Stabilize all fractures.
- Inspect and repair vascular, nervous, and tendinous lesions as early as possible.
- Obtain soft tissue coverage, keep in mind that subsequent approaches may be necessary (skin flaps preferred).
- "Second look" after 24 to 48 hours.
- Plan definitive treatment, if early total care not possible.

15.6 Conclusion

Management of wrist open fractures and bone defects is challenging due to the combination of bone and soft tissue injuries in different magnitudes. These fractures should be treated as an emergency and may require sophisticated reconstructive techniques. Contamination and tissue damage predispose to a higher risk of infection. The principles of local treatment include prompt diagnosis, irrigation, debridement, skeletal stabilization with reduction and fixation of fractures, soft tissue repair or reconstruction, and treatment of segmental bone loss. Damage control using an external fixation device is usually indicated in more complex settings. Situations that contraindicate reconstructive procedures are rare and usually related to the patient's clinical condition. Early specialized treatment carried out by skilled hand surgeons significantly improves outcomes, with decreased infection rates, shorter hospitalization time, and better functional and aesthetic results.

References

[1] Schädel-Höpfner M, Siebert H. [Operative strategies for hand injuries in multiple trauma. A systematic review of the literature]. Unfallchirurg 2005;108(10):850–857

[2] Ciclamini D, Panero B, Titolo P, Tos P, Battiston B. Particularities of hand and wrist complex injuries in polytrauma management. Injury 2014;45(2):448–451

[3] American College of Surgeons. Advanced Trauma Life Support (ATLS) for Doctors. 7th ed. Chicago, IL: American College of Surgeons; 2004

[4] Hildebrand F, Pape HC, Krettek C. [The importance of cytokines in the posttraumatic inflammatory reaction]. Unfallchirurg 2005;108(10):793–794, 796–803

[5] Giannoudis PV, Mallina R, Harwood P, Perry S, Sante ED, Pape HC. Pattern of release and relationship between HMGB-1 and IL-6 following blunt trauma. Injury 2010;41(12):1323–1327

[6] Giannoudis PV. Surgical priorities in damage control in polytrauma. J Bone Joint Surg Br 2003;85(4):478–483

[7] Green D, Hotchkiss R, Pederson WC. Green's Operative Hand Surgery. 5th ed. Philadelphia, PA: Churchill Livingstone; 2005

[8] Gustilo RB, Anderson JT. Prevention of infection in the treatment of one thousand and twenty-five open fractures of long bones: retrospective and prospective analyses. J Bone Joint Surg Am 1976;58(4):453–458

[9] Swanson TV, Szabo RM, Anderson DD. Open hand fractures: prognosis and classification. J Hand Surg Am 1991;16(1):101–107

[10] McLain RF, Steyers C, Stoddard M. Infections in open fractures of the hand. J Hand Surg Am 1991;16(1):108–112

[11] Duncan RW, Freeland AE, Jabaley ME, Meydrech EF. Open hand fractures: an analysis of the recovery of active motion and of complications. J Hand Surg Am 1993;18(3):387–394

[12] Capo JT, Hall M, Nourbakhsh A, Tan V, Henry P. Initial management of open hand fractures in an emergency department. Am J Orthop 2011;40(12):E243–E248

[13] Saint-Cyr M, Gupta A. Primary internal fixation and bone grafting for open fractures of the hand. Hand Clin 2006;22(3):317–327

[14] Bannasch H, Heermann AK, Iblher N, Momeni A, Schulte-Mönting J, Stark GB. Ten years stable internal fixation of metacarpal and phalangeal hand fractures-risk factor and outcome analysis show no increase of complications in the treatment of open compared with closed fractures. J Trauma 2010;68(3):624–628

[15] Ketonis C, Dwyer J, Ilyas AM. Timing of debridement and infection rates in open fractures of the hand: a systematic review. Hand (N Y) 2017;12(2):119–126

[16] Gustilo RB, Merkow RL, Templeman D. The management of open fractures. J Bone Joint Surg Am 1990;72(2):299–304

[17] Fitzgerald RH Jr, Cooney WP III, Washington JA II, Van Scoy RE, Linscheid RL, Dobyns JH. Bacterial colonization of mutilating hand injuries and its treatment. J Hand Surg Am 1977;2(2):85–89

[18] Sanger JR, Yousif NJ, Matloub HS. Aeromonas hydrophila upper extremity infection. J Hand Surg Am 1989;14(4):719–721

[19] Callaham M. Controversies in antibiotic choices for bite wounds. Ann Emerg Med 1988;17(12):1321–1330

[20] Griego RD, Rosen T, Orengo IF, Wolf JE. Dog, cat, and human bites: a review. J Am Acad Dermatol 1995;33(6):1019–1029

[21] Brook I. Human and animal bite infections. J Fam Pract 1989;28(6):713–718

[22] Arons MS, Fernando L, Polayes IM. Pasteurella multocida--the major cause of hand infections following domestic animal bites. J Hand Surg Am 1982;7(1):47–52

[23] Gonzales MH, Bach HG, Elhassan BT, Graft CN, Weinzweig N. Management of Open fractures. J Am Soc Surg Hand 2003;3(4):208–218

[24] Nylén S, Carlsson B. Time factor, infection frequency and quantitative microbiology in hand injuries: a prospective study. Scand J Plast Reconstr Surg 1980;14(2):185–189

[25] Sloan JP, Dove AF, Maheson M, Cope AN, Welsh KR. Antibiotics in open fractures of the distal phalanx? J Hand Surg [Br] 1987;12(1):123–124

[26] Peacock KC, Hanna DP, Kirkpatrick K, Breidenbach WC, Lister GD, Firrell J. Efficacy of perioperative cefamandole with postoperative cephalexin in the primary outpatient treatment of open wounds of the hand. J Hand Surg Am 1988;13(6):960–964

[27] Suprock MD, Hood JM, Lubahn JD. Role of antibiotics in open fractures of the finger. J Hand Surg Am 1990;15(5):761–764

[28] Cooney WP. The Wrist: Diagnosis and Operative Treatment. 2nd ed. Philadelphia, PA: Lippincott Williams & Wilkins; 2010

[29] Hoffman RD, Adams BD. The role of antibiotics in the management of elective and post-traumatic hand surgery. Hand Clin 1998;14(4):657–666

[30] Patzakis MJ, Wilkins J. Factors influencing infection rate in open fracture wounds. Clin Orthop Relat Res 1989;(243):36–40

[31] Freeland AE, Jabaley ME, Burkhalter WE, Chaves AM. Delayed primary bone grafting in the hand and wrist after traumatic bone loss. J Hand Surg Am 1984;9A(1):22–28

[32] Freeland AE. External fixation for skeletal stabilization of severe open fractures of the hand. Clin Orthop Relat Res 1987;(214):93–100

[33] Roberts CS, Pape HC, Jones AL, Malkani AL, Rodriguez JL, Gionnoudis PV. Damage control orthopaedics. evolving concepts in the treatment of patients who have sustained orthopedic trauma. J Bone Joint Surg Am 2005;87:434–449

[34] Braakenburg A, Obdeijn MC, Feitz R, van Rooij IA, van Griethuysen AJ, Klinkenbijl JH. The clinical efficacy and cost effectiveness of the vacuum-assisted closure technique in the management of acute and chronic wounds: a randomized controlled trial. Plast Reconstr Surg 2006;118(2):390–397, discussion 398–400

[35] Birch R, Raji AR. Repair of median and ulnar nerves. Primary suture is best. J Bone Joint Surg Br 1991;73(1):154–157

[36] Paul JS. Lister's: The Hand: Diagnosis and Indications. 4th ed. Philadelphia, PA: Churchill Livingstone; 2002

[37] Hernandez JD, Stern PJ. Complex injuries including flexor tendon disruption. Hand Clin 2005;21(2):187–197

[38] Strickland JW. Delayed treatment of flexor tendon injuries including grafting. Hand Clin 2005;21(2):219–243

[39] Bakri K, Moran SL. Initial assessment and management of complex forearm defects. Hand Clin 2007;23(2):255–268, vii

[40] Wei FC, Chang YL, Chen HC, Chuang CC. Three successful digital replantations in a patient after 84, 86, and 94 hours of cold ischemia time. Plast Reconstr Surg 1988;82(2):346–350

[41] Sagraves SG, Toschlog EA, Rotondo MF. Damage control surgery—the intensivist's role. J Intensive Care Med 2006;21(1):5–16

16 Radiocarpal Dislocation

Mark Henry

Abstract

Radiocarpal fracture-dislocations are far more common than pure dislocations; both are easily reduced but may then be underappreciated by a subsequent provider. Complete dislocation between the carpus and the radius requires intrasubstance rupture or bony avulsion of all the extrinsic ligaments of the wrist, both volar and dorsal. Incongruent radiocarpal subluxation may occur with subtotal failure of the extrinsic ligaments. Radiocarpal incongruity with extrinsic ligament failure may occur in combination with intrinsic ligament rupture or distal radius fracture. Key elements of the initial assessment include the mechanism of injury, localization of trauma signs on examination, and plain radiographs demonstrating subtle radiocarpal incongruity or small marginal fracture fragments. When appropriate, further assessment may include CT scan (with or without arthrogram) to reveal incongruity, small marginal fragments, or sites of intrasubstance ligament rupture. The most complete and accurate means of assessing wrist trauma is arthroscopy, but in the setting of complete extrinsic rupture, axial distraction force must be minimized. Because the extrinsic ligaments will heal well as long as all skeletal relationships are accurately maintained, most radiocarpal dislocations can be treated entirely arthroscopically. When a bone fragment carrying a critical ligament attachment will not reduce arthroscopically, a limited open approach for direct fixation is appropriate. Fixation consists of radiocarpal pinning combined with pinning or screw fixation of marginal fragments. The radiocarpal pin may be removed by 4 weeks, with 6 weeks total splint or cast immobilization prior to initiating wrist range of motion therapy. Strengthening exercises progress gradually from 8 weeks onward.

Keywords: radiocarpal, extrinsic, ligaments, wrist, dislocation, subluxation, arthroscopy, fixation, pinning, fracture, rupture

16.1 Introduction

Pure radiocarpal dislocations are extremely rare, requiring intrasubstance failure of all wrist extrinsic ligaments, volar and dorsal. Dorsal dislocations are far more common than volar.[1,2,3,4] More common are radiocarpal fracture-dislocations where some of the ligament failures occur through their bony origin on the radius combined with the other extrinsic ligaments experiencing intrasubstance rupture (▶Fig. 16.1).[5,6,7,8,9] The volar extrinsic ligaments are the most important stabilizers resisting translation both dorsally (61% of total restraint) and

volarly (48% of total). The dorsal extrinsic ligaments contribute very little to restraining translation both dorsally (2% of total) and volarly (6% of total).[10] These are high-energy traumas typically associated with high falls, violent sports impact, or vehicular accidents.[6,11] The wrist specialist is usually not the first medical provider to encounter the patient, and the emergency responder will have often reduced the dislocation on site or soon thereafter.[4,12] Consequently, it is possible to underappreciate the gravity of the injury and fail to recognize the major ligament disruption that has actually occurred (▶Fig. 16.2).[13] The greatest risk of missing the extrinsic ligament failure is when it accompanies a more obvious distal radius fracture, carpal fracture (lunate mostcommon),or intercarpal dislocation (▶Fig. 16.3).[5,14,15,16,17] Treatment of the more obvious injury without stabilizing the radiocarpal exact positional relationships may then lead to chronic subluxation, instability, and eventually posttraumatic arthritis (▶Fig. 16.4).[18] The long-term direction of instability and subluxation is typically ulnar translocation for pure ligamentous injuries or combined with volar when associated with unhealed volar marginal fragments (▶Fig. 16.5).[2,14,19,20] All wrist traumas must be thoroughly assessed, proactively seeking evidence of any ligament injury patterns to ensure that the appropriate treatment is rendered.

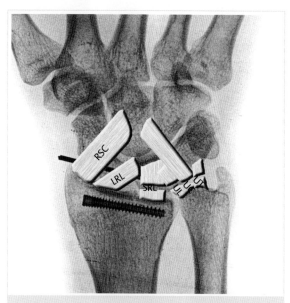

Fig. 16.1 Radiocarpal fracture-dislocations can occur with a larger radial styloid fragment controlling the origins of the radioscaphocapitate (RSC) and long radiolunate (LRL) ligaments with midsubstance rupture of the remaining volar extrinsics: short radiolunate (SRL), ulnolunate (UL), ulnocapitate (UC), and ulnotriquetral (UT).

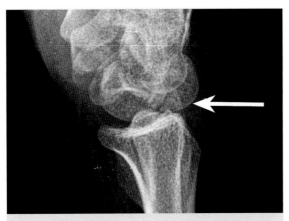

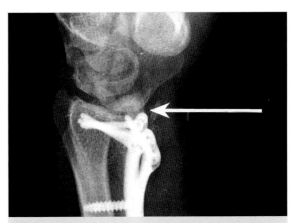

Fig. 16.2 Plain radiographs must be examined carefully to check all congruent relationships. Radiologist read this film as normal, but the proximal scaphoid (*arrow*) can easily be seen displaced over the dorsal rim of the radius in this combined radiocarpal and perilunate dislocation.

Fig. 16.3 Although the most frequently recognized location for small volar fragment displacement leading to carpal subluxation is the volar lip of the lunate fossa, isolated scaphoid subluxation (*arrow*) despite a congruent lunate is also possible.

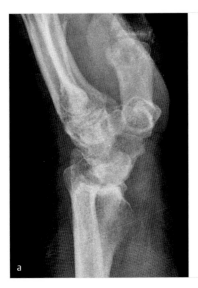

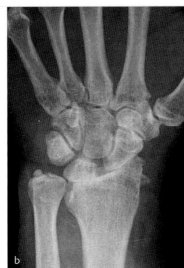

Fig. 16.4 Late sequelae of radiocarpal dislocation without distal radius fracture includes **(a)** volar and ulnar subluxation of the lunate and **(b)** hyaline cartilage loss throughout the radiocarpal interface with preservation of the midcarpal joint in distinct contrast to the pattern seen with scapholunate advanced collapse.

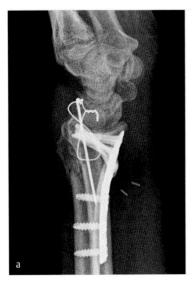

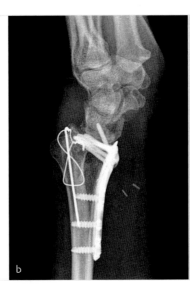

Fig. 16.5 Late avascular necrosis of key volar marginal fragments that appear **(a)** healed at 6 weeks postoperatively can ultimately lead to **(b)** late carpal subluxation when other intrasubstance ruptures of extrinsic ligaments fail to heal well.

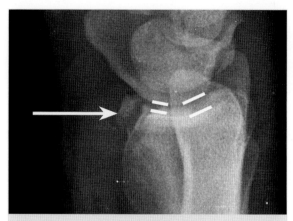

Fig. 16.6 The proximal carpal row is incongruent relative to the distal radius articular surface (*brackets*), having volarly subluxed with the displaced distal radius marginal fragment (*arrow*) representing the extrinsic ligament anchor.

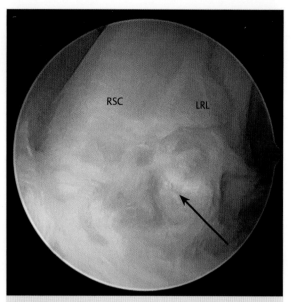

Fig. 16.7 Combined methods of failure exist, most commonly where the radioscaphocapitate (RSC) retains its attachment to a fragment of distal radius but the long radiolunate (LRL) avulses its origin (*arrow*).

16.2 Indications

Radiocarpal dislocations and fracture-dislocations are fundamentally surgical problems; casting alone is insufficient.[21] The indication to act surgically is simply ample evidence from the preoperative assessment that demonstrates the injury pattern.[11] Apart from taking the full history including mechanism of injury and conducting a full examination focusing on local signs of wrist trauma, the surgeon should carefully scrutinize the plain radiographs. In the rare event of a set of films obtained while the wrist is still dislocated, the pathology is clear. Most of the time, the surgeon is viewing postreduction radiographs.[4,13] The specific indications being sought are subtle degrees of incongruence in the radiocarpal relationship and small marginal fragments around the rim of the distal radius (►Fig. 16.6).[14] In a pure dislocation with no fracture fragments, the radiocarpal relationship may appear perfectly congruent. In this event, further investigation is warranted. Local anesthetic injection into the wrist joint can reduce posttraumatic pain, allowing the examiner to perform manual ligament stress testing. Computed tomography (CT) scanning can reveal subtle incongruity or marginal fractures not appreciated on two-dimensional films. Arthrogram contrast may be added to demonstrate sites of complete ligament rupture. The ultimate assessment tool for defining the pattern and extent of wrist trauma is arthroscopy (►Fig. 16.7).[22,23]

16.3 Surgical Technique

Although in the historical literature, surgeons advocated wide open approaches with substantial tissue dissection to reach the deep injury site, there is no benefit gained in doing so.[6,24] Likewise, direct suturing of ligament tissue

(with or without anchors) is an unnecessary action provided that the precise spatial relationships between the radius and carpals are restored and securely fixated during the early healing interval.[9,24,25] Assessment, reduction, and stabilization can all be done arthroscopically, reserving limited open approach for larger bone fragment fixation with screws or plates.[22,23,26]

Each surgeon will have a preferred basic arthroscopy set-up. The ideal working environment allows unobstructed access circumferentially, using light traction to an overhead boom rather than an on-table traction tower. If all extrinsic ligaments are ruptured, longitudinal distraction forces should be minimized to avoid traction injury to nerves (►Fig. 16.8). For a large patient, the 2.3-mm arthroscope is appropriate, whereas the 1.9-mm arthroscope should be used for a smaller patient to avoid iatrogenic injury to hyaline cartilage. Once hematoma and clot have been cleared from the joint, either wet or dry arthroscopy can be used according to surgeon preference, but caution should be exercised in the setting of complete extrinsic ligament rupture to avoid excessive fluid extravasation.[27] Inflow pressure settings should be kept to a minimum or gravity only. Midcarpal arthroscopy (using the midcarpal radial and midcarpal ulnar portals) checks for hyaline cartilage injury, continuation of extrinsic ligament injury more distally, and stress testing of scapholunate and lunotriquetral interosseous intrinsic ligaments to avoid missing associated injuries. Radiocarpal arthroscopy is used to confirm or identify marginal fractures of the radius and guide reduction of articular congruence and fragment approximation

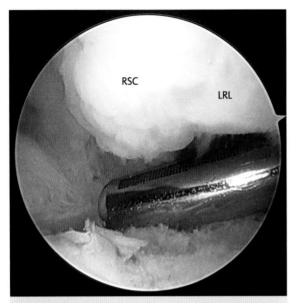

Fig. 16.8 When all volar extrinsics are ruptured, wide separation of the thick robust ligaments will be seen to pull away from the margin of the radius: radioscaphocapitate (RSC), long radiolunate (LRL).

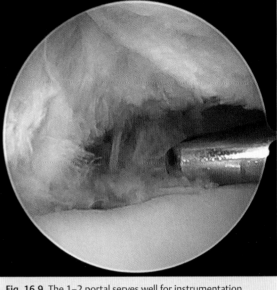

Fig. 16.9 The 1–2 portal serves well for instrumentation used to manipulate marginal fragments and to sweep ruptured ligament tissue out from becoming interposed into the joint.

followed by fixation. Ligament tissue interposed to the joint can be swept out with arthroscopic instruments to avoid the impingement blocking a congruent reduction and to return the ruptured ends to the proper location for subsequent healing (▶Fig. 16.9). Various portals are useful including the standard 3–4 and 4–5 portals, the 1–2 portal, and the flexor carpi radialis (FCR) portal. The standard portals are used for viewing the volar extrinsic ligaments and volar marginal fragments (▶Fig. 16.10). The FCR portal is used for viewing dorsal extrinsic ligaments and dorsal marginal fragments (▶Fig. 16.11). The 1–2 portal is the most useful operative portal for manipulating ligament tissue and reducing marginal fragments during fixation (▶Fig. 16.12). The 1–2 portal can also be used to view dorsal extrinsic ligaments in lieu of the FCR portal.

Most marginal fragments are so small as to only accommodate 0.7- to 1-mm Kirschner wires (K-wires) for fixation, such that even the smallest screws available prove too large. Fracture-dislocations with a larger radial styloid fragment, which carries the origins of the radioscaphocapitate and long radiolunate ligaments, benefit from more robust screw fixation (▶Fig. 16.1).[8,9] When occurring in association with articular distal radius fractures, select cases will have a large enough fragment at the volar margin of the lunate fossa for small plate and screw fixation (▶Fig. 16.13).[7] In the remainder, the limited fixation of small bone fragments is compensated by the fact that the overall maintenance of reduction for the dislocation is not dependent on the small fragments but rather the relationship between the carpals and the radial metaphysis (▶Fig. 16.14). The larger caliber (1.4 mm)

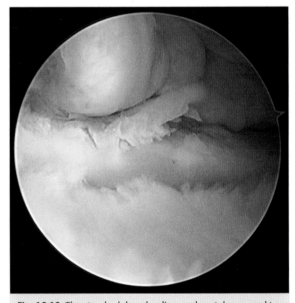

Fig. 16.10 The standard dorsal radiocarpal portals are used to visualize volar marginal radius fragments that carry the origins of the volar extrinsic ligaments.

K-wire placed obliquely from radius to proximal row is responsible for preventing displacement of the reduction and can easily be combined with fixation for associated intrinsic ligament injury (▶Fig. 16.15).

Screw fixation is permanent. K-wires are typically removed by 4 weeks but can be left until 6 weeks as the total time of cast or splint continuous immobilization should be 6 weeks.[3] At that point in time, range of

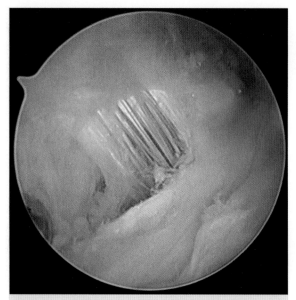

Fig. 16.11 The flexor carpi radialis (FCR) volar portal well visualizes the dorsal extrinsic ligaments, but only after the synovial lining has first been cleared away.

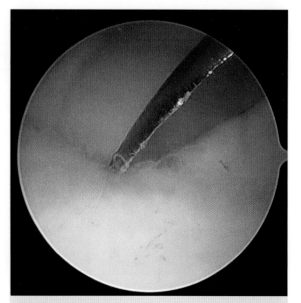

Fig. 16.12 Triangulating the surgical target by viewing from the opposing approach aids in marginal fragment reduction using sharp-tipped angled or curved instruments, typically working via the 1–2 portal.

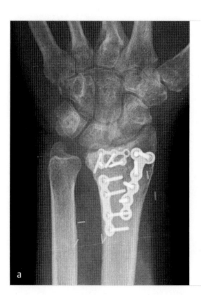

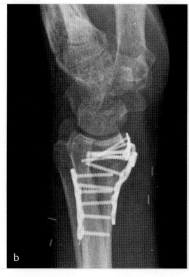

Fig. 16.13 (a, b) When maintenance of a congruent radiocarpal reduction depends on very small fragments distal to the watershed line, unique applications of smaller individual plates are required for sufficient stability.

motion therapy for the wrist begins. Light strengthening commences by 8 weeks, with progression to higher forces thereafter. More vigorous sports and heavy labor are not resumed until after 12 weeks.

16.4 Results

One of the largest series from a wrist specialty practice identified 27 cases (4 volar and 23 dorsal) over a 23-year capture period, attesting to the relative rarity of this injury pattern.[1] The authors classified the injury pattern as type I (pure dislocation or with only a small tip of radial styloid) or type II (singular bone fragment of greater than one-third the width of the radial styloid). At 27-month follow-up, seven type I patients demonstrated a mean of 27-kg grip strength and ranges of motion: pronation 76°, supination 66°, flexion 54°, and extension 54°. At 51-month follow-up, 13 type II patients demonstrated 38-kg grip strength and ranges of motion: pronation 53°, supination 76°, flexion 51°, and extension 56°.[1]

Another series of 20 dorsal radiocarpal fracture-dislocations yielded a mean grip strength of 85% contralateral with ranges of motion: pronation 87°, supination

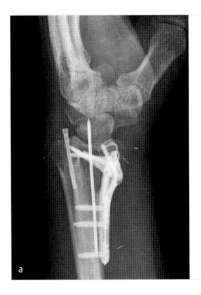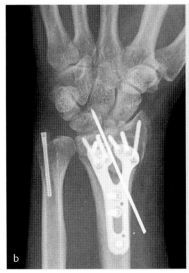

Fig. 16.14 (a, b) When radiocarpal dislocation combines with a highly comminuted distal radius fracture, even specialized fixation methods such as the hook plate extension may not be able to resist subluxation such that transarticular pinning with a 1.4-mm Kirschner wire (K-wire) is needed to maintain congruence.

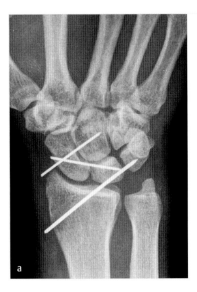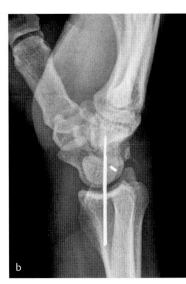

Fig. 16.15 (a, b) When radiocarpal dislocation combines with intrinsic ligament complete rupture, maintenance of congruent reduction depends on a 1.4-mm Kirschner wire (K-wire) for control of the radiocarpal relationship and 1.1-mm K-wires for the intercarpal relationships.

85°, flexion 59°, extension 56°; mean DASH (Disabilities of the Arm, Shoulder, and Hand) score 15; and modified Mayo wrist score 75.[5]

A major tertiary teaching institution was able to identify 26 cases over a search period spanning 31 years, noting that of the 17 patients who could be tracked to 6-month follow-up, 6 had already ended up requiring a fusion.[28]

16.5 Pitfalls and Contraindications

Radiocarpal dislocations and fracture-dislocations are major destabilizing traumas of the wrist joint that require treatment. The only contraindications to performing stabilization would be a patient whose extreme medical infirmity poses major anesthetic risk or a mentally ill patient expected to create a worse final outcome from surgical complications than the original problem.

The major pitfall associated with this injury pattern is simply missing it. Rarely does the surgeon get the opportunity to see the radiographs of the wrist in a dislocated position. Once reduced, the radiographic findings can be quite subtle. A complete clinical evaluation and judicious use of ancillary imaging will allow the surgeon to recognize the extrinsic ligament injury. The risk of missing the extrinsic ligament injury is greater when paired with a more obvious distal radius fracture or intrinsic ligament injury, as the surgeon's attention is drawn to the latter, which seems to fully satisfy the mechanism of injury and explain the trauma signs on examination (▶ Fig. 16.3).

Tips and Tricks

The two most familiar portals in wrist arthroscopy are the 3–4 and 4–5, both of which are useful portals for viewing the mid to volar portion of the radiocarpal joint (▶Fig. 16.10). However, they are too close together and point in relatively similar directions to function as surgical portals when viewing through the other. Manipulating tissue is best accomplished when the viewing portal and surgical portal are well distanced from each other and approach the target from more widely converging angles. Marginal radius fragments are best reduced using an instrument with a narrow curve or hook contour leading to a sharp tip that can capture and control the bone effectively, usually introduced through the 1–2 portal (▶Fig. 16.12). Reduced fragments can then be trapped and held in place by small (0.7–1 mm) K-wires. In the setting of a radiocarpal dislocation coincident to a complete articular distal radius fracture, carpal instability relative to the radius is solved by transfixing the anatomically correct articular relationship between the proximal carpal row and the reference landmark of the radius metaphysis with a 1.4-mm K-wire (▶Fig. 16.14).

References

[1] Dumontier C, Meyer zu Reckendorf G, Sautet A, Lenoble E, Saffar P, Allieu Y. Radiocarpal dislocations: classification and proposal for treatment. A review of twenty-seven cases. J Bone Joint Surg Am 2001;83-A(2):212–218

[2] Freeland AE, Ferguson CA, McCraney WO. Palmar radiocarpal dislocation resulting in ulnar radiocarpal translocation and multidirectional instability. Orthopedics 2006;29(7):604–608

[3] Obafemi A, Pensy R. Palmar radiocarpal dislocation: a case report and novel treatment method. Hand (N Y) 2012;7(1):114–118

[4] Singisetti K, Konstantinos M, Middleton A. Volar radiocarpal dislocation: case report and review of literature. Hand Surg 2011;16(2): 173–175

[5] Lozano-Calderón SA, Doornberg J, Ring D. Fractures of the dorsal articular margin of the distal part of the radius with dorsal radiocarpal subluxation. J Bone Joint Surg Am 2006;88(7):1486–1493

[6] Mudgal CS, Psenica J, Jupiter JB. Radiocarpal fracture-dislocation. J Hand Surg [Br] 1999;24(1):92–98

[7] Souer JS, Davis JS, Marent M, Ring D. Case reports: volar marginal articular fractures with loss of articular apposition. Hand (N Y) 2010;5(2):195–199

[8] Takase K, Morohashi A. A case of acute dorsal radiocarpal dislocation with radial styloid fracture. Eur J Orthop Surg Traumatol 2013;23(2, Suppl 2):S197–S201

[9] Watanabe K, Nishikimi J. Transstyloid radiocarpal dislocation. Hand Surg 2001;6(1):113–120

[10] Katz DA, Green JK, Werner FW, Loftus JB. Capsuloligamentous restraints to dorsal and palmar carpal translation. J Hand Surg Am 2003;28(4):610–613

[11] Ilyas AM, Mudgal CS. Radiocarpal fracture-dislocations. J Am Acad Orthop Surg 2008;16(11):647–655

[12] Woon CY, Baxamusa T. A stepwise approach to management of open radiocarpal fracture-dislocations: a case report. J Hand Surg Asian Pac Vol 2017;22(3):366–370

[13] Ilyas AM, Williamson C, Mudgal CS. Radiocarpal dislocation: is it a rare injury? J Hand Surg Eur Vol 2011;36(2):164–165

[14] Apergis E, Dimitrakopoulos K, Chorianopoulos K, Theodoratos G. Late management of post-traumatic palmar carpal subluxation: a case report. J Bone Joint Surg Br 1996;78(3):419–421

[15] Enoki NR, Sheppard JE, Taljanovic MS. Transstyloid, translunate fracture-dislocation of the wrist: case report. J Hand Surg Am 2008;33(7):1131–1134

[16] Garcia-Paredero E, Cecilia D, Sandoval E. Acute dorsal radiocarpal dislocation associated with scapholunate ligament avulsion: a proposal for surgical treatment. Plast Reconstr Surg 2010;125(1): 24e–25e

[17] Shunmugam M, Phadnis J, Watts A, Bain GI. Lunate fractures and associated radiocarpal and midcarpal instabilities: a systematic review. J Hand Surg Eur Vol 2018;43(1):84–92

[18] Jebson PJ, Adams BD, Meletiou SD. Ulnar translocation instability of the carpus after a dorsal radiocarpal dislocation: a case report. Am J Orthop 2000;29(6):462–464

[19] Arslan H, Tokmak M. Isolated ulnar radiocarpal dislocation. Arch Orthop Trauma Surg 2002;122(3):179–181

[20] Maschke SD, Means KR Jr, Parks BG, Graham TJ. A radiocarpal ligament reconstruction using brachioradialis for secondary ulnar translation of the carpus following radiocarpal dislocation: a cadaver study. J Hand Surg Am 2010;35(2):256–261

[21] Naranja RJ Jr, Bozentka DJ, Partington MT, Bora FW Jr. Radiocarpal dislocation: a report of two cases and a review of the literature. Am J Orthop 1998;27(2):141–144

[22] Hardy P, Welby F, Stromboni M, Blin JL, Lortat-Jacob A, Benoit J. Wrist arthroscopy and dislocation of the radiocarpal joint without fracture. Arthroscopy 1999;15(7):779–783

[23] Smith DW, Henry MH. Comprehensive management of associated soft tissue injuries in distal radius fractures. J Am Soc Surg Hand 2002;2:153–164

[24] Potter MQ, Haller JM, Tyser AR. Ligamentous radiocarpal fracture-dislocation treated with wrist-spanning plate and volar ligament repair. J Wrist Surg 2014;3(4):265–268

[25] Brown D, Mulligan MT, Uhl RL. Volar ligament repair for radiocarpal fracture-dislocation. Orthopedics 2013;36(6):463–468

[26] Kamal RN, Bariteau JT, Beutel BG, DaSilva MF. Arthroscopic reduction and percutaneous pinning of a radiocarpal dislocation: a case report. J Bone Joint Surg Am 2011;93(15):e84

[27] del Piñal F, García-Bernal FJ, Pisani D, Regalado J, Ayala H, Studer A. Dry arthroscopy of the wrist: surgical technique. J Hand Surg Am 2007;32(1):119–123

[28] Yuan BJ, Dennison DG, Elhassan BT, Kakar S. Outcomes after radiocarpal dislocation: a retrospective review. Hand (N Y) 2015;10(3): 367–373

17 Common Errors of Volar Plate Fixation

Robert J. Medoff, James M. Saucedo

Abstract

Treatment of distal radius fractures has changed dramatically since the introduction of the volar locking plate. As the number of volar plate procedures has increased, the type and frequency of complications have changed as well. Many of these complications are avoidable and result from technical errors related to the surgical approach, misinterpretation of the pattern or mechanism of fracture, incomplete reduction, or errors in surgical technique. Inadequate or inappropriate exposure may cause nerve injury, malreduction, poor positioning of implants, joint penetration, protruding hardware, or inadequate fixation. Applying a plate too distal can result in joint penetration, plate irritation, and tendon problems; whereas placing the plate too proximal can result in loss of fixation from inadequate support and plate lift-off. Errors in the position or length of screws or pegs is another frequent source of complications leading to patient morbidity. In addition, relying too much on the implant for reduction or stretching volar plate indications to include all complex patterns, small rim fragments, extensive comminution, and certain shear fractures may set the stage for catastrophic failure. While the volar locking plate can be a versatile and effective tool for many distal radius fractures, appropriate exposure, reduction, and surgical technique are essential to avoid errors that compromise outcomes.

Keywords: distal radius fractures, volar plate, errors, complications, morbidity, failure, tendon rupture, retained hardware, protrusion, nerve injury, malreduction, pain, secondary surgery

> "We cannot solve our problems with the same thinking we used when we created them."
>
> – Albert Einstein

The treatment of distal radius fractures has changed dramatically in the past 15 years as volar plate fixation has become a new standard of care. Not surprisingly, as the number of patients treated with open reduction and volar plate fixation have increased, both the character and frequency of complications have changed as well. Although some morbidity associated with distal radius fractures is clearly related to the pattern and complexity of the injury itself, many clinical failures are avoidable and simply caused by errors in the approach or technique of volar plate fixation.

17.1 Background

Several clinical studies have compared clinical outcomes of volar plate fixation to other "more traditional" methods of treatment. Although most show improvement in clinical outcomes in the early postoperative period (the initial 12 weeks postoperatively), few demonstrate superiority of volar plate fixation in long-term outcomes. Wei et al prospectively randomized patients to either volar plate fixation, external fixation, or radial column fixation and found early improvement in the two internal fixation groups at 6 weeks but no difference in outcome scores at 1 year.[1]

Zhang et al performed a meta-analysis on 6 studies totaling 445 patients comparing external fixation and volar plate fixation.[2] Although volar plate fixation showed better early clinical outcomes, results were equivalent at 12 months. In addition, the number of reoperations for complications was higher in the volar plate group.

Karatana et al prospectively randomized 130 patients to percutaneous treatment or volar plate fixation. Although volar plate fixation showed better early clinical scores with improved grip strength, clinical outcomes at 1 year were not significantly different.[3] Volar plate complications included extensor pollicis longus rupture, plate removal due to flexor tendinopathy, and late articular collapse with intra-articular penetration.

Finally, Arora et al prospectively randomized 73 patients aged 65 years or older to either volar plate fixation or nonoperative management.[4] Although operatively managed patients had better disabilities of arm, shoulder and hand (DASH) and patient-rated wrist evaluation (PRWE) scores in the first 6 weeks, no difference was demonstrated after 6 weeks. Complications were nearly three times higher in the volar plate group (36%). These studies underscore the technical complications associated with volar plate fixation.

A variety of errors may expose patients to complications and morbidity with volar locking plate fixation of distal radius fractures. Many are avoidable, with some related to surgical technique and others to design limitations of the plate itself. Specific categories of errors include inadequate or inappropriate surgical exposure, hardware-related issues, tendinopathies, and inadequate reduction and/or fixation problems (▶ Table 17.1). Recognizing these pitfalls can help avoid complications and morbidity.

17.2 Errors of Surgical Exposure

Most distal radius fractures are exposed with a volar approach.[5,6,7] The palmar cutaneous branch of the median nerve in the subcutaneous tissues between the flexor carpi radialis (FCR) tendon and palmaris longus is at risk of injury with incisions placed too far ulnar, resulting in

Table 17.1 Categories of errors with volar plate fixation

- Errors of surgical approach
  - Inadequate exposure
  - Nerve injury
  - Inadequate reduction
- Flexor tendinopathy/rupture
  - Plate design features
  - Plate position distal or volar to pronator insertion ridge or volar rim
  - Inadequate subchondral support/migration of distal fragment
  - Protruding hardware
  - Retained instrumentation
- Protruding screw tips
  - Attempt to lag dorsal fragments
  - Incorrect screw length
  - Improper interpretation of intraoperative X-rays
- Complex, distal, multiarticular fracture pattern
  - Complex intra-articular pathology not amenable to volar plate fixation
  - Very distal fracture lines with inadequate buttress by volar plate
  - Associated ulnar column injuries
- Excessive or inadequate plate width
- Inadequate reduction
  - Intra-articular incongruity
  - Radial shortening
  - Coronal malalignment
- Inadequate plate length or placement
  - Subchondral screws/pegs too far from subchondral bone
  - Plate of insufficient length
- Patient/biologic issues
  - Noncompliant patient
  - Functional quadruped
  - Severe osteoporosis

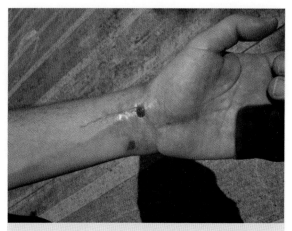

Fig. 17.1 Combining an flexor carpi radialis approach with a standard carpal tunnel exposure results in transection of the palmar cutaneous branch of the median nerve and neuroma.

A volar ulnar approach between the digital flexor tendons and the ulnar neurovascular bundle is another option for visualization of the intermediate column (▶Fig. 17.2). This approach should be considered when direct access to the volar ulnar corner is required, whether planned preoperatively or required intraoperatively because of inadequate visualization.

Some injury patterns, such as extensive comminution of the radial column, dorsal comminution, extremely distal fracture components, or fragmentation of the sigmoid notch, are not adequately fixed with a volar plate and may require alternate or additional exposures.

17.3 Hardware-Related Errors

Although safe and adequate exposure is essential for open treatment of distal radius fractures, appropriate implant selection and positioning are also important. Applying a plate in the wrong position may result in morbidity, ranging from minor hardware irritation to major complications such as tendon rupture or fracture collapse. A position that is too far proximal places locking screws in softer metaphyseal bone and not buttressing the dense subchondral surface. Especially in patients with osteoporosis, subsidence of the distal fragment can result in loss of reduction, shortening, and dorsal angulation. In addition, the distal fragment may drift away from the distal end of the plate resulting in plate "lift-off," which may, in turn, lead to abrasive wear of flexor tendons against the distal edge of the plate and eventual rupture (▶Fig. 17.3). In addition, distal radioulnar joint (DRUJ) dysfunction may occur, resulting in loss of forearm rotation or early arthrosis.[8]

Misinterpretation of radiographs may also result in inadvertent joint penetration. The 10 degree lateral radiograph should be routinely used to confirm proper position of locked distal screws behind the subchondral

painful neuromas and palmar numbness. Combining an FCR incision with a traditional carpal tunnel approach crosses this nerve, which may result in transection and patient morbidity (▶Fig. 17.1). Radially, neuropraxia or injury of the sensory nerves may be caused by overzealous retraction or extension of the skin incision radially.

Inadequate exposure, especially in large patients or those with extensive swelling, can result in problems with reduction, plate position, and secure fixation. In addition, overzealous retraction to visualize the ulnar corner may result in iatrogenic injury to the median nerve. Releasing the FCR distally or using the interval ulnar to the FCR tendon may help provide full visualization of distal radius fragmentation.

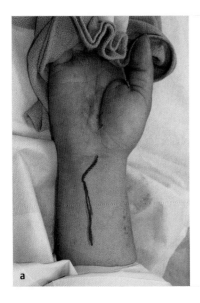
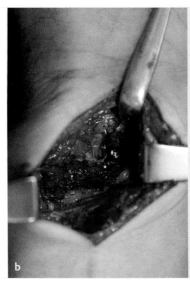

Fig. 17.2 Volar ulnar approach. **(a)** Skin incision. **(b)** Direct access to volar ulnar corner with fixation using a volar buttress pin (TriMed).

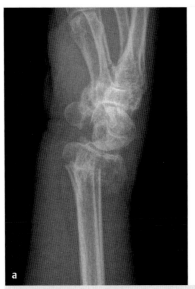
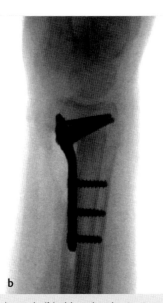
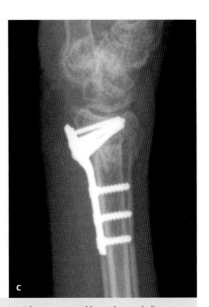

Fig. 17.3 Positioning error. **(a)** Lateral injury radiograph. **(b)** Although reduction is anatomic with near normal lateral carpal alignment and teardrop axis, locked distal fixation is too far proximal from the subchondral bone, resulting in an ineffective buttress of the joint surface. **(c)** Distal fragment has drifted proximally and shifted dorsally away from the plate (dorsal shift of capitate center, depression of teardrop angle), exposing flexor tendons to abrasive wear against plate edge.

bone, especially along the ulnar two-thirds of the joint surface (▶Fig. 17.4).[9]

Screw penetration of the radiocarpal or even DRUJ is another error of technique (▶Fig. 17.5). Standard fixed-angle plates have a single, specific geometry for the footprint of the locking pegs, and optimal subchondral support only occurs when placed in a single, specific location on the volar surface of the radius. The shape of a particular plate can affect the position of distal fixation screws since variation in the curve of the metaphyseal flare determines where a specific plate design sits naturally on the bone. As a result, standard fixed-angle plates require more precise placement to position fixed-angle screws against subchondral bone. In contrast, plate designs with polyaxial locking screws allow more flexibility, since the surgeon can individually orient each distal locking screw optimally against the subchondral surface. This may also allow more uniform subchondral support over a wider range of plate positions (▶Fig. 17.6).

Although more forgiving in terms of plate position, variable-angle locking designs come with their own set of problems. With a greater range of insertion angles, additional care is needed to avoid radiocarpal or even DRUJ penetration. Additional views such as the axial tangential view and pronation oblique views can help identify violation of the sigmoid notch and DRUJ (▶Fig. 17.7).[10,11]

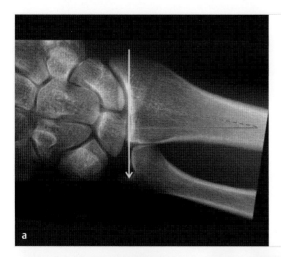
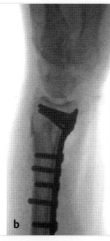

Fig. 17.4 10 degree lateral radiograph. (a) Elevating the forearm about 10 degree aligns the ulnar two-thirds of the radiocarpal joint to the axis of the beam. (b) This view provides accurate assessment of the proximity of the locked distal fixation to the subchondral bone.

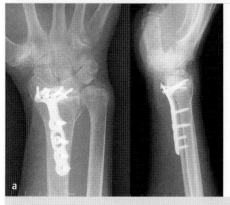
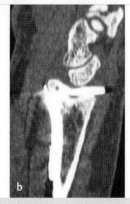
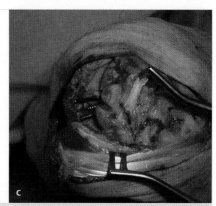

Fig. 17.5 Positioning error resulting in articular penetration by distal locking screws. (Courtesy of Jesse Jupiter, MD). (a) Anteroposterior and lateral X-ray images after surgery show plate applied too distal and too radial with articular penetration by distal pegs and screws. (b) Confirmation of articular penetration on CT scan. (c) Articular penetration confirmed at time of surgery by direct exposure of joint.

In addition, intraoperative clinical evaluation of DRUJ for stability and crepitance helps avoid unrecognized residual joint instability, articular incongruity, and inadvertent hardware penetration.

Patients vary in bone size and shape, and no single plate can be expected to fit the complete range of morphologies in a given population. In large patients, standard implants can leave significant portions of the distal radius uncovered, requiring wider plate designs or additional fixation. In contrast, in petite individuals, standard plate sizes may protrude beyond the edge of the bone leading to hardware irritation (▶Fig. 17.8). These problems are easily avoided by detailed preoperative assessment and ensuring that a range of implant sizes is available at the time of surgery.

17.4 Tendon Complications

17.4.1 Flexor Tendon Rupture and Irritation

Prior to 1998, few articles described flexor tendon complications associated with distal radius fractures; Rymaszewski in 1987 stated that "attritional ruptures of flexor tendons to the fingers following Colles' fractures are very rare."[12,13,14,15] Tendinopathy is now well recognized as a complication of volar plate fixation.[16,17,18,19,20,21,22,23,24,25,26,27,28,29,30,31,32] Although Orbay suggested in 2000 that the volar approach allows "safe application of internal fixation devices," long-term clinical experience has confirmed that it is by no means free from iatrogenic tendon complications (▶Fig. 17.9).[6]

Soong et al studied the relation of tendon complications to plate position either palmar or distal to the distal ridge in a series of distal radius fractures treated with volar locked plates.[33] These authors concluded that placement in these positions contributed to a higher risk of flexor tendinopathy and rupture. Several other studies have supported this correlation between plate position and flexor tendinopathy and rupture.[25,32] As a result, volar plates should avoid extending volar or distal to the volar ridge; subsequent removal should be planned if placement in this position is necessary for fixation. In addition, very distal plates with proximal obliquity of the locking screws may allow the distal fragment to slide off with wrist dorsiflexion and do not provide the same degree of subchondral support as plates with distal obliquity to the locking screws (▶Fig. 17.10).

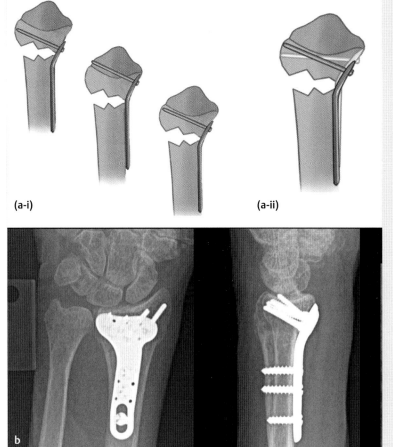

Fig. 17.6 Variable locking volar plate design. **(a-i)** Standard fixed-angle plates orient the pegs in a position in the distal fragment based on the location of the plate. Plate position too proximal may not provide adequate subchondral support. Positions too distal risk joint penetration. **(a-ii)** Variable-angle locking design allows independent positioning of each distal support peg over range of plate locations. **(b)** Variable-angle locking plate with uniform subchondral support.

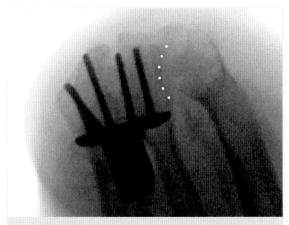

Fig. 17.7 Axial tangential view for assessing position and dorsal penetration of the distal locking screws; this view also provides some visualization of the sigmoid notch.

Although these studies have underscored the importance of plate position, the etiology of flexor tendon irritation, attrition, and rupture is probably not simple. Specific plate designs as well as the quality of fracture reduction have also been suggested as important compounding factors correlated with flexor tendinopathy. Limthongthang et al studied the proximity of five plate designs to the flexor tendons and concluded that all raised concerns regarding prominence to the flexor pollicis longus.[34] Selvan et al examined the relation of plate position and fracture reduction on plate prominence in three different fixed-angle plate designs; they concluded that both fracture reduction and plate position have a statistically and clinically significant effect on plate prominence.[30]

Mehrzad and Kim reviewed the rate of complications between one group of 60 patients treated with Stryker (Stryker Inc., Mahwah, NJ) or Acu-Loc (Acumed Inc., Hillsboro, OR) fixed-angle plates and another group of 148 patients treated with a TriMed (TriMed Inc., Santa Clarita, CA) variable-angle locking plate. There was a statistical difference in reoperation rates for hardware-related complications with 12% requiring repeat surgery in the Stryker/Acu-Loc group and 0% requiring reoperations in the TriMed variable-angle locking plate. They concluded that polyaxial locking plates were more forgiving and avoided flexor tendon problems.[35] Although Cross et al presented two cases of flexor tendon rupture after volar plating and concluded that both healed in

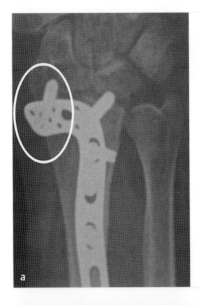
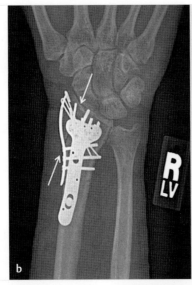

Fig. 17.8 Inappropriate plate size. **(a)** Too wide of a plate may cause soft-tissue irritation if protruding radially (*oval*), and interference with distal radioulnar joint (DRUJ) function if protruding against the ulnar head. (Courtesy of David Ruch, MD). **(b)** Plates that are too small may leave fragments unsupported; in this case, a radial column plate was necessary to secure an unstable radial column fragment (*arrows*).

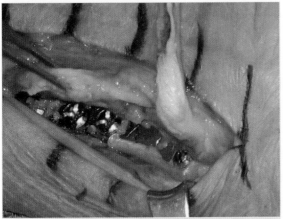

Fig. 17.9 Flexor rupture due to abrasive wear against a prominent plate edge.

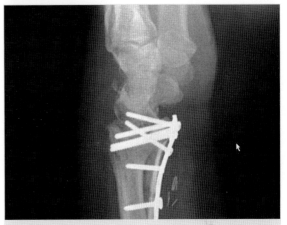

Fig. 17.10 Plate and screw position. Plates positioned distal to the distal ridge of pronator quadratus insertion may produce abrasive wear of flexor tendons and so should be removed after bone healing. In addition, plates that direct distal locking screws proximally are at a biomechanical disadvantage for resisting dorsal shift with dorsiflexion; this can result in loss of reduction and screw penetration. (This image is provided courtesy of David Ruch, MD.)

"anatomic position" without plate lift-off, close evaluation of one radiograph shows a design extending past the volar rim and dorsal migration of the distal fragment exposing the edge of the plate in the other.[25]

Kara et al suggested that plates extending to the volar rim are at high risk of causing tendinitis and rupture, and should be removed.[36] Tokunaga et al reviewed 32 patients treated for distal radius fractures; all 5 cases of flexor tendon erosion occurred in the 16 patients who were treated with an Acu-Loc plate.[37] Even in the article by Soong et al which correlated plate position with flexor tendon pathology, all flexor ruptures occurred in the 72 patients treated with an Acu-Loc plate compared to none in the 93 patients treated with a DVR (DePuy Synthes Trauma, West Chester, PA) plate. These studies suggest that plate design may also be a significant contributing factor related to flexor tendinopathy.

The quality of reduction and stability of fixation is also important in avoiding flexor problems. Locking pegs positioned too far from the articular surface may result in the distal fragment settling to a position of stability; plates with sharp distal edges may result in abrasive wear as the distal fragments drift proximally and dorsally. Residual dorsal subluxation of the carpus, unreduced teardrop angle, and lateral carpal malalignment also contribute to plate "lift-off."

Other less common technical errors can cause flexor tendinopathy. Yamazaki et al reported a case of delayed flexor rupture from a prominent screw head.[23] Bhattacharyya and Wadgaonkar reported three patients with retained mini drill guides requiring secondary surgery, one with complete flexor tendon rupture.[38]

17.4.2 Extensor Tendon Injury and Rupture

Although it has been suggested that volar plates avoid extensor tendon complications, clinical studies have shown these complications occur as well. Dorsal tendons have been injured from overpenetration by drills or screws of excessive length, with injury to the extensor pollicis longus as the most frequent injury (▶ Fig. 17.11).[39]

Relying on a single lateral radiograph can result in error when assessing screw length.[11,39,40] Since the dorsal surface of the distal radius is trapezoidal, a screw protruding past the cortex may give an appearance of being inside the bone on a lateral radiograph. Screws placed near Lister tubercle are especially prone to this error and may protrude as much as 4 mm before being identified by X-ray.[41] To address this shortcoming, live fluoroscopy or an axial

tangential view should be considered (▶ Fig. 17.7).[11] In addition, Wall et al suggested from biomechanical studies that only 75% of the anteroposterior distance is required for fixation.[39]

Some patterns of distal radius fractures include fracture elements that simply cannot be stabilized from the volar side alone (▶ Fig. 17.12). Attempts to lag a dorsal fragment with a lag screw inserted from the volar side typically result in overpenetration of the dorsal cortex, leaving a prominent screw tip with sharp cutting flutes adjacent to gliding tendons. Patterns such as dorsal shearing fractures or sigmoid notch comminution often cannot be stabilized from a volar approach; dorsal fixation may be necessary in such cases.

Problems from prominent dorsal hardware are not isolated to locked subchondral screws. Excessively long screws in the radial shaft may cause irritation, synovitis, and pain (▶ Fig. 17.13). Using an implant system that provides proximal shaft screws with single millimeter increments can help avoid this problem.

17.5 Inadequate Reduction and Fixation

Not all distal radius fractures can be treated with a volar plate, and it is a mistake to assume this method will address all injuries. When accurately positioned behind the subchondral surface, the distal tilt of the subchondral locking screws or pegs provides articular support, maintaining radial length and preventing dorsal migration and subsidence. However, not all fractures behave like the typical dorsally angulated, extra-articular fracture pattern. Fractures with palmar instability displace by a different mechanism (i.e., volar shear), a mechanism that is not stabilized by subchondral support pegs.

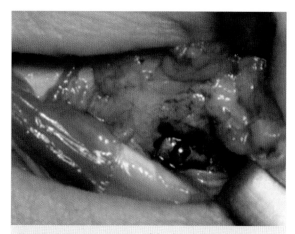

Fig. 17.11 Screw penetration of the dorsal cortex causing extensor tendon rupture. (This image is provided courtesy of David Ruch, MD.)

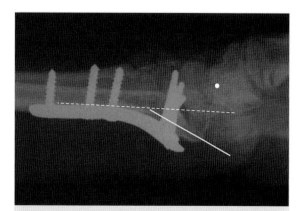

Fig. 17.12 Inadequate stabilization of dorsal fragmentation with volar plate. Note the dorsal shift of the capitate center to the reference line extended from the volar cortex of the radial shaft (dotted line) and the marked depression of the teardrop angle. Supplemental dorsal fixation or a bridge plate should be considered if dorsal stability is not controlled by a volar plate.

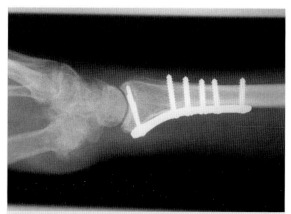

Fig. 17.13 Protruding proximal bone screws. Accurate measurement and using a system that provides increments of 1 mm lengths should avoid this problem.

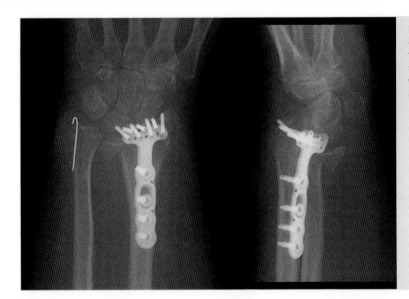

Fig. 17.14 Failure from migration of the critical corner fragment over the edge of the plate. Insufficient palmar support over the volar rim of the lunate facet, especially with small volar rim fragments, can lead to catastrophic failure of the critical corner.

In these circumstances, other types of fixation should be considered. If a volar plate is used, it should be positioned distal enough to provide a palmar buttress to the distal fragment, effectively sandwiching it between the distal locked screws and the distal edge of the plate. If a very distal position is required, subsequent surgery for plate removal should be considered to avoid soft-tissue complications related to prominent hardware. Extremely distal fractures involving a small portion of the volar rim, such as fragmentation of the critical corner, are at high risk of migration over the edge of the plate, which could result in catastrophic palmar instability and loss of reduction. In these cases, a different approach to treatment should be considered (▶Fig. 17.14 and ▶Fig. 17.15).[42]

Fractures with severe comminution may not be adequately controlled by a volar plate alone. In these highly unstable, polyarticular injuries, fixation of individual fracture elements, such as the radial column, dorsal rim and wall, intermediate column, and the DRUJ, may be needed. Fractures that include extensive comminution into the radial column may not be adequately stabilized by one or two screws from a volar plate and may require adjunctive fixation with a dedicated radial column plate, pins, or bone graft. Residual loss of lateral carpal alignment may indicate the need for dedicated stabilization of dorsal fracture elements. In these complex cases, the surgeon should be prepared for alternative or supplemental approaches such as bone grafting, fragment-specific fixation, external fixation, or bridge plating (▶Fig. 17.16).

Avoiding complications related to inadequate fixation starts with careful recognition of various indicators that raise concern for a fracture at risk. Accurate assessment of radiographs, as suggested by Medoff, includes essential radiographic measurements such as the teardrop angle, uniform carpal intervals on both anteroposterior and lateral radiographs, lateral carpal alignment, anteroposterior distance, and adjunctive study with computed

tomography as needed. Taken together, these measures are invaluable in helping to predict injuries at risk in multiple planes of instability.[9,43]

One of the benefits of the volar locking plate has been to simplify the fixation of many distal radius fractures. For better or worse, it has also been advocated as a reduction tool, and this has sometimes led to reductions that rely too much on the plate. Some malreductions are obvious, such as incompletely corrected dorsal tilt, insufficient restoration of radial height or inclination and inadequate articular surface reduction. The effects of malreduction in these parameters have been well described.

Coronal malreduction, however, may go unrecognized (▶Fig. 17.17). A widened joint interval at the DRUJ on the anteroposterior view or radial translation of the distal fragment(s) and offset of the cortical alignment along the lateral column may indicate this problem. If uncorrected, the normal resting tension in the interosseous membrane that helps stabilize the DRUJ is lost, potentially resulting in DRUJ instability.[44,45] Occasionally, coronal malalignment may also result in impaction of a metaphyseal spike against the ulnar head, producing pain, a physical "clunk" with forearm rotation, and limited motion.

Several methods can be used to correct coronal malalignment. A simple option is to supplement fixation with a radial column plate to restore a congruent radial border. Another method is to loosen the plate proximally, disengage fragments with traction, and use a clamp to push the radial side of the plate to the ulnar border of radial shaft. Alternatively, a lamina spreader can distract the radial and ulnar shaft away from each other while longitudinal traction is applied. Whichever method is used to correct medialization of the shaft and restoration of the normal radial bow, all require recognition as a first step.

Axial instability of the volar rim can be overlooked and it can compromise clinical outcomes. In this pattern, depression of the teardrop angle is present, combined

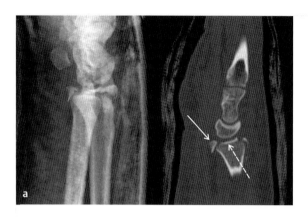
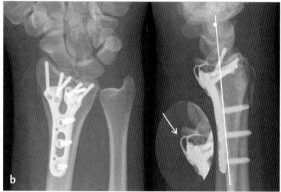
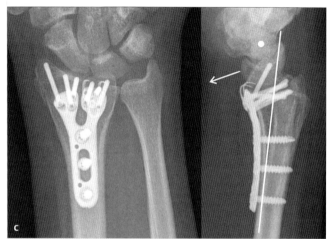
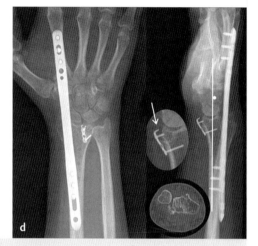

Fig. 17.15 Inappropriate volar plate indication. Other methods of treatment, such as bridge plating or fragment-specific fixation, should be considered for extremely distal or communited fractures. **(a)** Injury: CT scan shows that subchondral position of distal locking screws with a volar plate only supports the uninjured bone (*dashed arrow*); the unstable volar rim fragment (*solid arrow*) is too far distal for fixation with a volar plate. **(b)** Initial fixation: A volar plate was applied, in this case augmenting with a hook attachment from the surface of the plate. Reduction of lateral carpal alignment has been obtained (capitate center aligned with reference axis). However, the design of this hook augmentation from the surface of the plate leaves the palmar surface of the volar rim unsupported and affords only marginal penetration of the fragment (*inset arrow*). **(c)** Follow-up: The carpus and volar rim fragment have shifted palmar to settle into the unsupported defect (*arrow*); note the significant palmar shift in lateral carpal alignment (capitate center palmar to reference axis). Patient presented with pain and restricted motion. **(d)** Revision surgery: The previous volar plate has been removed and a bridge plate and small fragment plate applied. The bridge plate has restored normal lateral carpal alignment (capitate center aligned with reference axis); however, inadequate buttress and fixation of the volar rim fragment persists (*top inset, arrow*). As a result, the volar rim fragment migrated (*bottom inset*), clinically resulting in complete loss of supination from the bony block within the sigmoid notch.

with dorsal shift of the lateral carpal alignment and an adaptive instability pattern of the carpus.[46,47] These subtle patterns of malreduction suggest an incomplete restoration of the articular surface, with residual abnormalities of carpal alignment. A volar locking plate may not adequately treat these types of complex instabilities involving the volar rim and thus a more aggressive approach with supplementary or alternate fixation, such as a volar buttress pin, hook plate, dorsal fixation, bone graft, external fixation, or bridge plate, may be required to restore articular congruency and carpal alignment.

17.6 Conclusion

There is little doubt that volar plate fixation has significantly changed the management of distal radius fractures

in the past two decades. Though long-term studies, especially in the elderly population, question whether clinical outcomes are superior with volar plate fixation, many studies however seem to confirm that volar plate fixation results in acceleration of recovery when compared to more traditional methods of treatment.

Despite these benefits, increasing evidence shows that volar plate fixation is not without problems. Although volar plates show better early postoperative clinical results, comparative studies have shown complications and secondary procedures higher than with traditional treatment methods. In many cases, complications are caused by errors in technique or inappropriate indications. Mistakes related to surgical approaches, fracture reduction, misapplication, and inadequate or inappropriate use often contribute to reported complications. A thorough understanding of the anatomy, surgical

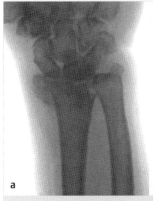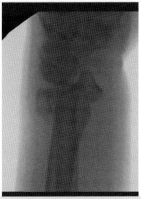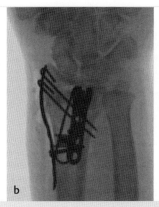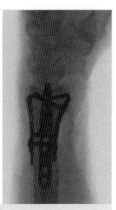

Fig. 17.16 Complex articular fragmentation. **(a)** Elderly patient presented 3 weeks after sustaining this highly unstable, distal multiarticular fragmentation. Attempts to stabilize with volar plate at time of surgery were unsuccessful. **(b)** Treatment with fragment-specific fixation using radial column fixation, volar hook plate, dorsal buttress pin and bone graft; bridge plating and external fixation are alternate options.

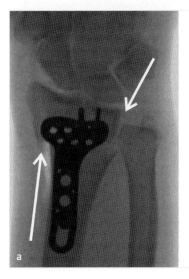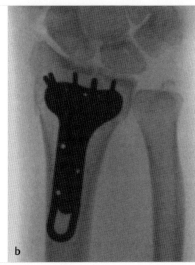

Fig. 17.17 Coronal malreduction. **(a)** Coronal malalignment can be recognized by offset of the cortical margins and widening of the distal radioulnar joint (DRUJ) (*arrows*). If left untreated, it can contribute to DRUJ dysfunction and instability. **(b)** Coronal malalignment corrected at time of surgery.

approaches, patterns of injury, and biomechanical principles of this method of internal fixation is essential for optimum clinical results, and it underscores that distal radius fixation is more than just simple placement of a plate and screws on the palmar surface of the radius.

References

[1] Wei DH, Raizman NM, Bottino CJ, Jobin CM, Strauch RJ, Rosenwasser MP. Unstable distal radial fractures treated with external fixation, a radial column plate, or a volar plate. A prospective randomized trial. J Bone Joint Surg Am 2009;91(7):1568–1577

[2] Li-hai Z, Ya-nan W, Zhi M, et al. Volar locking plate versus external fixation for the treatment of unstable distal radial fractures: a meta-analysis of randomized controlled trials. J Surg Res 2015;193(1):324–333

[3] Karantana A, Downing ND, Forward DP, et al. Surgical treatment of distal radial fractures with a volar locking plate versus conventional percutaneous methods: a randomized controlled trial. J Bone Joint Surg Am 2013;95(19):1737–1744

[4] Arora R, Lutz M, Deml C, Krappinger D, Haug L, Gabl M. A prospective randomized trial comparing nonoperative treatment with volar locking plate fixation for displaced and unstable distal radial fractures in patients sixty-five years of age and older. J Bone Joint Surg Am 2011;93(23):2146–2153

[5] Henry AK. Extensile Exposures, 2nd ed. Edinburgh: Chirchill Livingstone; 1973: 90–110

[6] Orbay JL. The treatment of unstable distal radius fractures with volar fixation. Hand Surg 2000;5(2):103–112

[7] Orbay JL, Fernandez DL. Volar fixation for dorsally displaced fractures of the distal radius: a preliminary report. J Hand Surg Am 2002;27(2):205–215

[8] Nishiwaki M, Welsh M, Gammon B, Ferreira LM, Johnson JA, King GJW. Distal radioulnar joint kinematics in simulated dorsally angulated distal radius fractures. J Hand Surg Am 2014;39(4):656–663

[9] Medoff RJ. Radiographic evaluation and classification of distal radius fractures. In: Slutsky D, Osterman AL, eds. Distal Radius Fractures and Carpal Injury: The Cutting Edge. Philadelphia, PA: Elsevier; 2009:19–31

[10] Klammer G, Dietrich M, Farshad M, Iselin L, Nagy L, Schweizer A. Intraoperative imaging of the distal radioulnar joint using a modified skyline view. J Hand Surg Am 2012;37(3):503–508

[11] Rausch S, Marintschev I, Graul I, et al. Tangential view and intraoperative three-dimensional fluoroscopy for the detection of screw-misplacements in volar plating of distal radius fractures. Arch Trauma Res 2015;4(2):e24622

[12] Rymaszewski LA, Walker AP. Rupture of flexor digitorum profundus to the index finger after a distal radial fracture. J Hand Surg [Br] 1987;12(1):115–116

[13] Ashall G. Flexor pollicis longus rupture after fracture of the distal radius. Injury 1991;22(2):153–155

[14] Lugger LJ, Pechlaner S. Tendon rupture as a complication after osteosynthesis of distal radius. Unfallchirurgie 1984;10(5):266–270

[15] Takami H, Takahashi S, Ando M. Attritional flexor tendon ruptures after a malunited intra-articular fracture of the distal radius. Arch Orthop Trauma Surg 1997;116(8):507–509

[16] Bell JS, Wollstein R, Citron ND. Rupture of flexor pollicis longus tendon: a complication of volar plating of the distal radius. J Bone Joint Surg Br 1998;80(2):225–226

[17] Valbuena SE, Cogswell LK, Baraziol R, Valenti P. Rupture of flexor tendon following volar plate of distal radius fracture. Report of five cases. Chir Main 2010;29(2):109–113

[18] Lifchez SD. Flexor pollicis longus tendon rupture after volar plating of a distal radius fracture. Plast Reconstr Surg 2010;125(1):21e–23e

[19] Ishii T, Ikeda M, Kobayashi Y, Mochida J, Oka Y. Flexor digitorum profundus tendon rupture associated with distal radius fracture malunion: a case report. Hand Surg 2009;14(1):35–38

[20] Berglund LM, Messer TM. Complications of volar plate fixation for managing distal radius fractures. J Am Acad Orthop Surg 2009;17(6):369–377

[21] Casaletto JA, Machin D, Leung R, Brown DJ. Flexor pollicis longus tendon ruptures after palmar plate fixation of fractures of the distal radius. J Hand Surg Eur Vol 2009;34(4):471–474

[22] Adham MN, Porembski M, Adham C. Flexor tendon problems after volar plate fixation of distal radius fractures. Hand (N Y) 2009;4(4):406–409

[23] Yamazaki H, Hattori Y, Doi K. Delayed rupture of flexor tendons caused by protrusion of a screw head of a volar plate for distal radius fracture: a case report. Hand Surg 2008;13(1):27–29

[24] Suppaphol S, Woratanarat P, Channoom T. Flexor tendon rupture after distal radius fracture. Report of 2 cases. J Med Assoc Thai 2007;90(12):2695–2698

[25] Cross AW, Schmidt CC. Flexor tendon injuries following locked volar plating of distal radius fractures. J Hand Surg Am 2008;33(2):164–167

[26] Duncan SF, Weiland AJ. Delayed rupture of the flexor pollicis longus tendon after routine volar placement of a T-plate on the distal radius. Am J Orthop 2007;36(12):669–670

[27] Arora R, Lutz M, Hennerbichler A, Krappinger D, Espen D, Gabl M. Complications following internal fixation of unstable distal radius fracture with a palmar locking-plate. J Orthop Trauma 2007;21(5):316–322

[28] Satake H, Hanaka N, Honma R, et al. Complications of distal radius fractures treated by volar locking plate fixation. Orthopedics 2016;39(5):e893–e896

[29] Monaco NA, Dwyer CL, Ferikes AJ, Lubahn JD. Hand surgeon reporting of tendon rupture following distal radius volar plating. Hand (N Y) 2016;11(3):278–286

[30] Selvan DR, Machin DG, Perry D, Simpson C, Thorpe P, Brown DJ. The role of fracture reduction and plate position in the aetiology of flexor pollicis longus tendon rupture after volar plate fixation of distal radius fractures. Hand (N Y) 2015;10(3):497–502

[31] Selvan DR, Perry D, Machin DG, Brown DJ. The role of postoperative radiographs in predicting risk of flexor pollicis longus tendon rupture after volar plate fixation of distal radius fractures—a case control study. Injury 2014;45(12):1885–1888

[32] Kitay A, Swanstrom M, Schreiber JJ, et al. Volar plate position and flexor tendon rupture following distal radius fracture fixation. J Hand Surg Am 2013;38(6):1091–1096

[33] Soong M, Earp BE, Bishop G, Leung A, Blazar P. Volar locking plate implant prominence and flexor tendon rupture. J Bone Joint Surg Am 2011;93(4):328–335

[34] Limthongthang R, Bachoura A, Jacoby SM, Osterman AL. Distal radius volar locking plate design and associated vulnerability of the flexor pollicis longus. J Hand Surg Am 2014;39(5):852–860

[35] Mehrzad R, Kim DC. Complication rate comparing variable angle distal locking plate to fixed angle plate fixation of distal radius fractures. Ann Plast Surg 2016;77(6):623–625

[36] Kara A, Celik H, Oc Y, Uzun M, Erdil M, Tetik C. Flexor tendon complications in comminuted distal radius fractures treated with anatomic volar rim locking plates. Acta Orthop Traumatol Turc 2016;50(6):665–669

[37] Tokunaga S, Abe Y. Asymptomatic flexor tendon damages after volar locking plate fixation of distal radius fractures. J Hand Surg Asian Pac Vol 2017;22(1):75–82

[38] Bhattacharyya T, Wadgaonkar AD. Inadvertent retention of angled drill guides after volar locking plate fixation of distal radial fractures. A report of three cases. J Bone Joint Surg Am 2008;90(2):401–403

[39] Wall LB, Brodt MD, Silva MJ, Boyer MI, Calfee RP. The effects of screw length on stability of simulated osteoporotic distal radius fractures fixed with volar locking plates. J Hand Surg Am 2012;37(3):446–453

[40] Thomas AD, Greenberg JA. Use of fluoroscopy in determining screw overshoot in the dorsal distal radius: a cadaveric study. J Hand Surg Am 2009;34(2):258–261

[41] Maschke SD, Evans PJ, Schub D, Drake R, Lawton JN. Radiographic evaluation of dorsal screw penetration after volar fixed-angle plating of the distal radius: a cadaveric study. Hand (N Y) 2007;2(3):144–150

[42] Beck JD, Harness NG, Spencer HT. Volar plate fixation failure for volar shearing distal radius fractures with small lunate facet fragments. J Hand Surg Am 2014;39(4):670–678

[43] Pienaar G, Anley C, Ikram A. Restoration of teardrop angle (TDA) in distal radius fractures treated with volar locking plates. SA Ortho J. 2013;12(3):32–34

[44] Riggenbach MD, Conrad BP, Wright TW, Dell PC. Distal oblique bundle reconstruction and distal radioulnar joint instability. J Wrist Surg 2013;2(4):330–336

[45] Ross M, Di Mascio L, Peters S, Cockfield A, Taylor F, Couzens G. Defining residual radial translation of distal radius fractures: a potential cause of distal radioulnar joint instability. J Wrist Surg 2014;3(1):22–29

[46] Lichtman DM, Wroten ES. Understanding midcarpal instability. J Hand Surg Am 2006;31(3):491–498

[47] Taleisnik J, Watson HK. Midcarpal instability caused by malunited fractures of the distal radius. J Hand Surg Am 1984;9(3):350–357

18 Distal Ulna Fractures

Christopher Klifto, David Ruch

Abstract

Distal ulna fractures are often encountered in conjunction with distal radius fractures and can result in poor outcomes if not treated. Fractures of the distal ulna may be classified as ulnar styloid, head, and metaphysis fractures. Methods of fixation can include K-wires, plates, and compression screws. If a malunion or nonunion develops, salvage procedures such as the Sauve-Kapandji or the Darrach procedure may be utilized. If salvage procedures fail, then ulnar head arthroplasties can be attempted for future salvage. Overall, outcomes are promising for properly treated ulna fractures.

Keywords: distal radius fracture, distal radius malunion, intra-articular osteotomy, arthroscopy, wrist pain

18.1 Introduction

Untreated fractures of the base of the ulnar styloid, head, and metaphysis result in high rates of nonunion and have been associated with distal radioulnar joint (DRUJ) instability. These injuries are often undertreated and overlooked compared to distal radius fractures. The role of internal fixation of the ulnar styloid is debated. Some surgeons feel that routine repair limits the risk of symptomatic instability or nonunion, and others feel that the added surgical time, scar, risks, and implant prominence are not justified, given the low risk of problems—at least when the distal radius fracture is managed with open reduction and internal fixation.

Untreated distal ulna fractures, specifically ulna styloid fractures may lead to nonunions and DRUJ instability. While most distal ulna fractures infrequently lead to long-term issues, recent literature has been dedicated to investigating which distal ulna fractures require surgical management and long-term outcomes.

Distal ulna fractures most often occur by falls on an extended and supinated wrist. Due the complex anatomy of the distal ulna and the DRUJ, these injuries can become symptomatic. Understanding how to optimally treat ulna fractures begins with a detailed knowledge of the complex anatomy of the DRUJ. The DRUJ is stabilized by boney congruence and soft tissue constraints that intricately work in conjunction. The boney congruence comprises the ulnar head and the sigmoid notch of the radius. Because of the need for rotation through the DRUJ, there is a mismatch between radius of curvature between the radius and ulna, with the radius possessing a larger arc than the ulnar head. This allows for volar translation of the ulnar head with supination and dorsal translation of the ulnar head with pronation.

Standard radiographs including posteroanterior, lateral, and oblique radiographs often reveal the pathology; however, computed tomography may be useful in examining the articular surface and magnetic resonance imaging may be used to examine the integrity of the triangular fibrocartilage complex (TFCC). Treatment of distal ulna fractures can be difficult and may be categorized into ulnar styloid fractures, articular ulnar head fractures, and distal ulnar neck/shaft fractures and malunions.

18.2 Indications

18.2.1 Ulnar Styloid Fractures/ Nonunions

It is critical to evaluate the DRUJ for stability in these injuries as an unstable joint affects the outcomes. Fractures could be avulsion fractures which often do not influence the stability of the DRUJ or ulnar base fractures which are more likely to affect stability. If the radioulnar ligament is attached to the fragment then the joint will demonstrate instability. If fractures through the base of the ulnar styloid are displaced more than 2 mm, then operative intervention may be necessary whereas fractures through the tip are more likely to be stable.[1] Radial translation of the fractured ulna indicates detachment of the radioulnar ligament which often causes instability of the DRUJ.

Indications for repair of nonunions include reattachment of the nonunited fragment if the fragment is large and instability is present. If the fragment is small, it may be excised and the radioulnar ligament may be reattached directly to the fovea. If pain is the main complaint and there is no concomitant instability, then the fragment may be removed with the assistance of wrist arthroscopy to evaluate the TFCC and ligamentous structures.

Fractures of the ulnar head involve the articular surface. They may be seen in isolation or may occur concomitantly with ulnar styloid fractures and ulnar shaft fractures. Distal ulnar neck/shaft fractures occur within 4 cm of the articular surface of the ulnar head. Often occurring with distal radius fractures, these fractures can be treated nonoperatively if reducible and stable after correction of the distal radius fracture, but may require stabilization due to instability.

Malunited distal radius fractures or distal ulna fractures may cause degeneration at the DRUJ. Indications for salvage procedures include pain with forearm rotation, swelling, decreased grip strength, stiffness, and failure of conservative treatment which includes injections and bracing. Salvage procedures are designed to eliminate the articulation between the distal ulna and radius by resecting the distal ulna, fusing the joint, or replacing the ulna.

Indications for distal ulna arthroplasty include highly comminuted fractures of the distal ulna that are not amenable to repair. Posttraumatic indications include symptomatic DRUJ arthritis. Arthroplasty should only be indicated after failure of conservative treatment such as physical therapy which includes a splinting program for at least 4 to 6 months before considering surgery for post-traumatic arthritis.

18.3 Surgical Technique

18.3.1 Approach

Most distal ulna pathology can be addressed through the same approach. The distal ulna is approached through a dorsal zig zag incision centered over the DRUJ. The dorsal sensory branches of the ulnar nerve should be identified and protected. The extensor retinaculum of the fifth compartment is identified and incised. Next, an ulnar based interval is developed between the extensor retinaculum and the separate dorsal sheet of the extensor carpi ulnaris (ECU) tendon without compromising the ECU tendon sheath. Next, the dorsal capsule is opened by creating a ulnar based flap raised from the 4–5 septum. The capsular incision begins at the neck of the ulna and is extend to the 4,5 intercompartmental artery. The incision is continued along the radiocarpal joint where it extends distally and ulnarly along the dorsal radiotriquetral ligament to the triquetrum while preserving the dorsal ligaments. The TFCC is identified next and the ulnar styloid, ulnocarpal joint, and ulnar neck can be visualized.

18.3.2 Ulnar Styloid Fractures Technique

There are multiple options to fix ulnar styloid base fractures which include conservative management in a supination brace, Kirschner wires (K-wires), tension band wiring, suture or screw fixation, and radial lengthening. Patients may be treated in a supination brace for 6 weeks if intraoperative assessment reveals instability when the forearm is in the neutral or pronated position but stability with forearm supination. The above arm supination brace is often customized by occupational therapy and is worn full time for 6 weeks. K-wires may be placed percutaneously or with a small incision to protect the dorsal sensory branch of the of the ulnar nerve. They are typically left outside of the skin and are removed after 6 weeks. Tension band fixation uses one or two oblique K-wires which are passed through the tip of the ulnar styloid. A 24-gauge stainless steel wire or suture is passed around the tip of the wire and through a drill hole in the ulnar neck in a figure of eight fashion. A suture anchor may be used in a similar fashion. The suture anchor is placed in the defect created by the ulnar styloid fracture and looped around the ulnar styloid or through the styloid if the fragment is large enough to pass a suture though without fragmenting the styloid. A subsequent drill hole is placed through the ulna proximally and the suture is passed through the hole and tied (▶ Fig. 18.1).

The styloid may be also be secured with a headless compression screw. The styloid may be reduced percutaneously with a K-wire or a mini open incision may be made for protecting the dorsal ulnar sensory branch. The screw is then inserted over the K-wire stabilizing the fracture fragment (▶ Fig. 18.2).

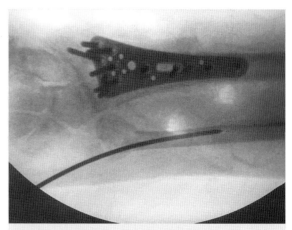

Fig. 18.1 Kirschner wires (K-wires) used for stabilization of the ulnar styloid and distal ulna.

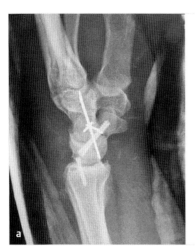
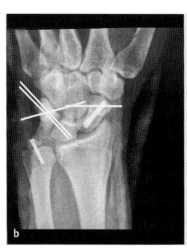

Fig. 18.2 (a, b) Headless compression screw used for fixation of the ulnar styloid.

Radius lengthening is a newer technique for instability that involves a standard volar Henry approach with provisional fixation of the distal radius first distal to the fracture. The radius is then lengthened and fixed proximally distracting it and tightening the TFCC.

18.3.3 Ulnar Head Fractures

Ulnar head fractures that are displaced or unstable may be treated with a buried headless compression screw or K-wires. Ulnar head fractures with extension into the ulnar shaft may be treated with condylar blade plates whereas fractures that include the ulnar styloid which can be treated with tension band wiring. Distal ulnar neck and shaft fractures that are irreducible or unstable may be treated with a condylar blade plate or a tension band wiring with added fixation with intrafragmentary screws.

18.3.4 Comminuted Intra-articular Distal Ulnar Fractures

Comminuted intra-articular distal ulnar fractures may be treated with any of the abovementioned treatment options if the fracture pattern is amendable. Occasionally these fractures are best treated conservatively with an above-elbow cast immobilization in supination or supplemented with removable K-wires. If the ulna is unable to be salvaged or if future malunion/arthritis develops, treatment can include distal head replacements, a total/partial excision of the ulnar head, DRUJ arthrodesis with distal ulnar neck resection (Sauve-Kapandji procedure), or distal ulnar resection (Darrach procedure). There are many options for salvage procedures but the Sauve-Kapandji and the Darrach procedures are most commonly utilized.

The Sauve-Kapandji procedure is typically approached dorsally with an incision made over the fifth extensor compartment extending from the level of the ulna styloid extending proximally. The extensor digiti quinti (EDQ) is retracted and the extensor retinaculum and DRUJ capsule are raised as an ulnar based flap. Multiple options are available for fixation but it is the author's preference to use two parallel K-wires placed beneath the ECU sheath which are subsequently replaced with two 3.5-mm cannulated screws with the ulnar head in neutral rotation. 1 cm of the ulna neck is resected and bone graft is placed in the arthrodesis site. A distally based strip of the flexor carpi ulnaris (FCU) may be used to stabilize the proximal ulna stump.

The Darrach procedure is another alternative to the Sauve-Kapandji technique. The same approach is utilized and the distal 3 cm of the ulna is exposed while maintaining the attachments of the ulnar styloid. The ulnar styloid is osteotomized at its base and left in situ, and a periosteal sleeve is used to close the incision to help stabilize

the ulnar stump. Soft-tissue stabilization procedures utilizing the ECU or FCU tendon may be used to secure the free proximal ulna (▶Fig. 18.3).

Occasionally, fractures of the distal ulna are not amendable to repair and are best suited to be treated with arthroplasty. Arthroplasty may also be used for patients with posttraumatic arthritis/contractures of the DRUJ. It is an attractive option due to the unpredictable results of soft-tissue stabilization procedures. Arthroplasty procedures offer the benefit of restoring load transmission and preventing radioulnar impingement. Various implants are available such as total ulnar head replacements with or without a collar partial ulnar head replacement, unlinked total DRUJ arthroplasty, and linked DRUJ arthroplasty.

The dorsal approach as described above is utilized for ulnar head arthroplasty. If a malunited distal radius is encountered then a corrective osteotomy should be done at the same time of the arthroplasty. Regardless of the type of implant used, soft-tissue tensioning without overstuffing the joint must be balanced. Once the head is exposed, Hohmann retractors are placed beneath the ulnar shaft to present the canal and serial reamers are used to prepare the canal. A cutting guide is placed on the reamer and the ulnar head is resected using a sagittal saw. Once the head is resected, it is measured and trial implants are inserted to find the appropriate size. The DRUJ capsule and retinaculum are then closed in layers.

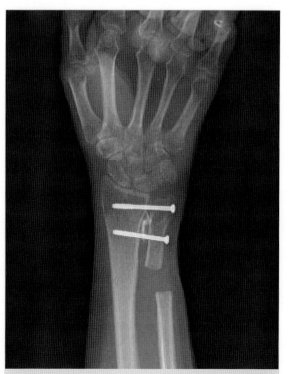

Fig. 18.3 Sauve-Kapandji technique for salvage of the distal radioulnar joint (DRUJ).

18.4 Results

Frykman reported that 61% of all distal radius fractures had concomitant ulnar styloid fracture.[2] Satisfactory outcomes have been demonstrated in ulnar styloid fractures, and fractures that go on to nonunion often have not demonstrated postoperative ulnar-sided wrist pain when instability is not present.[3] However, it is critical to evaluate the DRUJ for stability in these injuries as an unstable joint affects outcomes. If the radioulnar ligament is attached to the fracture, then the joint will demonstrate instability. If fractures through the base of the ulnar styloid are displaced more than 2 mm, then operative intervention may be necessary whereas fractures through the tip are more likely to be stable.[1] Radial translation of the fractured ulna indicates detachment of the radioulnar ligament which often causes instability of the DRUJ. Regardless of the of the method of treatment, fracture union is not always consistently achieved but a fibrous union with adequate position is generally consistent with resolution of symptoms and DRUJ instability. Newer studies have evaluated radial lengthening for DRUJ instability and the results have been promising; however, there are no long-term outcomes at this point for the technique.[4]

Sauve-Kapandji procedures are effective for malunited distal radius and ulna fractures. Guo et al looked at 15 patients with posttraumatic arthritis and found that 13 patients had excellent results and there were no major complications.[5] Taleisnik reported on 24 patients with elimination of pain, few complications, and improved range of motion with the Sauve-Kapandji procedure and very few complications regarding the proximal stump[6] while Stern has reported unpredictable results.[7]

The results of the Darrach procedure are less predictable than the Sauve-Kapandji procedure and results are not as consistent. The procedure is typically used for patients who are low functioning without rheumatoid arthritis and who have incongruous or posttraumatic degenerative changes from a sequalae of an intra-articular fracture. Results are correlated with the stability of the proximal stump in the anterior, posterior, and coronal planes which can lead to substantial weakness and pain. Outcomes are worse in patients who are higher functioning.[8] Dingman evaluated extraperiosteal or subperiosteal resection, the obliquity of the cut, whether to remove the styloid, and the amount of bone resected and found that none of these factors with the exception of the bone resection correlated with patient outcomes. He advised that only the ulna adjacent to the sigmoid notch be resected and that subperiosteal resection was ideal because patients who had regeneration had improved results.[9]

There are no long-term results for ulnar head replacements. Biomechanical studies have shown excellent restoration of kinematics and early clinical results are promising. Van Schoonhoven analyzed the results of 23 patients treated with a ceramic and a titanium stem and found optimistic results which included only two revisions in the cohort and improved symptoms and stability.[10]

Due to the recent development of ulnar head replacements, there are no long-term outcome studies. Much of the literature for ulnar head replacements is in the inflammatory arthritis population which showed substantial improvements in pain and range of motion.[11] Studies have shown that the index procedure affects outcomes, as primary arthroplasty has superior results than arthroplasty after previous reconstructive procedures. Lack of soft-tissue constraints prevents use of standard ulnar head arthroplasties and linked prosthesis may be utilized. Again, there are only few outcome studies on linked prosthesis but early studies are promising. Studies have shown good outcomes with few complications and no implant failures.[12] Long-term follow-up studies need to be completed to understand survivorship and complications.

18.5 Pitfalls

The most preventable pitfall in ulnar fractures is failure to recognize the instability. If it is adequately diagnosed and treated, then patients typically have good outcomes. Failure to stabilize the proximal stump in distal ulnar replacements can lead to complications including impingement and tendon ruptures. Partial ulnar head replacements are contraindicated in patients with substantial ulnar positive variance and in patients with previous ulnar head resections. It is critical to evaluate the soft-tissue constraints as if there is substantial tissue loss than unconstrained ulnar head replacements will lack stability and constrained arthroplasties should be used.

Tips and Tricks

Ulnar styloid:
- Splinting in supination for 6 weeks often leads to good outcomes and stability. If further stabilization is needed, then K-wires or compression screws may be successfully used

Ulnar head:
- K-wire fixation often provides acceptable stabilization but plate fixation may be necessary for comminuted fractures

Ulnar shaft:
- Low profile plates often provide adequate fixation and if placed correctly maybe resolve asymptomatic implant and fracture union

Sauve-Kapandji:
- Stabilizing the ulna proximal to the fusion site may prevent future complications

Darrach:
- Cut the distal ulna obliquely from proximal ulnar to distal radial. Place a convergence stress on the ulna to see if it impinges on the radius

Distal ulna arthroplasty:
- Proper soft-tissue balancing and constraint are needed for successful outcomes

18.6 Conclusion

Distal ulna fractures are commonly encountered in conjunction with distal radius fractures. In the presence of instability, untreated fractures lead to worse outcomes and persistent symptoms that may require additional procedures. Fractures of the distal ulna may be classified as ulnar styloid, head, and metaphysis fractures. If fractures are not treated appropriately, they may go on to progress to nonunions or malunions. Treatment depends on the type of injury but methods of fixation include K-wires, plates, and compression screws. If a malunion or nonunion develops then salvage procedures, such as the Sauve-Kapandji procedure and the Darrach procedure, may be utilized. Sometimes fracture patterns are highly comminuted and not amendable to repair so ulnar head arthroplasty is used primarily. If salvage procedures fail then ulnar head arthroplasties can be attempted for future salvage. Overall, outcomes are promising for properly treated ulna fractures. Long-term studies are lacking for ulnar head arthroplasty implants but early studies are promising.

References

[1] May MM, Lawton JN, Blazar PE. Ulnar styloid fractures associated with distal radius fractures: incidence and implications for distal radioulnar joint instability. J Hand Surg Am 2002;27(6):965–971

[2] Frykman G. Fracture of the distal radius including sequelae—shoulder-hand-finger syndrome, disturbance in the distal radio-ulnar joint and impairment of nerve function. A clinical and experimental study. Acta Orthop Scand 1967; (Suppl 108):3

[3] Ozasa Y, Iba K, Oki G, Sonoda T, Yamashita T, Wada T. Nonunion of the ulnar styloid associated with distal radius malunion. J Hand Surg Am 2013;38(3):526–531

[4] Wang JP, Huang HK, Fufa D. Radial distraction to stabilize distal radioulnar joint in distal radius fixation. J Hand Surg Am 2018;43(5):493.e1–493.e4

[5] Guo Z, Wang Y, Zhang Y. Modified Sauve-Kapandji procedure for patients with old fractures of the distal radius. Open Med (Wars) 2017;12:417–423

[6] Taleisnik J. The Sauvé-Kapandji procedure. Clin Orthop Relat Res 1992; (275):110–123

[7] George MS, Kiefhaber TR, Stern PJ. The Sauve-Kapandji procedure and the Darrach procedure for distal radio-ulnar joint dysfunction after Colles' fracture. J Hand Surg [Br] 2004;29(6):608–613

[8] Hartz CR, Beckenbaugh RD. Long-term results of resection of the distal ulna for post-traumatic conditions. J Trauma 1979;19(4):219–226

[9] Dingman PV. Resection of the distal end of the ulna (Darrach operation); an end result study of twenty four cases. J Bone Joint Surg Am 1952;34 A(4):893–900

[10] van Schoonhoven J, Fernandez DL, Bowers WH, Herbert TJ. Salvage of failed resection arthroplasties of the distal radioulnar joint using a new ulnar head prosthesis. J Hand Surg Am 2000;25(3):438–446

[11] Galvis EJ, Pessa J, Scheker LR. Total joint arthroplasty of the distal radioulnar joint for rheumatoid arthritis. J Hand Surg Am 2014;39(9):1699–1704

[12] Kachooei AR, Chase SM, Jupiter JB. Outcome assessment after Aptis distal radioulnar joint (DRUJ) implant arthroplasty. Arch Bone Jt Surg 2014;2(3):180–184

19 Distal Radioulnar Joint Instability Associated with Distal Radius Fractures

Shohei Omokawa, Takamasa Shimizu, Kenji Kawamura, Tadanobu Onishi

Abstract

This chapter describes the pathomechanics, diagnosis, and treatment protocol of distal radioulnar joint (DRUJ) instability associated with distal radius fractures. The pathomechanics consist of: (1) rupture of the deep ligamentous portion of the triangular fibrocartilage complex (TFCC), (2) extra-articular metaphyseal displacement of the distal radius, (3) intra-articular step in the sigmoid notch, and (4) displaced ulnar styloid base fractures. Pre- and intraoperative assessments can be used to diagnose accompanying TFCC tears and DRUJ instability. DRUJ widening (> 4 mm) on prereduction posteroanterior view is an indicator of joint instability, and manual stress testing after distal radius fixation provides a practical screening test to differentiate the degree of DRUJ instability. Incomplete metaphyseal reduction of the distal radius does lead to DRUJ instability. The arthroscopic hook test at the radiocarpal joint can diagnose foveal detachment injury of the TFCC, and DRUJ arthroscopy with a 1.9-mm scope provides direct visualization of the ulnar attachment site for the radioulnar ligaments, which is deep ligamentous portion of the TFCC. DRUJ arthroscopy can also be used to assess the presence of articular step-off at the sigmoid notch. In the case where accompanying complete ligamentous tear of the TFCC is confirmed, we recommend open or arthroscopic repair of the torn ligament. In the case of a displaced ulnar styloid base fracture after accurate reduction of distal radius fractures, we recommend fixation of the fracture by a compression device (K-wire and wiring). Partial ligamentous tear of the TFCC can be treated by postoperative immobilization of upper arm casting for 3 weeks.

Keywords: distal radioulnar joint, instability, distal radius fractures

19.1 Introduction

A tear in the triangular fibrocartilage complex (TFCC) is the most frequent soft-tissue injury associated with fractures of the distal radius, and rupture of the deep ligamentous portion of the TFCC is considered to contribute to instability of the distal radioulnar joint (DRUJ).[1,2,3,4,5,6,7] Moreover, displacement of the fracture fragment(s) can affect the stability of the DRUJ. Extra-articular malalignment of the distal radius[8,9,10,11,12] and intra-articular step in the sigmoid notch[13,14] can change DRUJ kinematics, leading to DRUJ instability.

The purpose of this chapter is to describe the pathomechanics of DRUJ instability associated with distal radius fractures and discuss the strategies for evaluating and treating patients with acute or chronic instability of the DRUJ.

19.2 Pathomechanics of DRUJ Instability

19.2.1 Metaphyseal Fracture Displacement

Extra-articular malalignment of the distal radius can affect DRUJ kinematics and joint loading mechanics.[8,9,10,11,12] In vivo kinematic studies have found that a malunited distal radius with dorsal metaphyseal angulation can decrease the contact area of the DRUJ and result in lengthening of the dorsal radioulnar ligament (RUL).[8,9] Previous cadaveric studies investigating the effects of metaphyseal malalignment on DRUJ stability[10,11,12] found that 3 mm of radial shortening, 10 degrees of dorsal and volar angulation, or 2 mm of radial translation can lead to DRUJ instability. These biomechanical studies indicate that minimal metaphyseal malalignment can affect DRUJ stability, which may result in ulnar-sided wrist problems. Despite a lack of consensus regarding acceptable metaphyseal alignment, accurate anatomic restoration of the distal radius metaphysis is required to prevent residual DRUJ instability in the treatment of athletes and other active individuals.

19.2.2 Disruptions Accompanying TFCC (Radioulnar Ligament) Tears

The DRUJ is inherently unstable because the curvature of the sigmoid notch of the radius (18 mm) is twice as large as that of the ulnar head (8 mm).[15,16] The ligamentous and capsular structures thus play an important role in stabilizing this complex joint. The deep ligamentous portions of the TFCC are the primary stabilizers of the DRUJ.[7,17] These fibers, which attach to the ulnar fovea and lie on the axis of forearm rotation, are the most isometric and undergo the least length changes during pronosupination. Supplemental stability is provided by superficial fibers of the RUL, which attaches to the base of the ulnar styloid process, and these fibers may have a checkrein effect during forearm rotation. The other ligamentous structures include the ulnocarpal ligament (UCL) complex and the floor of the extensor carpi ulnaris (ECU) tendon sheath (the ulnar collateral ligament).[18,19]

In patients with distal radius fracture, when high-energy forces damage the ligamentous structures of the DRUJ and separate the radius from the ulnar head, the deep ligamentous portion of the TFCC usually detaches from the ulnar fovea with or without ulnar styloid fractures. Complete rupture of the ligaments contributes to DRUJ instability. The incidence of TFCC injury is correlated with intra-articular involvement and the severity of fracture displacement.[3] A long-term prospective cohort study revealed no significant adverse subjective outcomes over the natural course of untreated peripheral TFCC tears in distal radius fractures.[20] However, early recognition and treatment of DRUJ instability may lead to better clinical results rather than attempting to manage chronic instability.[3,21,22]

19.2.3 Ulnar Styloid Fractures

Ulnar styloid fractures accompany 51 to 65% of distal radius fractures, 25% of which result in nonunion.[23,24,25] Because of its close anatomical location with the TFCC, fractures of the ulnar styloid base may also be associated with a tear in the deep portion of the TFCC and result in DRUJ instability. However, previous studies suggest that ulnar styloid fractures are poor prognostic factors for DRUJ instability.[26,27,28,29,30,31] When the distal radius is treated by rigid plate fixation, most ulnar styloid fractures do not affect functional outcomes. Only displaced ulnar styloid base fractures following accurate reduction and rigid fixation of the distal radius may be associated with an unstable DRUJ, because these fractures are often associated with displacement of a torn TFCC.

19.2.4 Intra-articular Displacement of the Sigmoid Notch

In 55 to 65% of displaced distal radius fractures, the fracture line can extend into the sigmoid notch. Most frequently, this is associated with the dorsoulnar corner fragment of the distal radius that is best seen on oblique pronated radiographic views. Coronal plane fractures that enter into the sigmoid notch are difficult to identify on radiographs. Indeed, Rozental et al[13] identified fracture extension into the sigmoid notch in 65% of cases using computed tomography (CT) but it was observed only in 35% cases using radiographs. Nakanishi et al[32] analyzed fracture patterns and the magnitude of displacement in the DRUJ by 3D-CT and reported that 83% of intra-articular distal radius fractures had DRUJ involvement. In their study, 28% of wrists had multiple fragments, and fracture extending into the distal margin of the sigmoid notch was the most common type of longitudinal fracture. The authors suggested that surgical intervention for the DRUJ fragment(s) may be beneficial when there is remarkable intra-articular displacement.

Although previous studies have addressed the issue of intra-articular malunion involving the radiocarpal joint,[33,34] less attention has been paid to the residual gap and step in the DRUJ. Evidence is lacking as to how intra-articular malunion of the DRUJ affects clinical outcomes. When a displaced sigmoid notch fragment is left untreated, residual joint instability or incongruity may lead to degenerative arthritis of the DRUJ, resulting in symptomatic problems.[35,36] Future prospective studies can elucidate how residual malunion of the sigmoid notch would affect functional outcomes.

19.3 Case Presentation

A 27-year-old male sustained a volar rim fracture of the distal radius and underwent open reduction and palmar plating (▶Fig. 19.1). Six months postoperatively, the patient complained of ulnar wrist pain (VAS: 60, DASH 37, PRWE: 65) and restriction in forearm supination. The ulnar fovea and piano key signs of the ulnar head were positive. CT images showed an intra-articular step-off at the sigmoid notch, and we noted dorsal subluxation of the ulna. Magnetic resonance imaging (MRI) revealed a high signal intensity lesion at the ulnar fovea and fluid collection in the DRUJ on fat-suppressed T2-weighted images.

DRUJ arthroscopy was undertaken and was followed by open TFCC repair and resection of a bony prominence in the DRUJ. This bony prominence (intra-articular step-off) obstructed the ulnar head from moving within the palmar aspect of the sigmoid notch and was the cause of limited forearm supination. Marked synovitis and intra-articular scar formation was noted in the DRUJ. The TFCC was reattached to the ulnar fovea using a suture anchoring system. Three years postoperatively, the patient has minimum wrist pain and disability (VAS:7, DASH 10, PRWE: 19) with improvement in forearm supination.

19.4 Diagnosis of Accompanying TFCC Tears and DRUJ Instability

Although it is difficult to accurately diagnose RUL tears, pre- and intraoperative assessments can diagnose accompanying TFCC tears and DRUJ instability. Evidence of preoperative DRUJ widening on prereduction posteroanterior plain radiography can be used to identify DRUJ instability. Manual stress testing after distal radius fixation can provide a practical screening test to differentiate DRUJ instability. However, surgeons should notice that the most important reason of instability is

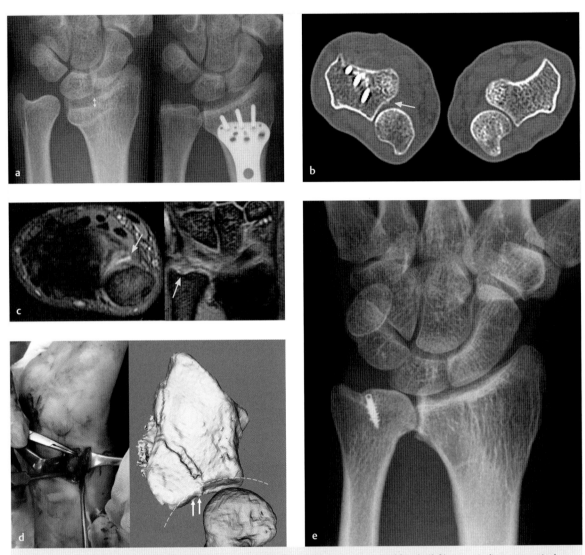

Fig. 19.1 **(a)** Anteroposterior X-ray of a volar rim fracture of the distal radius in a 27-year-old male (*left*). *Arrow* indicates an articular step-off of volar rim fragment. Postsurgical X-ray after open reduction and internal fixation by palmar plating (*right*). **(b)** Computed tomography (CT) image showing an intra-articular step-off at the sigmoid notch and dorsal subluxation of the ulna (*left*) compared with the contralateral side (*right*). *Arrow* indicates a bony prominence in the intra-articular displacement site. **(c)** Magnetic resonance imaging shows fluid collection in the distal radioulnar joint (distal radioulnar joint [DRUJ]; *left arrow*) and a high signal intensity lesion at the ulnar fovea (*right arrow*) on fat-suppressed T2-weighted images. **(d)** Open triangular fibrocartilage complex (TFCC) repair and resection of the bony prominence in the DRUJ (*left*). *Arrows* in the CT image (*right*) indicate a bony prominence obstructing the ulnar head from moving into the palmar aspect of the sigmoid notch during forearm supination. **(e)** Postoperative X-ray showing reattachment of the TFCC to the ulnar fovea using a suture anchoring system.

incomplete metaphyseal reduction of the distal radius fractures. Not only residual shortening and dorsal tilt angle, but radial translation of the distal fragment can also lead to DRUJ instability.[37]

The arthroscopic hook test at the radiocarpal joint can be used to accurately diagnose foveal detachment injury of the TFCC. Finally, DRUJ arthroscopy can provide direct visualization of the RUL attachment to the ulna. Here, we outline these preoperative and intraoperative assessments in detail.

19.4.1 Preoperative Assessment

Plain X-Ray

Fujitani et al[38] prospectively treated patients with unstable distal radius fractures with the volar locking plating system. Complete RUL tears representing DRUJ instability were present in 11 (6.7%) of 163 distal radius fracture cases. Using a multivariate logistic regression analysis, the authors identified a radiographic finding of normalized DRUJ gap as a significant risk factor, with the relative risk of instability increasing by 50% when the ratio of DRUJ widening increases by 1%. A cutoff value of 15% for the normalized gap showed the highest diagnostic accuracy rate. Because the normalized DRUJ gap was calculated as the fraction of the DRUJ gap distance relative to the radioulnar width of the proximal fracture fragment, the substantial DRUJ gap was equivalent to 3.0 mm in the patient who had 20 mm of the radioulnar width of the proximal fracture fragment ($20 \times 0.15 = 3.0$ mm). The authors found that a 1-mm increase in the DRUJ gap increases the risk of RUL tear by five times (▶Fig. 19.2 and ▶Fig. 19.3).

CT and CT Arthrography

As described above, 3D-CT can provide a precise evaluation of fractures extending into the sigmoid notch. Although CT can be used to evaluate DRUJ congruency,[13,32] the normal range for DRUJ translation and joint congruity vary substantially among patients, and this can make it difficult to use CT to evaluate symptomatic patients.[39,40,41] Moritomo et al[42] classified TFCC foveal lesions based on CT arthrography in the radial plane. The authors showed that, for the detection of foveal tears, CT arthrography had high specificity (90 and 100%) and positive predictive value (89 and 100%) for type 3 (a roundish defect at the fovea) and type 4 (a large defect at the overall ulnar insertion) tears, respectively, whereas the sensitivity was only 35% for type 3 tears and 22% for type 4 tears. They concluded that radial plane CT arthrography can enhance the specificity of tear detection as compared with conventional methods.

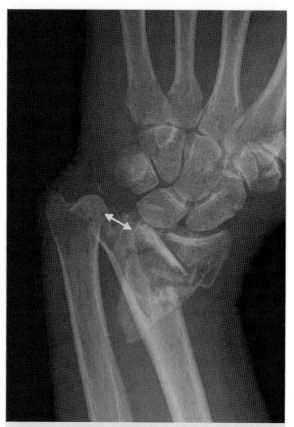

Fig. 19.2 Posteroanterior (PA) X-ray image indicating distal radioulnar joint (DRUJ) widening (*arrow*). A DRUJ gap larger than 4 mm is indicative of a radioulnar ligament (RUL) tear.

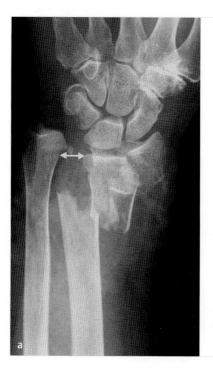
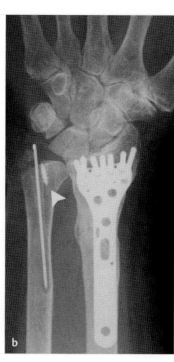

Fig. 19.3 (a) Preoperative posteroanterior (PA) view indicating a widening of distal radioulnar joint (DRUJ) (*arrow*).
(b) Postoperative PA view demonstrating open reduction and plating associated with suturing of radioulnar ligaments by anchoring system (*arrow head*).

Magnetic Resonance Imaging

MRI can be used to evaluate ligamentous tears in the TFCC and the presence of focal lesions at the ulnar fovea, defined as a high signal intensity in the coronal plane on fat saturated T2-weighted images.[43] However, diagnostic test sensitivities and specificities are variable across studies, ranging from 17 to 94% and from 75 to 94%, respectively.[44,45,46,47] The absence of continuity of a low-signal band between the rim of the radius and the ulnar fovea may distinguish complete from partial TFCC ligament tears.

Subluxation of the ulnar head can predict RUL tears on transaxial MRIs with the wrist in pronation. A retrospective study evaluating ulnar head subluxation in patients with foveal TFCC tears revealed a mean dorsal subluxation of 16%, whereas the control subjects had a subluxation of 4%.[48]

19.4.2 Intraoperative Assessment

Provocative Test

Preanesthetic Assessment (Ulnar Foveal Sign)

The ulnar fovea is the depression between the ulnar styloid base and the flexor carpi ulnaris tendon, and it is the deep portion to which the TFCC attaches. When there is no ulnar styloid fracture, a positive ulnar fovea sign (exquisite tenderness in the ulnar fovea) may suggest a TFCC foveal tear; the degree of tenderness can be compared with the contralateral side. The sensitivity of detecting foveal disruptions and/or ulnotriquetral ligament injuries using the ulnar foveal sign is 95%, and its specificity is 87%.[49]

Postplating Assessment (DRUJ Ballottement)

Once the radius fracture is fixed by plate fixation, surgeons can then assess DRUJ instability by manual stress tests. A previous biomechanical study using cadaveric wrists demonstrated that, as compared with other manual stress tests, the DRUJ ballottement test, was the most accurate for evaluating instability.[50] The DRUJ ballottement test is a passive mobility test that examines dorso-palmar laxity of the DRUJ with the forearm in neutral rotation.[51,52] The sensitivity of the DRUJ ballottement test as a means of diagnosing a complete peripheral tear of the TFCC is 59% and the specificity is 96%.[2]

Nakamura[53] proposed criteria for assessing DRUJ instability using the DRUJ ballottement test. Instability is rated as a grade 3 when there is gross instability without end point in both the palmar and dorsal directions. Grade 2 instability is when the examiner identifies instability with a lack of end point in either palmar or dorsal direction, and grade 1 instability is when the

instability of the affected side is greater than that of the contralateral side with solid end points. Grade 2 and 3 instability may suggest complete RUL tears. Onishi et al[54] recommend that the carpal bones should be manually held against the radius during the ballottement test to improve accuracy and reliability; this was confirmed in their biomechanical study investigating the reliability of the DRUJ ballottement test using cadaveric specimens (▶Fig. 19.4).

Provocative tests to the DRUJ conducted separately during forearm pronation or supination can detect which part of the RUL (palmar or dorsal part) is disrupted. When abnormal translation of the ulnar head to the palmar side is positive during maximum forearm supination, a tear in the dorsal deep part of the RUL is suspected, and when dorsal translation during maximum pronation is positive, a palmar deep RUL tear is suspected.[17] A previous cadaveric biomechanical study[55] revealed that wrist position significantly influenced DRUJ laxity: the DRUJ was more stable in wrist extension than in a neutral position before UCL

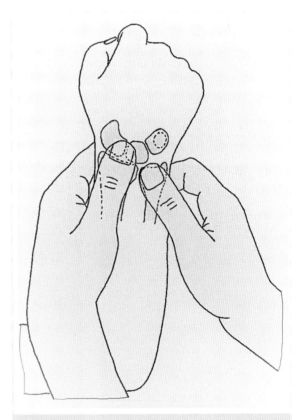

Fig. 19.4 Schematic diagram demonstrating distal radioulnar joint (DRUJ) ballottement test. Note that examiner holds the radiocarpal unit by one hand and mobilizes the ulna by the other hand.

sectioning. After UCL sectioning, there were no significant differences in laxity. These results suggest that the ballottement test in wrist extension may detect UCL tears. After sectioning the RUL, DRUJ laxity in radial deviation was significantly lower than when in a neutral position. After sectioning the ECU floor, there were no significant differences. The DRUJ is stabilized in radial deviation due to tightening of the ECU floor. Thus, the ballottement test with the wrist in radial deviation may also be used to detect disruption to the ECU floor. When an examiner identifies DRUJ laxity during testing conducted with the wrist in radial deviation, a tear in the ECU floor can be suspected.

Arthroscopy

Radiocarpal Arthroscopy

A tear in the foveal attachment site of the TFCC (foveal lesion) can be indirectly assessed using radiocarpal arthroscopy. Based on a cadaveric study, the hook test seems to be highly sensitive, specific, and reliable for the diagnosis of TFCC foveal detachment.[56] This and two other tests are discussed further.

- *Trampoline sign*: The trampoline test, described by Hermansdorfer and Kleinman,[56] examines the elasticity of the articular disc. The test is performed with a probe in the 4–5 or 6R portal and the arthroscope in the 3–4 portal. The elasticity of the articular disc is tested with the probe by applying a compressive load to the TFCC, and a positive test is the loss of normal tissue tautness and a "trampoline effect." A cadaveric assessment showed that the interobserver reliability Cohen kappa for the trampoline test is low (0.16), and the sensitivity and specificity for diagnosing foveal detachment are 43 and 83%, respectively.
- *Hook test*: The arthroscopic hook test, described by Ruch et al,[5] applies a radially directed traction force to the prestyloid recess of the TFCC by hooking a probe in the 6R portal. A positive hook test is judged as excessive movement of the TFCC disc proper by the probe. A cadaveric assessment revealed that the hook test has high sensitivity and specificity for isolated foveal detachment diagnoses (90 and 90%, respectively), and an interobserver reliability Cohen kappa of 0.87.
- *Floating sign*: The floating sign, described Takeuchi and Fujio,[57] applies a suction force to the TFCC disc using an arthroscopic full-radius shaver. A positive finding is judged as floating of the TFCC disc proper during suction. The authors reported the test sensitivity at 98%, specificity at 91%, and interobserver reliability Cohen kappa at 0.87.

DRUJ Arthroscopy

DRUJ arthroscopy with a 1.9-mm arthroscope directly visualizes the undersurface of the TFCC and can diagnose foveal tears.[58,59] Once the 1.9-mm arthroscope is inserted into the joint, the TFCC disc proper can be lifted over the ulnar head using a 21-G needle to create space between the disc proper and the ulnar head, and to observe the RUL at the foveal insertion site. When the RUL is torn, the remnant of the torn ligament may be retracted to the palmar aspect of the ulnar head (▶ Fig. 19.5). Surgeons can observe the articular surface of the sigmoid notch to confirm displacement of the fracture line and the presence of any free fracture fragments in the DRUJ.

19.4.3 DRUJ Arthrography

Shigematsu et al[60] reported the efficacy of intraoperative DRUJ arthrography in patients with distal radius fractures. The diagnostic accuracy for complete RUL tears was 77%, with a positive finding defined as the presence of contrast medium pooling in the ulnar fovea.

19.5 Treatment for TFCC Tears and DRUJ Instability

Although untreated peripheral TFCC tears are not a cause of adverse outcomes over the long term, early recognition

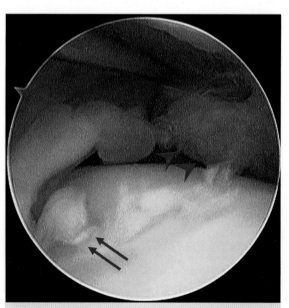

Fig. 19.5 Abnormal arthroscopic view of the distal radioulnar joint (DRUJ) indicates complete detachment of the radioulnar ligament (RUL). *Arrows* show the ulnar fovea and torn ligament. *Arrow heads* depict the retracted remnant of the torn palmar RUL.

and treatment of acute DRUJ instability may lead to better clinical results rather than attempting to manage chronic instability.[61] If surgeons can confirm displaced complete RUL tears during distal radius fracture surgeries, primary TFCC repair may be an adequate treatment option to enhance patient's postoperative recovery during hand therapy.

19.5.1 Authors' Preferred Method

Complete Ligamentous Tear

Refer to Fig. 19.6 for treatment strategy. When the DRUJ gap is more than 4 mm on initial posteroanterior wrist radiographs, surgeons may suspect a complete RUL tear. If a positive diagnosis of complete RUL tear at the fovea can be made by MRI, we suggest suturing the torn ligament. During the intraoperative manual stress test, when the DRUJ is grossly unstable without end point, we suggest using radiocarpal or DRUJ arthroscopy to confirm complete ligamentous tear of the TFCC. When confirmed, we recommend opening the joint to repair the RUL or arthroscopically suturing the torn ligament. When the injury is accompanied by a displaced ulnar styloid base fracture, we recommend fixing the fracture site using a Kirschner wire and compression wire. Postoperative upper arm casting for 3 weeks and the use of a wrist brace for 2 months is also recommended.

Partial Ligamentous Tear of TFCC

When the DRUJ is unstable but with end point during the manual stress test after rigid distal radius fixation, we suggest using radiocarpal or DRUJ arthroscopy to confirm a partial ligamentous tear of the TFCC. When confirmed, we recommend upper arm casting for 3 weeks and the use of a wrist brace for 2 months.

19.6 Summary

- The pathomechanics of DRUJ instability associated with distal radius fractures consists of: (1) rupture of the deep ligamentous portion of the TFCC, (2) extra-articular metaphyseal displacement of the distal radius, (3) intra-articular step in the sigmoid notch, and (4) displaced ulnar styloid base fractures.
- Although it is difficult to accurately diagnose RUL tears, pre- and intraoperative assessments can be used to diagnose accompanying TFCC tears and DRUJ instability. DRUJ widening (> 4 mm) on prereduction posteroanterior view is an indicator of joint instability, and manual stress testing after distal radius fixation provides a practical screening test to differentiate the degree of DRUJ instability. Incomplete metaphyseal reduction of the distal radius does lead to DRUJ instability. The arthroscopic hook test at the radiocarpal joint can accurately diagnose foveal detachment injury of the TFCC, and DRUJ arthroscopy provides direct visualization of the ulnar attachment site for the RUL.
- In the case where accompanying complete ligamentous tear of the TFCC is confirmed, we recommend open or arthroscopic repair of the torn ligament. In the case of a displaced ulnar styloid base fracture, we recommend fixation of the fracture by a compression device.

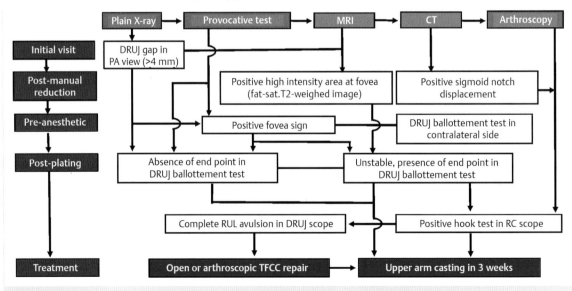

Fig. 19.6 Flow chart of a treatment strategy for acute DRUJ instability associated with distal radius fracture.

References

[1] Geissler WB, Freeland AE, Savoie FH, McIntyre LW, Whipple TL. Intracarpal soft-tissue lesions associated with an intra-articular fracture of the distal end of the radius. J Bone Joint Surg Am 1996;78(3):357–365

[2] Lindau T, Adlercreutz C, Aspenberg P. Peripheral tears of the triangular fibrocartilage complex cause distal radioulnar joint instability after distal radial fractures. J Hand Surg Am 2000;25(3):464–468

[3] Richards RS, Bennett JD, Roth JH, Milne K Jr. Arthroscopic diagnosis of intra-articular soft tissue injuries associated with distal radial fractures. J Hand Surg Am 1997;22(5):772–776

[4] Varitimidis SE, Basdekis GK, Dailiana ZH, Hantes ME, Bargiotas K, Malizos K. Treatment of intra-articular fractures of the distal radius: fluoroscopic or arthroscopic reduction? J Bone Joint Surg Br 2008;90(6):778–785

[5] Ruch DS, Yang CC, Smith BP. Results of acute arthroscopically repaired triangular fibrocartilage complex injuries associated with intra-articular distal radius fractures. Arthroscopy 2003;19(5):511–516

[6] Böhringer G, Schädel-Höpfner M, Junge A, Gotzen L. Primary arthroscopic treatment of TFCC tears in fractures of the distal radius Handchir Mikrochir Plast Chir 2001;33(4):245–251

[7] Hagert E, Hagert CG. Understanding stability of the distal radioulnar joint through an understanding of its anatomy. Hand Clin 2010;26(4):459–466

[8] Xing SG, Chen YR, Xie RG, Tang JB. In vivo contact characteristics of distal radioulnar joint with malunited distal radius during wrist motion. J Hand Surg Am 2015;40(11):2243–2248

[9] Crisco JJ, Moore DC, Marai GE, et al. Effects of distal radius malunion on distal radioulnar joint mechanics—an in vivo study. J Orthop Res 2007;25(4):547–555

[10] Saito T, Nakamura T, Nagura T, Nishiwaki M, Sato K, Toyama Y. The effects of dorsally angulated distal radius fractures on distal radioulnar joint stability: a biomechanical study. J Hand Surg Eur Vol 2013;38(7):739–745

[11] Nishiwaki M, Welsh M, Gammon B, Ferreira LM, Johnson JA, King GJ. Volar subluxation of the ulnar head in dorsal translation deformities of distal radius fractures: an in vitro biomechanical study. J Orthop Trauma 2015;29(6):295–300

[12] Dy CJ, Jang E, Taylor SA, Meyers KN, Wolfe SW. The impact of coronal alignment on distal radioulnar joint stability following distal radius fracture. J Hand Surg Am 2014;39(7):1264–1272

[13] Rozental TD, Bozentka DJ, Katz MA, Steinberg DR, Beredjiklian PK. Evaluation of the sigmoid notch with computed tomography following intra-articular distal radius fracture. J Hand Surg Am 2001;26(2):244–251

[14] Omokawa S, Abe Y, Imatani J, Moritomo H, Suzuki D, Onishi T. Treatment of intra-articular distal radius fractures. Hand Clin 2017;33(3):529–543

[15] Daneshvar P, Willing R, Pahuta M, Grewal R, King GJ. Osseous anatomy of the distal radioulnar joint: an assessment using 3-dimensional modeling and clinical implications. J Hand Surg Am 2016;41(11):1071–1079

[16] De Smet L, Fabry G. Orientation of the sigmoid notch of the distal radius: determination of different types of the distal radioulnar joint. Acta Orthop Belg 1993;59(3):269–272

[17] Kleinman WB. Stability of the distal radioulna joint: biomechanics, pathophysiology, physical diagnosis, and restoration of function what we have learned in 25 years. J Hand Surg Am 2007;32(7):1086–1106

[18] Nakamura T, Yabe Y, Horiuchi Y. Functional anatomy of the triangular fibrocartilage complex. J Hand Surg [Br] 1996;21(5):581–586

[19] Moritomo H. Anatomy and clinical relevance of the ulnocarpal ligament. J Wrist Surg 2013;2(2):186–189

[20] Mrkonjic A, Geijer M, Lindau T, Tägil M. The natural course of traumatic triangular fibrocartilage complex tears in distal radial fractures: a 13–15 year follow-up of arthroscopically diagnosed but untreated injuries. J Hand Surg Am 2012;37(8):1555–1560

[21] Geissler WB, Fernandez DL, Lamey DM. Distal radioulnar joint injuries associated with fractures of the distal radius. Clin Orthop Relat Res 1996(327):135–146

[22] May MM, Lawton JN, Blazar PE. Ulnar styloid fractures associated with distal radius fractures: incidence and implications for distal radioulnar joint instability. J Hand Surg Am 2002;27(6):965–971

[23] Sammer DM, Shah HM, Shauver MJ, Chung KC. The effect of ulnar styloid fractures on patient-rated outcomes after volar locking plating of distal radius fractures. J Hand Surg Am 2009;34(9):1595–1602

[24] Buijze GA, Ring D. Clinical impact of united versus nonunited fractures of the proximal half of the ulnar styloid following volar plate fixation of the distal radius. J Hand Surg Am 2010;35(2):223–227

[25] Ozasa Y, Iba K, Oki G, Sonoda T, Yamashita T, Wada T. Nonunion of the ulnar styloid associated with distal radius malunion. J Hand Surg Am 2013;38(3):526–531

[26] Zenke Y, Sakai A, Oshige T, Moritani S, Nakamura T. The effect of an associated ulnar styloid fracture on the outcome after fixation of a fracture of the distal radius. J Bone Joint Surg Br 2009;91(1):102–107

[27] Kim JK, Koh YD, Do NH. Should an ulnar styloid fracture be fixed following volar plate fixation of a distal radial fracture? J Bone Joint Surg Am 2010;92(1):1–6

[28] Almedghio S, Arshad MS, Almari F, Chakrabarti I. Effects of ulnar styloid fractures on unstable distal radius fracture outcomes: a systematic review of comparative studies. J Wrist Surg 2018;7(2):172–181

[29] Mulders MAM, Fuhri Snethlage LJ, de Muinck Keizer RO, Goslings JC, Schep NWL. Functional outcomes of distal radius fractures with and without ulnar styloid fractures: a meta-analysis. J Hand Surg Eur Vol 2018;43(2):150–157

[30] Wijffels MM, Keizer J, Buijze GA, et al. Ulnar styloid process nonunion and outcome in patients with a distal radius fracture: a meta-analysis of comparative clinical trials. Injury 2014;45(12):1889–1895

[31] Sawada H, Shinohara T, Natsume T, Hirata H. Clinical effects of internal fixation for ulnar styloid fractures associated with distal radius fractures: a matched case-control study. J Orthop Sci 2016;21(6):745–748

[32] Nakanishi Y, Omokawa S, Shimizu T, Nakano K, Kira T, Tanaka Y. Intra-articular distal radius fractures involving the distal radioulnar joint (DRUJ): three dimensional computed tomography-based classification. J Orthop Sci 2013;18(5):788–792

[33] Forward DP, Davis TR, Sithole JS. Do young patients with malunited fractures of the distal radius inevitably develop symptomatic post-traumatic osteoarthritis? J Bone Joint Surg Br 2008;90(5):629–637

[34] Mehta JA, Bain GI, Heptinstall RJ. Anatomical reduction of intra-articular fractures of the distal radius. An arthroscopically-assisted approach. J Bone Joint Surg Br 2000;82(1):79–86

[35] Del Piñal F, Studer A, Thams C, Moraleda E. Sigmoid notch reconstruction and limited carpal arthrodesis for a severely comminuted distal radius malunion: case report. J Hand Surg Am 2012;37(3):481–485

[36] del Piñal F, Klausmeyer M, Moraleda E, et al. Vascularized graft from the metatarsal base for reconstructing major osteochondral distal radius defects. J Hand Surg Am 2013;38(10):1883–1895

[37] Ross M, Allen L, Couzens GB. Correction of residual radial translation of the distal fragment in distal radius fracture open reduction. J Hand Surg Am 2015;40(12):2465–2470

[38] Fujitani R, Omokawa S, Akahane M, Iida A, Ono H, Tanaka Y. Predictors of distal radioulnar joint instability in distal radius fractures. J Hand Surg Am 2011;36(12):1919–1925

[39] Park MJ, Kim JP. Reliability and normal values of various computed tomography methods for quantifying distal radioulnar joint translation. J Bone Joint Surg Am 2008;90(1):145–153

[40] Lo IK, MacDermid JC, Bennett JD, Bogoch E, King GJ. The radioulnar ratio: a new method of quantifying distal radioulnar joint subluxation. J Hand Surg Am 2001;26(2):236–243

[41] Wechsler RJ, Wehbe MA, Rifkin MD, Edeiken J, Branch HM. Computed tomography diagnosis of distal radioulnar subluxation. Skeletal Radiol 1987;16(1):1–5

[42] Moritomo H, Arimitsu S, Kubo N, Masatomi T, Yukioka M. Computed tomography arthrography using a radial plane view for the detection of triangular fibrocartilage complex foveal tears. J Hand Surg Am 2015;40(2):245–251

[43] Zimmermann R, Rudisch A, Fritz D, Gschwentner M, Arora R. MR imaging for the evaluation of accompanying injuries in cases of distal forearm fractures in children and adolescents. Handchir Mikrochir Plast Chir 2007;39(1):60–67

[44] Oneson SR, Timins ME, Scales LM, Erickson SJ, Chamoy L. MR imaging diagnosis of triangular fibrocartilage pathology with arthroscopic correlation. AJR Am J Roentgenol 1997;168(6):1513–1518

[45] Haims AH, Schweitzer ME, Morrison WB, et al. Limitations of MR imaging in the diagnosis of peripheral tears of the triangular fibrocartilage of the wrist. AJR Am J Roentgenol 2002;178(2):419–422

[46] Blazar PE, Chan PS, Kneeland JB, Leatherwood D, Bozentka DJ, Kowalchick R. The effect of observer experience on magnetic resonance imaging interpretation and localization of triangular fibrocartilage complex lesions. J Hand Surg Am 2001;26(4):742–748

[47] Anderson ML, Skinner JA, Felmlee JP, Berger RA, Amrami KK. Diagnostic comparison of 1.5 Tesla and 3.0 Tesla preoperative MRI of the wrist in patients with ulnar-sided wrist pain. J Hand Surg Am 2008;33(7):1153–1159

[48] Ehman EC, Hayes ML, Berger RA, Felmlee JP, Amrami KK. Subluxation of the distal radioulnar joint as a predictor of foveal triangular fibrocartilage complex tears. J Hand Surg Am 2011;36(11):1780–1784

[49] Tay SC, Tomita K, Berger RA. The "ulnar fovea sign" for defining ulnar wrist pain: an analysis of sensitivity and specificity. J Hand Surg Am 2007;32(4):438–444

[50] Moriya T, Aoki M, Iba K, Ozasa Y, Wada T, Yamashita T. Effect of triangular ligament tears on distal radioulnar joint instability and evaluation of three clinical tests: a biomechanical study. J Hand Surg Eur Vol 2009;34(2):219–223

[51] King G, McMurtry RY. Physical examination of the wrist and hand. In: Gilula LA, Yin Y. eds. Imaging of the Wrist and Hand. Philadelphia: WB Saunders; 1996:5–18

[52] Cooney WP, Bishop AT, Linscheid RL. Physical examination of the wrist. In: Cooney WR, Linscheid RL, Dobyns JH, eds. The Wrist, 1st ed. Philadelphia: Lippincott Williams and Wilkins: 1998:236–261

[53] Nakamura T. Pathology, diagnosis and treatment of distal radioulnar joint instability. J Jpn Orthop Assoc 2008;80(2):90–90

[54] Onishi T, Omokawa S, Iida A, et al. Biomechanical study of distal radioulnar joint ballottement test. J Orthop Res 2017;35(5):1123–1127

[55] Trehan SK, Wall LB, Calfee RP, et al. Arthroscopic diagnosis of the triangular fibrocartilage complex foveal tear: a cadaver assessment. J Hand Surg Am 2018;43(7):680.e1–680.e5

[56] Hermansdorfer JD, Kleinman WB. Management of chronic peripheral tears of the triangular fibrocartilage complex. J Hand Surg Am 1991;16(2):340–346

[57] Takeuchi H, Fujio K. Diagnostic accuracy and reliability of arthroscopic "floating sign" for ulnar foveal avulsion injury of the TFCC. The Journal of Japanese Society for Surgery of the Hand 2014;31(3):173–175

[58] Nakamura T, Matsumura N, Iwamoto T, Sato K, Toyama Y. Arthroscopy of the distal radioulnar joint. Handchir Mikrochir Plast Chir 2014;46(5):295–299

[59] Yamamoto M, Koh S, Tatebe M, et al. Importance of distal radioulnar joint arthroscopy for evaluating the triangular fibrocartilage complex. J Orthop Sci 2010;15(2):210–215

[60] Shigematsu K, Omokawa S, Takaoka T, Suzuki J, Okuda M. Efficacy of DRUJ arthrography for detecting deep portion tears of triangular fibrocartilage complex. The Journal of Japanese Society for Surgery of the Hand 2001;17(5):558–561

[61] Gong HS, Cho HE, Kim J, Kim MB, Lee YH, Baek GH. Surgical treatment of acute distal radioulnar joint instability associated with distal radius fractures. J Hand Surg Eur Vol 2015;40(8):783–789

20 Distal Radius Fracture in the Elderly

Rohit Arora, Markus Gabl

Abstract

Distal radius fractures (DRFs) are typical fractures seen in relatively fit persons with osteoporotic bone. Considering the increasing life expectancy of the elderly population, appropriate management of these fractures is of growing importance. Generally, tolerance for anatomical deviations is higher, mostly due to decreased functional needs. Surgical indication should include factors such as patient's age, functional demand (return to sport activities), patient's comfort (short immobilization time), preinjury daily activity level, lifestyle requirements (cosmetically appearance), current medical conditions, and stage of osteoporosis. If decision for surgery is made, volar locking plate fixation for dorsally displaced DRFs is the appropriate treatment option. Distraction plate, hemiarthroplasty, and initial shortening and palmar plate fixation of DRF with primary Sauve-Kapandji procedure are alternative treatment possibilities.

Keywords: distal radius fracture, osteoporosis, elderly, treatment, geriatric trauma

20.1 Introduction

Distal radius fractures (DRFs) are typical fractures seen in relatively fit persons with osteoporotic bone. Traditionally, DRFs in older patients have been treated with closed reduction and cast immobilization.[1] Considering the increasing life expectancy of the elderly population, appropriate management of these fractures is of growing importance. Restoration of wrist function, allowing a rapid return to an active and independent lifestyle is the major goal of treating elderly.

Decision-making for surgical or nonsurgical approach to osteoporotic DRFs is difficult. These decisions are often made on the basis of data from treatments of much younger patients.[2] Some authors have suggested that unstable DRFs should be managed nonoperatively because fracture reduction and anatomical alignment on X-rays are not correlated with better functional outcomes in older adults. On the other hand, several case series have documented excellent results of internal fixation with very low complication rates of dorsally displaced DRF with the use of locking implants in older population.[3]

The impact on the function of an individual patient is variable and can be difficult to predict. Generally, tolerance for anatomical deviations is higher mostly due to decreased functional needs. DRFs are a good example illustrating how decision-making in older patients should differ considerably:

- Older patients are a heterogeneous group with diverse demands.
- Comorbidities contribute to increased perioperative risk.
- Consequences of malunited fractures are much less predictable and often clinically insignificant (►Fig. 20.1).

20.2 Indications

Currently there is no consensus regarding the best treatment for unstable DRFs in the older population.[4] Decision-making for operative or nonoperative treatment must involve patient's general health condition (e.g., comorbidities, daily activity level, independent living, taking care of somebody) and functional demand (e.g., sports activity, practiced yoga, using walking aids). Some patients require a cosmetically acceptable wrist posture without any visible deformity that should be included in the consideration for further treatment.

Apart from patient-related factors mentioned above, fracture-related factors might conduct to further treatment options. Primary reduction of the fracture is considered to be acceptable when dorsal tilt does not exceed 20 degrees, radial shortening is not more than 3 mm, and intra-articular step-off does not exceed 2 mm.[5] Fracture instability is also defined as a failure to hold the reduced position of the fracture within the forearm cast with a loss of reduction at 1 or 2 weeks. Osteoporosis weakens the metaphyseal bone by decreasing trabecular bone volume.[6] Therefore, osteoporotic DRFs very often show a large metaphyseal defect or void that increases fracture instability.[7] Nesbitt et al reported that the age was the only statistically significant risk factor in predicting secondary displacement and instability while treating DRFs by closed reduction and immobilization. The risk for displacement with an unacceptable radiographic result was found to increase in patients older than 58 years.[8] Sakai et al reported a significant correlation between increasing displacement of distal fracture fragment and lower bone mineral density (BMD).[9]

For palmarly displaced DRFs where the carpus follows the palmar fracture fragment leading to malalignment relative to the forearm shaft, for DRFs combined with distal ulnar fracture and involvement of all three columns that leads to a highly unstable situation, and for open fractures, we recommend standard operative fixation even in older adults.

20.3 Treatment Options

Spanning plate as a treatment option is mentioned in Chapter 10.

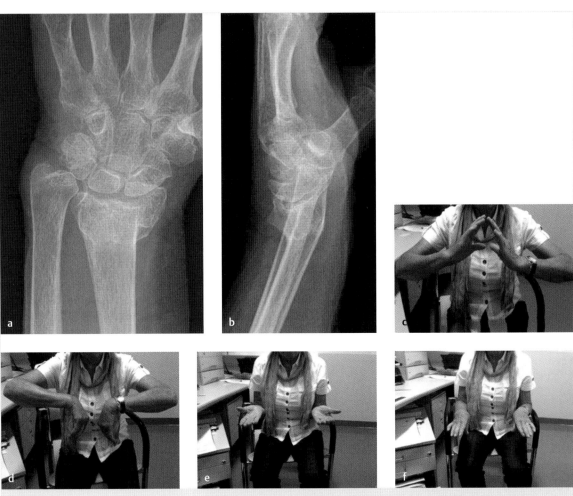

Fig. 20.1 A 77-year-old female with a malunited distal radius fracture (DRF). Anteroposterior (AP) **(a)** and lateral **(b)** X-ray after conservative treatment. **(c–f)** Despite malunion, satisfactory clinical result with good subjective outcome.

20.3.1 Closed Reduction and Cast Immobilization

Current protocol for nonoperative treatment of DRFs includes initial fracture reduction under local or general anesthesia in the emergency department and then immobilization with a below-forearm splint. After the primary swelling has decreased, the slab is converted to a complete below-elbow cast at 1 or 2 weeks. Secondary loss of primary reduction can occur up to 2 weeks after primary closed reduction. In these cases, repeated manipulation, especially in the osteoporotic bone, is insufficient and correlated with the incidence of complex regional pain syndrome (CRPS) type 1 and thus is not advised.[5] In total, the wrist is immobilized in a forearm cast in neutral position of the wrist for 5 weeks. Active and passive finger motion is encouraged early. A therapy program after cast removal including active assisted motion of the wrist and grip strengthening is started at 5 weeks.

20.3.2 Closed Reduction and Percutaneous Pinning

Pinning alone may not be enough to maintain articular and metaphyseal support, as Kirschner wires (K-wires) are not load-bearing devices. In addition, a forearm splint is necessary to neutralize the bending forces across the metaphysis. The wires are left up to 4 weeks and the forearm cast is worn for 6 weeks. Percutaneous pinning is a relatively simple method of fixation that is recommended for reducible extra-articular and simple intra-articular DRFs without metaphyseal comminution and with good bone quality. In multifragmented intra-articular fractures with impacted joint fragments, it is quite difficult to reduce these fragments by percutaneous pinning. Azzopardi et al concluded that percutaneous pinning of unstable, extra-articular DRFs provides only minimal improvement in the radiographic parameters compared with immobilization in a cast alone. This did not correlate with an improved functional outcome in older adults.[10]

20.3.3 External Fixation

External fixation (EF) as treatment option for DRFs was primary reserved for highly unstable and severely comminuted fractures. This technique relies on ligamentotaxis, which indirectly pulls the fracture fragments out to length through longitudinal traction. The joint spanning (wrist bridging) implant with fixation in the radius diaphysis and the metacarpal does not directly address the reduction and maintenance of the dorsal tilt and intra-articular fragments of the distal fracture fragment. The other option of application of EF in DRFs is the nonbridging technique where the distal pins are placed into the distal fracture fragment without spanning the wrist joint. This technique limits joint stiffness and maintains the reconstructed dorsal tilt but is only applicable where there is sufficient space in the distal fragment.

Complications associated with EF are pin-track infection and iatrogenic lesion of the superficial radial nerve. Overdistraction of the wrist joint may lead to CRPS. Usually the EF is applied for 6 weeks. Especially in osteoporotic bone quality with weak hold of the pins, loosening of the pins occurs quite early so they have to be removed before definitive bone healing. Adults with cognitive impairment do not easily tolerate and facilitate compliance with treatment using EF and weight bearing or range of motion (ROM) limitations, making complications due to EF more likely. Considering these issues, we no longer use percutaneous K-wire fixation or external fixation as definitive treatment option for treating unstable DRF in the elderly.

20.3.4 Volar Locking Plate Fixation

Volar locking plates are like an internal fixator unloading the usually comminuted dorsal metaphyseal bone. In a biomechanical study, the volar fixed-angle plate proved efficient in restoring the normal axial force distribution, superior to conventional palmar and dorsal T-plate fixation.[11] The fixed-angle screws lock into the plate and do not rely on engagement of the screw threads in bone leading to better fixation in osteoporotic bone. The other advantage of locking plates is the good subchondral support of the distal fragments even in very short distal fracture fragments. The latest generation of locking plates offer the option of variable locking screws that allow a total angulation of 30 degrees for screw placement.

The most appropriate plates should be selected to correspond with the fracture pattern. There is no single plate that is universally successful or devoid of any potential complications for all types of unstable DRFs, including intra-articular and extra-articular fracture patterns. Fragment-specific fixation and double-plate fixation techniques may be helpful to treat various fracture types, especially intra-articular fractures with a large metaphyseal void (▶ Fig. 20.2).

Surgical Technique

Surgery may be performed under a brachial plexus block or with use of general anesthesia and an upper arm tourniquet. The distal part of the radius is exposed through a Henry palmar approach between the flexor carpi radialis

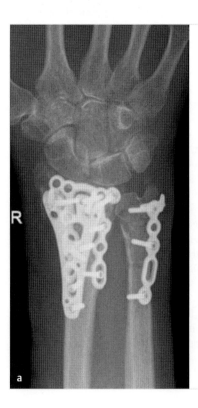
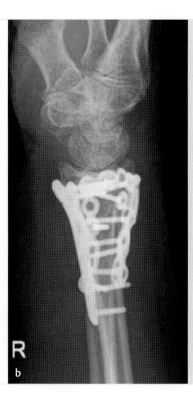

Fig. 20.2 Anteroposterior (AP) **(a)** and lateral **(b)** X-ray after palmar and dorsal plate fixation of the distal radius fracture (DRF). The unstable distal ulna fracture was fixed too to allow immediate postoperative mobilization.

tendon and the radial artery. After the release of the pronator quadratus muscle, the fracture site is exposed. Careful reduction of fracture fragments is performed, as poor bone quality can lead to iatrogenic fractures. Reduction is achieved with the assistance of an image intensifier and the fracture is temporarily stabilized with K-wires. The locking plate is placed on the palmar cortex and is first fixed at the gliding hole to allow appropriate positioning for the image-controlled subchondral placement of the locking screws. Care must be taken to place the plate proximal to the watershed line. In intra-articular fractures, wrist arthroscopy may be used to assess intra-articular steps and associated soft-tissue injuries. In comminuted intra-articular fractures, the locking screws are placed in the most distal subcortical position to act as a subcortical buttress against fracture subsidence. The subcortical bone plate retains greater loading capacity than the osteopenic compressed cancellous metaphyseal bone. Especially with variable locking plate systems, which allow approximately 30 degrees of screw insertion, intra-articular screw placement can be performed quite easily. If fracture instability demands distal placement of hardware, close follow-up investigations and hardware removal should be considered at first sign of flexor tendon irritation. Intraoperatively, the lateral tilt X-ray, with the wrist angulated 20 to 30 degrees, is performed to check the plate and screw position and it may detect intra-articular screw position or very distal plate position. The "dorsal horizon view" (▶ Fig. 20.3) is used to detect excessively long screws penetrating the

dorsal cortex.[12] If possible, the pronator quadratus muscle is reinserted to cover the plate.

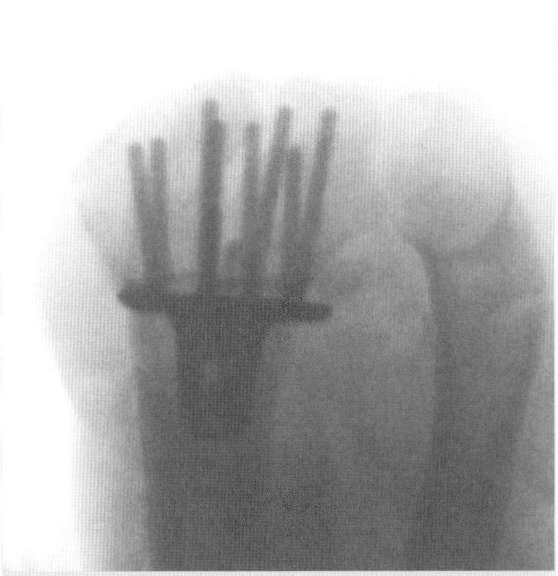

Postoperatively, the wrist is immobilized in a below-the-elbow splint for pain reduction. Active digital ROM is started immediately. Ten days after surgery, the sutures are removed and the wrist is placed in a removable splint for another week. At that time, physiotherapy with active and passive wrist mobilization out of the splint is started. No immobilization is necessary in extra-articular metaphyseal and in simple intra-articular DRFs as a stable fixation can be achieved intraoperatively.

20.3.5 Distal Radius Arthroplasty

Following the concept of primary hemi joint replacement in proximal and distal humeral fractures or neck of femur fractures in older adults, Herzberg et al[13] described the primary use of wrist hemiarthroplasty in multifragmented, impacted, and irreparable acute DRFs in an older cohort. Participants had an average age of 76 years and some comorbidities but were living at home and were independent in activities of daily living (ADLs). Hemiarthroplasty produced earlier return to preinjury independence in daily activities with shorter operative time and fewer complications compared to palmar plating (▶ Fig. 20.4).

20.3.6 Initial Shortening and Palmar Plate Fixation with Primary Sauve-Kapandji Procedure

In a complex DRF associated with a comminuted fracture of the ulna, the restoration of articular anatomy, neutral ulnar variance, and congruity of the distal radioulnar joint are critical to obtaining a good functional result and preventing posttraumatic arthritis. The wound in open fractures is usually close to the ulnar fracture. Thus, there is poor soft-tissue cover at the fracture site. The principles of open fracture management recommend sufficient soft-tissue cover of implants and preservation of the blood supply to bone. Although adjunctive corticocancellous iliac bone grafting in isolated closed DRFs may restore radial length, this is not the case with open fractures because of the need for an additional incision, a longer operation, and the limited amount of bone graft that can be obtained, especially in the elderly. Morbidity at the donor site can be high. In order to overcome these problems, we used internal fixation of the radius with shortening to obtain sufficient bone contact.[14] This concept of shortening is also described in the management of traumatic amputations of the forearm, where shortening of up to 2.5 cm has been reported.[15] In our study, an average forearm shortening of 12 mm showed no statistically significant correlation with ROM, grip strength, pain, disabilities of arm, shoulder and hand (DASH), or Green and O'Brien score.

Fig. 20.3 Skyline view. In this X-ray, palmar screws penetrating dorsal cortex can be detected and if needed changed immediately. The distal radioulnar joint (DRUJ) can be visualized too. In this case, the skyline views show that the palmar ulnar fragment is not addressed adequately.

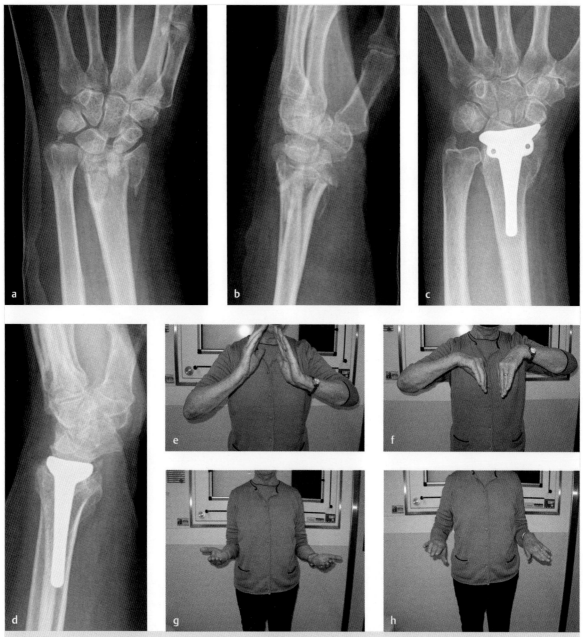

Fig. 20.4 Anteroposterior (AP) **(a)** and lateral **(b)** X-ray showing a multifragmented and irreparable distal radius fracture (DRF) in a 79-year-old female. Postoperative X-ray AP **(c)** and lateral **(d)** showing an implanted hemiprosthesis. **(e–h)** Follow-up at 2 months showing good functional outcome.

Fixation of the shortened radius without bone grafting and leaving the ulnar fracture untreated would cause the late development of posttraumatic arthritis, ulnar-sided wrist pain, distal radioulnar joint (DRUJ) instability, and limited rotation of the forearm. Fixation of the small distal ulnar fracture fragments with shortening to achieve neutral ulnar variance is technically difficult. Because unsatisfactory anatomical restoration of the DRUJ was inevitable, we performed the Sauvé-Kapandji procedure primarily to avoid complications and the need for

a secondary operation.[14] In contrast to a primary Darrach resection, the retained ulnar head provided ulnar-sided abutment to aid stability of the fixed radial fractures.

Instability and pain at the proximal ulnar stump might also be of concern following the Sauvé-Kapandji procedure. By keeping the proximal ulnar stump as long as possible and covering it with pronator quadratus, instability of the ulnar stump was not observed in our study. Symptoms of ulnar impingement are more relevant in manual workers than in elderly patients.

Due to the good clinical and radiological results and minor complications without the need for revision surgery, we believe that plating with shortening of the radius, combined with a primary Sauvé-Kapandji procedure, is a reasonable option for elderly patients with this complex injury (▶ Fig. 20.5).[14]

20.4 Complications

Chung et al[1] reported in a systematic review of the treatment options of DRFs in patients older than 60 years treated with five common techniques, i.e., volar locking plate system, nonbridging EF, bridging EF, percutaneous K-wire

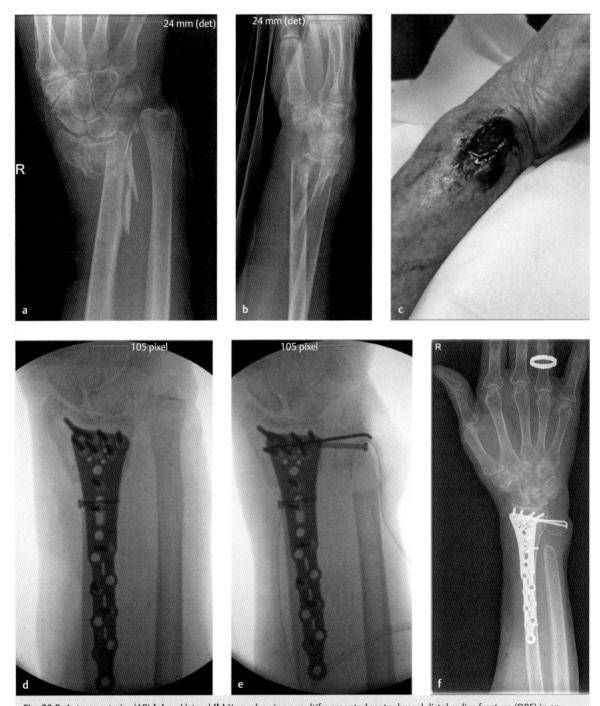

Fig. 20.5 Anteroposterior (AP) **(a)** and lateral **(b)** X-ray showing a multifragmented metaphyseal distal radius fracture (DRF) in an 82-year-old female. **(c)** Ulnar side wound. Intraoperative AP **(d)** showing the DRF plated in shortening with ulna-plus situation. **(e)** To avoid ulna impaction and to be able to close the ulna-sided wound without tension, the decision was made to perform an acute Sauve-Kapandji procedure. Follow-up at 13 months showing AP **(f)** and lateral.

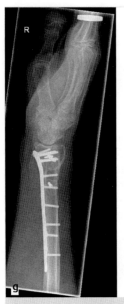
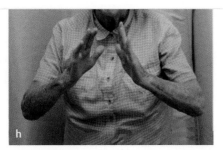
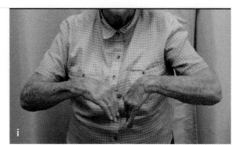
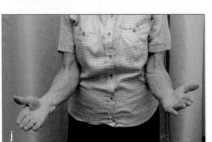
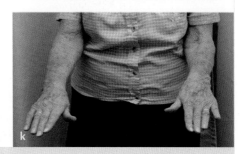

Fig. 20.5 (*Continued*) **(g)** X-rays and clinical results **(h–k)**.

fixation, and cast immobilization. The authors concluded worse radiographic results in the group with cast immobilization. Functional results were not different from those in the operatively treated groups. There were no significant differences for all five treatment groups regarding active ROM, grip strength, or the DASH scores though significantly better radiographic results were noticed in the group treated with volar locking plates. Major complications not requiring reoperation were mostly in the group of bridging EF, whereas major complications requiring secondary surgeries were found in the volar locking plate group.

Hinds et al[16] compared the short-term complication rates in geriatric versus nongeriatric cohorts following plate fixation of DRFs. The authors concluded increased rates of complications related to poor bone quality and poor health status among geriatric patients following osteosynthesis of DRFs.

20.5 Conclusion

For dorsally displaced DRFs, we published a prospective trial including 73 patients with a displaced and unstable DRF randomizing to open reduction and internal fixation (ORIF) with a volar locking plate or closed reduction and cast immobilization. There were no significant differences between the groups in terms of the ROM or pain relief during the entire follow-up period ($P > 0.05$). Patients in the operative group had lower DASH and patient-rated wrist/hand evaluation (PRWE) scores, indicating better wrist function in the early postoperative time period ($P < 0.05$), but there were no significant differences between the groups at 6 and 12 months. However, grip strength was significantly better at all times in the operative group ($P < 0.05$). Furthermore, dorsal radial tilt, radial inclination, and radial shortening were significantly better in the

operative than in the nonoperative treatment group at the time of the latest follow-up ($P < 0.05$). The number of complications was significantly higher in the operative treatment group (13 compared with 5, $P < 0.05$). At the 12-month follow-up examination, the ROM, pain rating, and the PRWE and DASH scores were not different between the operative and nonoperative treatment groups.[17] Achieving anatomical reconstruction did not produce any improvement in ROM or ability to perform ADLs.

The main goal of surgeons treating older adults with DRFs should be a pain-free patient with satisfactory functional hand and wrist motion for performance of ADLs, specifically in hygiene, feeding, and mobility. The poor correlation between the radiographic and functional outcomes in older adults might be related to decrease in functional demand on the wrist associated with aging.[18] But not every patient ages the same way. The chronological age is a number and the treating surgeon should also consider the biological age of the patient.

If there is no significant difference between functional outcomes in the long term after nonsurgical or surgical treatment of unstable DRFs in the elderly, various surgery factors such as patient's age, functional demand (return to sport activities), patient's comfort (short immobilization time), preinjury daily activity level, lifestyle requirements (cosmetically appearance), current medical conditions, and stage of osteoporosis should be included in the decision-making process.

20.6 Our Algorithm of Treatment

Surgery is recommended in following circumstances:
- Palmarly displaced DRFs.
- Distal forearm fractures.

- Open fractures.
- Associated fractures (e.g., lower extremity fractures that make use of crutches necessary).
- High functional demand (sport activities, independent living).
- Less perioperative anesthesiological risk.
- Less comorbidities.
- Early return to pretrauma activities.
- Patient comfort (no cast immobilization).
- High cosmetic demand.

20.7 Initial Treatment

Displaced DRFs are generally reduced under local or axial block in the emergency department and then immobilized with a below-forearm plaster cast. For us it is controversial if acute DRF should be reduced initially in older adults for the following reason: there is a high incidence of loss of reduction after cast treatment; 30% during the first 10 days and another 29% after 10 days.[8]

In a retrospective study, the value of fracture reduction and casting in the functionally low-demand patients or in patients with dementia living in nursing homes (i.e., patient age is 82 years) was assessed in a group of 60 patients. All fractures were initially reduced under regional or general anesthesia, with 53 fractures healing in a malunited position. There was no correlation identified between fracture classification, initial displacement, or final radiographic outcome.[5]

The risk for displacement with an unacceptable radiographic result increases in patients older than 58 years. Decreased BMD is associated with DRF instability and a 50% risk for secondary displacement after closed reduction and casting.[3]

Patient age correlates with fracture instability. Cumulative risk factors for the loss of reduction are as follows:
- Patient's age greater than 60 years.
- Dorsal angulation more than 20 degrees or 5 mm of radial shortening.
- Metaphyseal dorsal comminution.
- Additional ulnar fracture or intra-articular radiocarpal involvement.[9]

Considering these outcomes, the question arises whether reduction of displaced DRFs should be attempted. After reduction, the majority of these fractures will lose reduction and go on to radiological malunion, but without evidence that this reliably leads to poor functional outcome.

In our practice, closed fracture reduction by fracture manipulation is indicated only in specific situations such as:
- Simple fractures with dorsal angulation less than 20 degrees and radial shortening of less than 5 mm,

as fracture manipulation is more likely to lead to better anatomical fracture reduction.
- A polytraumatized patient presents.

In cases where nonoperative treatment and in cases where surgical treatment is planned in few days, painful fracture manipulations are avoided. Chinese finger trap traction and below-elbow cast application without any fracture manipulation as initial treatment option for acute DRF is suggested. In nonoperatively treated DRFs, after decrease of swelling, the cast is changed without any further manipulation. Wrists are immobilized in a short-arm cast in a neutral position for 5 weeks. Active finger exercises are started immediately. After cast removal, physiotherapy is recommended. In operatively treated DRFs, the cast is anyhow removed at the time of surgery.

References

[1] Chung KC, Shauver MJ, Birkmeyer JD. Trends in the United States in the treatment of distal radial fractures in the elderly. J Bone Joint Surg Am 2009;91(8):1868–1873

[2] McQueen M, Caspers J. Colles fracture: does the anatomical result affect the final function? J Bone Joint Surg Br 1988;70(4):649–651

[3] Rikli D, Goldhahn J, Käch K, Voigt C, Platz A, Hanson B. Erratum to: the effect of local bone mineral density on the rate of mechanical failure after surgical treatment of distal radius fractures: a prospective multicentre cohort study including 249 patients. Arch Orthop Trauma Surg 2015;135(7):1043

[4] Handoll HHG, Madhok R. WITHDRAWN: surgical interventions for treating distal radial fractures in adults. Cochrane Database Syst Rev 2009;(3):CD003209

[5] Beumer A, McQueen MM. Fractures of the distal radius in low-demand elderly patients: closed reduction of no value in 53 of 60 wrists. Acta Orthop Scand 2003;74(1):98–100

[6] Crilly RG, Delaquerrière Richardson L, Roth JH, Vandervoort AA, Hayes KC, Mackenzie RA. Postural stability and Colles' fracture. Age Ageing 1987;16(3):133–138

[7] Lafontaine M, Hardy D, Delince P. Stability assessment of distal radius fractures. Injury 1989;20(4):208–210

[8] Nesbitt KS, Failla JM, Les C. Assessment of instability factors in adult distal radius fractures. J Hand Surg Am 2004;29(6):1128–1138

[9] Sakai A, Oshige T, Zenke Y, Suzuki M, Yamanaka Y, Nakamura T. Association of bone mineral density with deformity of the distal radius in low-energy Colles' fractures in Japanese women above 50 years of age. J Hand Surg Am 2008;33(6):820–826

[10] Azzopardi T, Ehrendorfer S, Coulton T, Abela M. Unstable extra-articular fractures of the distal radius: a prospective, randomised study of immobilisation in a cast versus supplementary percutaneous pinning. J Bone Joint Surg Br 2005;87(6):837–840

[11] Leung F, Zhu L, Ho H, Lu WW, Chow SP. Palmar plate fixation of AO type C2 fracture of distal radius using a locking compression plate—a biomechanical study in a cadaveric model. J Hand Surg [Br] 2003;28(3):263–266

[12] Haug LC, Glodny B, Deml C, Lutz M, Attal R. A new radiological method to detect dorsally penetrating screws when using volar locking plates in distal radial fractures. The dorsal horizon view. Bone Joint J 2013;95-B(8):1101–1105

[13] Herzberg G, Burnier M, Marc A, Izem Y. Primary Wrist Hemiarthroplasty for Irreparable Distal Radius Fracture in the Independent Elderly. J Wrist Surg 2015;4(3):156–163

[14] Arora R, Gabl M, Pechlaner S, Lutz M. Initial shortening and internal fixation in combination with a Sauvé-Kapandji procedure for severely comminuted fractures of the distal radius in elderly patients. J Bone Joint Surg Br 2010;92(11):1558–1562

[15] Sabapathy SR, Venkatramani H, Bharathi RR, Dheenadhayalan J, Bhat VR, Rajasekaran S. Technical considerations and functional outcome of 22 major replantations (The BSSH Douglas Lamb Lecture, 2005). J Hand Surg Eur Vol 2007;32(5):488–501

[16] Hinds RM, Capo JT, Kakar S, Roberson J, Gottschalk MB. Early complications following osteosynthesis of distal radius fractures: a comparison of geriatric and nongeriatric cohorts. Geriatr Orthop Surg Rehabil 2017;8(1):30–33

[17] Arora R, Lutz M, Deml C, Krappinger D, Haug L, Gabl M. A prospective randomized trial comparing nonoperative treatment with volar locking plate fixation for displaced and unstable distal radial fractures in patients sixty-five years of age and older. J Bone Joint Surg Am 2011;93(23):2146–2153

[18] Young BT, Rayan GM. Outcome following nonoperative treatment of displaced distal radius fractures in low-demand patients older than 60 years. J Hand Surg Am 2000;25(1):19–28

21 Extra-articular Malunion

Karl-Josef Prommersberger

Abstract

Extra-articular malunion is still a common complication of the distal radius fractures (DRF). Also, not all nonanatomically aligned DRFs lead to a poor clinical outcome, many patients with a malunion of the distal radius have disabilities of arm and wrist. If ever indicated, corrective osteotomy is the best option to treat an extra-articular radial malunion. While in former times dorsal malunions were mostly approached dorsally, now with use of locking plates, designed to fix acute dorsally tilted fractures from the palmar side, palmar and dorsal malunions are routinely treated through a palmar approach. There is a discussion whether a structural or nonstructural bone graft should be used, and actually whether there is a need for a bone graft at all. Independent of whether a structural or nonstructural bone graft is used, in most cases the distal radius will heal quickly. The more anatomical relation between the distal radius and the distal ulna and the carpus improves wrist and forearm motion and grip strength and diminishes pain. The changes from pre- to postoperative are statistically significant. Furthermore, there is a correlation between functional and radiological outcome. If the radius is restored more anatomically, the clinical outcome will be better.

Keywords: distal radius fracture, extra-articular malunion, corrective osteotomy, palmar approach, dorsal approach, structural bone graft, nonstructural bone graft, locking plates

21.1 Introduction

Despite the advances in the treatment of distal radius fractures (DRFs), malunion remains one of the most common complications. Distal radius malunion (DRM) mostly occurs following conservative treatment. Now, that surgical fixation of DRF has become more commonplace, there is an increasing number of malunion following operative treatment.[1]

DRM may be extra-articular, intra-articular, or combined intra-extra-articular.[2] In most extra-articular malunion, a combination by an angulation in the sagittal and frontal plane with a loss of length relative to the ulna is found, while a pure sagittal rotational malunion is rare.[3] In addition, a rotational deformity of the distal fragment with respect to the diaphysis can be seen.[4] Moreover, there may be a translation of the distal fragment in either the sagittal and/or the frontal plane.[5] Isolated shortening of the radius is a rare condition. In our own experience, the amount loss of length is greater in dorsally tilted than in palmarly tilted malunion.

It may be true that not all nonanatomically aligned DRF result in a poor functioning outcome. However, many patients with a malunited DRF complain about a decreased range of wrist motion and forearm rotation, weakness, and pain. In palmar malunion, supination of the forearm is more affected than pronation. Due to a posttraumatic ulnar impaction, often the pain is located on the ulnar side of the wrist. Many patients, both women and men, are unhappy with the unpleasant appearance of the wrist with a prominent ulna head typically for malunited Colles type fractures and a bayonet deformity typically for a Smith type fracture. DRM can lead to a subclinical irritation of the median nerve, while a manifest carpal tunnel syndrome is less often seen.[6]

21.1.1 Biomechanics of Distal Radial Malunion

Normal wrist biomechanics depend upon maintenance of the anatomical position of the distal end of the radius with respect to the carpus and the distal end of the ulna. Normal wrist motion consists of greater than 120 degrees of wrist flexion and extension, 50 degrees of wrist radial and ulnar deviation, and 150 degrees of forearm rotation at the distal radioulnar joint (DRUJ). The distal radius carries 80% of the axial load through the wrist and the distal ulna carries 20%.[7]

The osseous deformity in DRM affects the normal mechanics of the radiocarpal joint producing a limitation of the extension–flexion arc of motion. In addition, the malalignment affects the normal load transmission not only through the radiocarpal joint, but also across the whole wrist joint. Dorsal tilting of radial surface decreases the joint contact area by shifting axial loading through the wrist dorsally and ulnarly. Therefore, the pressure distribution on the radial articular surfaces becomes more concentrated[7,8,9] and may represent a prearthritic condition of the wrist joint.[10] The force borne by the ulna increases with shortening of the radius and dorsal tilting of the articular surface. As the angulation of the distal radius fragment increases from 10 degree of palmar tilt to 45 degree of dorsal tilt, the load through the ulna increases from 21 to 67% of the total load.[11] Lengthening of the ulna by 2.5 mm relative to the radius increases the force borne by the ulna from 18.4 to 41.9% of the total axial load.[7]

Malalignment of the surface of the distal radius in both the sagittal and coronal planes may result in a decreased mechanical advantage of the flexor tendons as they pass through the carpal tunnel, diminishing the grip strength.[12] In addition, median nerve compression neuropathy can also be encountered as a result of the deformity of the distal radius.[6]

At the midcarpal level, dorsal tilt of the distal radius, as an adaptive response to the dorsally rotated proximal carpal row, may lead to a compensatory flexion deformity,[13] an extrinsic midcarpal dynamic instability,[14] and a fixed carpal malalignment in dorsiflexion.[15]

Tilting and shortening of the distal radius may cause incongruity of the DRUJ and reduction of radioulnar contact area.[16] Radial shortening in relation to the distal part of the ulna can increase the strain in the triangular fibrocartilage complex[17] and result in a disruption of the deep portion of the dorsal radioulnar ligament.[18] These factors may limit the arc of forearm rotation.[19]

Fellmann et al[20] showed that an anatomical reduction of acute DRF correlates with a significantly better range of motion, while McQueen and Caspers[21] found that motion was significantly worse in wrists with dorsal tilting of more than 12 degrees. Jenkins and Mintowt-Czyz,[22] and Cooney et al[23] reported a close relationship between decreased grip strength and the severity of residual fracture deformity. Aro and Koivunen[24] found that only 4% of patients with an acceptable anatomic result had an unsatisfactory functional end result, compared with 25% of the patients with minor shortening and 31% of patients with gross shortening of the radius.

21.1.2 Treatment Options

Treatment options for symptomatic DRM must take into account the functional demands of the patient, patient's motivation, and the anatomy of the deformity. Fixed-angle devices allowing a stable fixation even of osteoporotic bone have made the bone quality less important.

Intervention to correct symptomatic malunion may be categorized into four broad areas: procedures aimed at restoring anatomic relationships, procedures aimed solely at gaining a functional improvement, procedures aimed at eliminating pain, and procedures that combined two or more of the above approaches.

Procedures aimed at eliminating pain are wrist denervation[25] and arthrodesis. For extra-articular DRM, arthrodesis is rarely indicated. In the setting of an extra-articular malunion combined with a carpal collapse due to scapholunate dissociation, radioscapholunate fusion reduces pain and preserves a certain degree of wrist motion as long as the midcarpal joint is intact.[26] Otherwise a total wrist joint might be indicated.

From the different procedures aimed solely at gaining a functional improvement on forearm rotation, satisfactory results can be achieved with Bowers hemiresection interposition arthroplasty and ulnar head replacement.[27,28]

Procedures aimed at restoring anatomic relationships between the distal end of the radius and the carpus and the distal end of the ulna are primarily osteotomies of the distal radius and the ulna.

21.2 Indications and Contraindications

The indication for corrective osteotomy of an extra-articular radial malunion is symptomatic, rather than radiological. It depends on the limitation of function, the severity of pain, the presence of midcarpal instability, the associated problems of the DRUJ, and the displeasing appearance of the wrist.

From a radiological standpoint, there are no fixed parameters to indicate a radial corrective osteotomy (RCO). However, because any angular deformity in the sagittal plane affects the DRUJ, shortening of the ulna is only indicated for dorsal malunion with dorsal tilting less than 10 degree and palmar malunion with less than 20 degree palmar angulation.[29] In more severe multidirectional deformities, an open wedge osteotomy of the distal radius or a combined closed wedge osteotomy of the distal radius with an ulna shortening is needed to restore the anatomic relationships between the distal end of the radius and the carpus and the distal end of the ulna as base of an almost normal wrist and forearm function. Radial shortening up to 12 mm can often be managed by RCO alone. If there is a greater radial shorting, a combined closed wedge osteotomy of the radius and ulna shortening should be considered.[30]

Poor general health and marked degenerative changes of the radiocarpal joint are contraindications for RCO. Moreover, fixed carpal malalignment is a contraindication, because in this setting the carpus does not correct with the radius and the patient will have ongoing pain midcarpal, where the head of the capitate is sitting on the dorsal pole of the lunate. There is always a discussion, whether evidence of an acute sympathetic reflex dystrophy is a contraindication for RCO. If the reflex dystrophy is caused by an irritation of the median nerve by the malaligned distal fragment, RCO can address the problem. Patients with reduced finger function should undergo physiotherapy prior to the operative intervention. As locking plates allow a more rigid fixation of the distal radius, only a really severe osteoporosis is a contraindication for RCO.

A slight instability of the DRUJ is not a contraindication for radial osteotomy, because the restored anatomical relation between the distal radius and the distal ulna restabilize the DRUJ. In several patients, we observed a healing of a nonunited ulnar styloid following RCO without any procedure on the ulnar side of the wrist. Also, a marked instability of the DRUJ is no contraindication for RCO, but requires a simultaneous or a secondary procedure on the ulnar side of the wrist, such as an Adams procedure.[31]

The combination of a DRM with degenerative changes of the DRUJ, located either at the sigmoid notch or the ulnar head, can be addressed with RCO combined with Bowers procedure.[27] Due to persisting postoperative problems in some patients following Bowers hemiresection arthroplasty, ulnar head replacement in combination with RCO is preferred nowadays.[28]

Based on the overall good results after RCO, there is no longer an upper age limit for RCO, provided that there is good general health. Elderly people can benefit significantly from RCO, even though they do not recover as much as younger patients.[32] Due to the enormous remodeling capacity of the distal radius, there is rarely a need for osteotomy in children.[33] It is indicated if there is a growth arrest or if the time left for remodeling is too short for a complete spontaneous correction (▶ Fig. 21.1a–f).

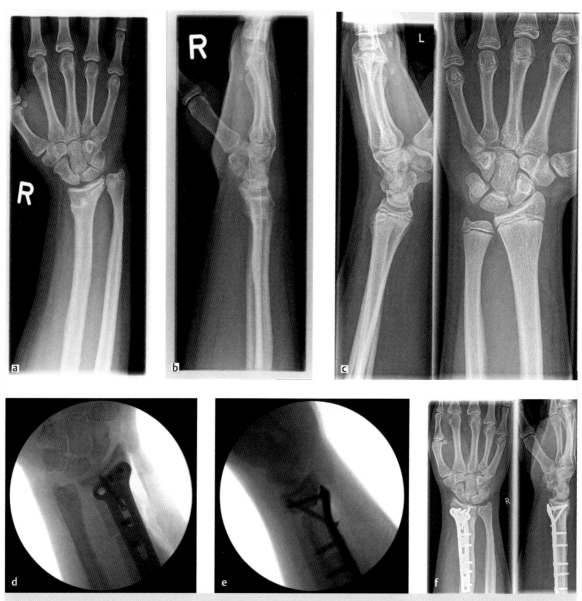

Fig. 21.1 A 15-year-old boy with a growth arrest of his right radius following Kirschner wires (K-wire) fixation of a dislocated fracture of radius and ulna at the age of 11 years. Extension-flexion injured wrist 30–0-40°, left side 60–0-55°; pro-/supination injured wrist 40–0-75°, left forearm 80–0-80°. **(a)** Anteroposterior radiograph of the injured right wrist showing the growth arrest of the radius with a negative ulnar inclination. **(b)** Lateral radiograph of the injured wrist preoperatively. **(c)** Radiographs of the uninjured left wrist showing an ulna minus of 2 mm, an ulna inclination of 20 degree, and 10-degree palmar tilt of the articular surface of the radius. **(d)** Intraoperative fluoroscopy in the anteroposterior plane. **(e)** Lateral intraoperative fluoroscopy showing the big structural bone graft necessary to restore the length of the radius. **(f)** Six months postoperative the bone graft is completely integrated, the radius is healed with a dorsal tilting of the radius articular surface of 5 degree, an ulnar inclination of 20 degree, and an ulna neutral.

21.3 Surgical Technique

21.3.1 Timing for Radial Correction Osteotomy in an Extra-articular Malunion

In patients who are still in work or retired but still very active, RCO should be performed after the fracture as soon as it is decided that the patient meets the criteria and the swelling is subsided. Jupiter and Ring retrospectively compared the results of 10 patients in whom DRM had been corrected within 6–14 weeks after the injury with the results of 10 patients with late RCO, i.e., 30–48 weeks after the injury.[34] They found that the results were comparable, early reconstruction is technically easier and reduces the overall period out of work.

For patients who are retired and less active, there is no need for early intervention. With respect to their individual demands many of these patients will achieve satisfied or even good clinical results. Those who suffer from persisting disabilities of the wrist can undergo a late RCO leading to the same good clinical outcome as with an early correction.

21.3.2 Preoperative Work-up

Patients with extra-articular DRM often present with associated concerns that can degrade the outcome. Therefore, a meticulous preoperative physical and radiographic evaluation is imperative. Physicians should identify the location of the discomfort, check the stability of the DRUJ, and measure both the range of motion of the wrist and forearm motion, and grip strength compared to that of the contralateral side. The disabilities of the arm, shoulder and hand (DASH) questionnaire can be used preoperatively to assess the subjective disabilities of the patients and quantify self-rated treatment effectiveness after surgery.

Standard biplanar radiographs of the injured and uninjured wrist are mostly adequate for planning the operative treatment of patients with an extra-articular DRM (▶ Fig. 21.2a). Comparison with the uninjured side is crucial to determine carpal alignment, ulnar variance, and inclination of the articular surface of the distal radius in the sagittal and frontal plane (▶ Fig. 21.2b). Computed tomography (CT) scanning may be helpful to detect degenerative changes and malalignment of the DRUJ and assess malrotation of the distal fragment with respect to the diaphysis. An arthroscopy of the wrist may be indicated to assess the ligaments and the articular cartilage, if a ligament tear is suspected. The lunate follows the articular surface of the radius in the malposition. There might be a scapholunate dissociation, if the tilting of the lunate is greater as 10 degree as the tilting of the distal radius in the sagittal plane.

Preoperative drawing of the planned surgical intervention showing the level of osteotomy, the angle of correction, the ulnar plus, and the size of the osteotomy gap is essential. Nowadays, the preoperative planning of the surgical intervention is often done on a computer.[35]

21.3.3 Technique

Approach

For decades most surgeons thought that the approach to expose the distal part of the radius for RCO of an extra-articular malunion depends on the direction of the deformity using a classic palmar Henry approach for palmarly tilted malunion[36,37] and a dorsal incision between the third and fourth dorsal compartments for dorsally angulated malunion.[38] In 1937, Campbell had already published an osteotomy technique approaching the radius radially.[39] In the 1970s, Lanz described a technique to correct dorsal malunion using a special plate and a radiopalmar approach.[40] Now that newer plates designed specifically for the palmar fixation of dorsally tilted DRF by incorporating buttress pins and screws that lock to the plate are available, the idea to correct dorsally tilted malunion through a palmar approach has become more popular.[41,42,43,44]

There are many facts influencing the approach to the distal radius for RCO. For dorsal malunion in spite of palmar plate fixation, the radius can easily be approached using the prior incision. If the distal fragment of the radius following dorsal plating is displaced in the direction opposite to the plate or if the fracture is overcorrected, a second approach on the palmar aspect of the radius may be needed. In the rare situation where an additional procedure on the ulnar side of the wrist or on the carpal ligaments simultaneous with the RCO of the radius is required, the radius should be approached dorsally.

RCO should include correction of malrotation of the radius along with correction of angular deformities and radial shortening. Correct rotational alignment of the distal radius with respect to the radial diaphysis can easily be achieved by application of a buttress plate on the palmar aspect of the radius.

In patients with a soft-tissue problem associated with DRM, such as flexor pollicis longus (FPL) laceration, the soft-tissue problem may influence the choice of the approach to the radius. If there is a manifest carpal tunnel syndrome together with the DRM, a separate approach over the carpal tunnel is beneficial. If radial lengthening is complicated by soft-tissue contracture, complete tenotomy or z-lengthening of the brachioradialis tendon may be helpful.[45]

Where and How to Osteotomize the Radius?

The osteotomy can be performed either at the prior fracture site or at a different site. In many cases, it is technically easier to perform the osteotomy proximal to the original fracture site. This can result in a severe humpback deformity of the

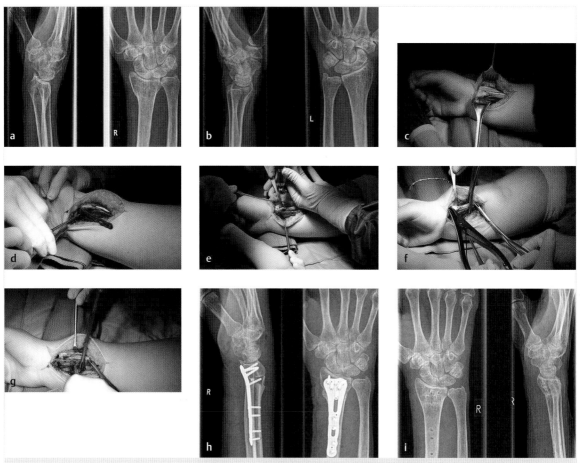

Fig. 21.2 Extra-articular malunion of the distal right radius of a 55-year-old ophthalmologist. Extension-flexion of the injured wrist 60–0–40°, pro-/supination 70–0–80°; limitation while performing eye surgery. Extension-flexion of the uninjured side 80–0–80°, pro-/supination 90–0-90°. **(a)** Preoperative radiographs of the injured wrist showing the extra-articular malunion of the distal radius with a severe dorsal tilt of 45 degrees. **(b)** Radiograph of the uninjured left wrist showing a palmar tilt of the articular surface of the radius of 10 degrees. **(c)** Author's technique for corrective osteotomy of a dorsal tilted distal radius malunion: the radius is approached radiopalmarly by a Y-shaped incision with the long leg of the Y overlying the radial artery. The first extensor compartment and any additional subcompartment are released. The third dorsal compartment is opened and the extensor pollicis longus tendon is transposed subcutaneously. The tendon of the brachioradialis muscle is partially, or if necessary, totally detached from the radius. The pronator quadratus together with the flexor pollicis longus muscle and the radial artery is retracted from the radius to the ulnar side. **(d)** The used special radius correction plate is positioned as far distally as possible and fixed by locking screws. After distal fixation of the plate, the stem of the plate sticks out from the radius. The angle between the shaft of the radius and the stem of the plate corresponds to the necessary correction of the radius in the sagittal plane. **(e)** The osteotomy is carried out with use of an oscillating saw. The angle of osteotomy in both planes in relation to the long axis of the radial shaft should be half of the planned angle of correction. **(f)** The osteotomy gap is opened up with a spreader. This brings the stem of the plate in contact with the shaft of the radius as soon as the distal fragment has reached its proper position of correction. **(g)** With two plate-holding forceps the plate is fixed temporarily to the radial shaft. The osteotomy gap—seen distally—will be filled with a structural bone graft from the iliac crest.
(h) Postoperative radiograph of the right wrist in two planes after removal of the drainage showing the iliac bone graft. The radius is restored in length and shape. **(i)** 1 year after the radial corrective osteotomy the hardware is removed.

distal radius and/or a dislocation of the DRUJ. The hump-back deformity with the long axis of the carpus palmar to the long axis of the radius may disturb force transmission and can lead to a refracture after hardware removal.

Such problems can be avoided by locating the osteotomy as close to the original fracture site as possible and by exact preoperative planning of the center of rotation. The center of rotation can lie in, on, or outside the margins of the radial cortex.[46] When a limited lengthening is needed, the center of rotation lies on the bone margins and an incomplete open wedge osteotomy is enough. This situation is encountered in many palmar malunions. When the radius needs to be largely lengthened, the center of rotation is away from the bone and a complete osteotomy is required. This situation is given in most dorsal malunion. Radial shortening up to 12 mm can be corrected with an open wedge osteotomy of the radius alone. Radial shortening over 12 mm requires a closed wedge osteotomy of the radius together with an ulna shortening.

How to Deal with the Osteotomy Gap?

For a long time the defect created by the open wedge osteotomy was filled with bi- or tricorticocancellous bone graft from the iliac crest. Ring et al found that the use of a cancellous bone graft do not impair the radiographic and functional results.[47] Recently, several authors reported about unproblematic healing of the radius leaving the osteotomy gap alone by using a locking plate.[48,49] Others found that not grafted trapezoid voids are significantly associated with nonunion.[50,51] Some investigators reported about the use of bone substitute.[52,53] Callotaxis can successfully be used for correction of the radial deformity, especially in young patients with growth arrest.[54]

If a bone graft is interposed in the void, most surgeons harvest the bone graft from the iliac crest. In 1988, Watson[55] picked by a technique described by Durman[56] cutting the graft longitudinally from the distal end of the proximal fragment of the radius. Campbell harvested the graft from the distal ulna.[38]

How to Fix the Radius in an Extra-articular Corrective Osteotomy?

Every technique used to fix an acute DRF, such as plating or pinning, can also be used to stabilize the distal radius in RCO. By deciding how to fix the radius the quality of the bone stock, the quality of the bone graft, and the interval between the injury and the RCO should be taken into account. To avoid implant failure, the used plate should be strong, especially in a longstanding malunion and if the bone graft is very tiny.[57] Using an external fixator with pins placed in the distal fragment allows postoperative adjustment if the restoration of length or alignment proves to be inadequate.[54]

Author's Preferred Technique of Corrective Osteotomy for Dorsal Malunion of the Distal Radius

A Y-shaped incision with the long leg of the Y overlying the radial artery is made over the distal radiopalmar aspect of the radius. The oblique leg of the Y on the palmar side extends to the middle crease of the wrist where it crosses the flexor carpi radialis tendon. The dorsal leg of the Y ends at the radial border of the extensor carpi radialis longus tendon. Throughout the whole procedure, care is taken to protect the superficial branch of the radial nerve which remains attached to the subcutaneous flap. The first extensor compartment and any additional subcompartments are released. The third dorsal compartment is opened and the extensor pollicis longus tendon is transposed subcutaneously. The tendon of the brachioradialis muscle is partially, or if necessary, totally detached from its insertion. The pronator quadratus together with the FPL muscle and the radial artery is retracted from the radius to the ulnar side (▶ Fig. 21.2c).

The used special radius correction plate is positioned as far distally as possible and fixed by a locking screw through the middle of the three distal holes. The plate must be positioned according to the angle of correction of the ulnar inclination. Therefore, the plate is pivoted around the middle of the three distal holes until the angle between the radial border of the radius and the radial border of the proximal part of the plate corresponds to the angle of correction of the ulnar inclination. After positioning of the plate, the radial and ulnar distal locking screws are inserted. After distal fixation of the plate, the stem of the plate forms an angle with the shaft of the radius that corresponds to the necessary correction in the dorsopalmar plane (▶ Fig. 21.2d).

With the plate in place, the site of the osteotomy is marked with an osteotome. It should be as close to the original fracture site as possible and lie just proximal to the three distal screws. The osteotomy is carried out with use of an oscillating saw (▶ Fig. 21.2e). The angle of osteotomy in both planes in relation to the long axis of the radial shaft should be half of the planned angle of correction. This has proved to be advantageous; while opening up the osteotomy a double trapezoid gap is created which eases the fitting and wedging in of the bone graft. If a smaller angle is chosen, the distal fragment needs to be tilted more with the result that the long axis of the carpus lies palmar to the axis of the forearm. Therefore, the load transmission through the radiocarpal joint is still affected. If one chooses a greater angle for the osteotomy, the distal fragment becomes longer. This, in turn, results in a posterior humpback when the fragments are spread.

The osteotomy gap is opened up with a spreader inserted between the posterior cortices of the fragments (▶ Fig. 21.2f). This brings the stem of the plate in contact with the shaft of the radius as soon as the distal fragment has reached its proper position of correction. With two plate-holding forceps the plate is fixed temporarily to the radial shaft (▶ Fig. 21.2g). A double trapezoid, bicortical bone graft harvested from the iliac crest is now inserted into the widened gap (▶ Fig. 21.2h). However, the use of cancellous bone graft will be enough. The plate is then fixed definitively to the radius. If a structural bone graft is used, the bone graft and the distal fragment are fixed by two screws from the second screw row. The extensor retinaculum will not be sutured and the tendon of the extensor pollicis longus remains subcutaneously. The pronator quadratus muscle is loosely sutured to the tendon of the brachioradialis muscle. After a careful hemostasis the wound is closed. The wrist is immobilized in a palmar plaster splint until the wound has healed properly.

The patient begins active exercises of the fingers immediately after surgery. The day after surgery, elbow motion and forearm rotation start. The suction drain is removed on the second day after operation and the sutures are removed after 2 weeks. Usually this coincides with the removal of the plaster splint. Physiotherapy includes wrist motion as well as forearm rotation. The plate is only removed if it causes problems (▶ Fig. 21.2i).

21.4 Results

More than 200 papers on RCO have been published. Those who include data show that RCO improves wrist and forearm motion as well as grip strength, and diminishes pain. Furthermore, the changes from pre- to postoperative are statistically significant. In addition, there is a correlation between the radiological and clinical outcome. Patients with no or only a minor residual deformity after RCO have significantly better results than those with a gross residual deformity as shown for wrist extension and forearm supination.[58] Even elderly patients benefit from RCO of DRM.[32]

A study on long-term outcomes of RCO for the treatment of DRM with 12 Dutch patients and 10 patients from the Unites States showed that RCO can improve wrist function and radiographic appearance, but the early results can deteriorate over time because of radiocarpal arthritis and the small but possible occurrence of radiocarpal and/or carpal malalignment over time.[59] The study has several limitations: there was a mix of extra-articular and intra-articular RCO, there was a lack of presurgical data, neither the surgical technique nor the postoperative regiment was standardized due to the retrospective character of the study and the inclusion of patients from at least two institutions, and no locking plates were used. Pillukat et al published the preoperative, short-term follow-up (7–44 months) and long-term follow-up (120–254 months) data of 17 patients, who had RCO of extra-articular DRM in one institution in a standardized manner.[60] The comparison of the short-term and long-term results revealed no deterioration of the results but a further statistically significant improvement in grip strength, even when 5 patients developed osteoarthritis.

Bauer et al retrospectively compared the results of 31 patients who underwent RCO performed conventionally with 25 patients treated with a computer-assisted method using patient-specific instrumentation.[61] The results demonstrate that the computer-assisted method facilitates shorter operation times while providing similar clinical results.

21.4.1 Own Results

Between 1975 and 1999, we performed 195 RCOs for dorsal DRM; 181 were carried out using the above-described technique. Preoperative radiographs revealed an average dorsal tilt of the articular surface of 24 degree, an average ulnar inclination of 13 degree, and an average ulnar variance of plus 6 mm. Preoperatively, extension of the wrist averaged 44 degree (range 30–50 degree), flexion of the wrist averaged 34 degree (range 25–50 degree), supination of the forearm was on average 66 degrees with a range of 55 to 90 degree, and forearm pronation ranging from 60 to 90 degree, averaged 64 degrees. The average grip strength was 29 kg compared with 69 kg in the contralateral hand.

At an average of 54 months after the osteotomy, extension and flexion of the wrist had improved on average to 49 degrees with extension of the wrist ranging from 45 to 55 degrees and flexion ranging from 40 to 60 degrees. Supination of the forearm had improved on average to 78 degree (range 70–90 degrees) and pronation on average to 77 degrees (range 65–90 degrees). The average grip strength had increased to 40 kg. Postoperative measurements of the radiographs showed on average a palmar tilt of the articular surface of 7 degree, a radial inclination of 22 degree, and an ulnar plus variance of less than 1 mm.[44]

21.5 Pitfalls

Every complication seen in the treatment of acute DRF can also happen in RCO of extra-articular DRM—tendon and nerve irritation, hematomas, infection, persisting malalignment, loss of reduction, etc. With the number of nonunion frequently higher in RCO as in acute DRF, nonunion following RCO is a severe and major complication.[62]

21.6 Conclusion

Still malunion is major complication following DRF. For extra-articular malunion, RCO is a well-accepted option. In the majority of cases, RCO of an extra-articular malunion leads to an improved wrist and forearm motion, improved grip strength, and diminished pain. The clinical outcome correlates with the radiological result. The more anatomically the radius is restored, the better is the clinical outcome.

Tips and Tricks

- Decision-making about operating or not operating a patient with an extra-articular DRM depends on the clinical findings. In other words: do not operate the radiographs, operate the patient.
- Decision about how to operate on an extra-articular malunion is primarily based on radiographs of both wrists, but it is good to get the original fracture radiographs.
- If the radial styloid looks very prominent in the anteroposterior radiographs, there might be an additional rotational deformity of the distal fragment. Think about a special CT to analyze rotation of the distal fragment, especially if you will approach the radius dorsally.
- Look for associated injuries of the carpus and the DRUJ and address them.
- If the radiolunate angle is more than 10 degrees greater as the dorsal tilting of the articular surface of the radius, there might be scapholunate dissociation.
- A fixed carpal malalignment will not correct with the radius. The patient will have ongoing pain.
- Hand function is more important as wrist function. Patients with limited finger function should undergo physiotherapy before RCO. Because pain is mostly on the ulnar side, unload the ulna by overlengthening the radius a little bit compared to the opposite side. If you have to lengthen the radius a lot (> 1 cm), the fingers will be stiff the next day. Do not worry, muscles and tendons will adapt. If you use a corticocancellous bone graft in a dorsal malunion and the bone graft is much thinner as compared to the radius, put it more dorsally in the osteotomy gap. There is more load transmitted in the dorsal part of the articular surface.

References

[1] Gradl G, Jupiter J, Pillukat T, Knobe M, Prommersberger KJ. Corrective osteotomy of the distal radius following failed internal fixation. Arch Orthop Trauma Surg 2013;133(8):1173–1179

[2] Buijze GA, Prommersberger KJ, González Del Pino J, Fernandez DL, Jupiter JB. Corrective osteotomy for combined intra- and extra-articular distal radius malunion. J Hand Surg Am 2012;37(10): 2041–2049

[3] Del Piñal F, García-Bernal FJ, Studer A, Regalado J, Ayala H, Cagigal L. Sagittal rotational malunions of the distal radius: the role of pure derotational osteotomy. J Hand Surg Eur Vol 2009;34(2):160–165

[4] Prommersberger KJ, Froehner SC, Schmitt RR, Lanz UB. Rotational deformity in malunited fractures of the distal radius. J Hand Surg Am 2004;29(1):110–115

[5] Bilić R, Zdravković V, Boljević Z. Osteotomy for deformity of the radius. Computer-assisted three-dimensional modelling. J Bone Joint Surg Br 1994;76(1):150–154

[6] Megerle K, Baumgarten A, Schmitt R, van Schoonhoven J, Prommersberger KJ. Median neuropathy in malunited fractures of the distal radius. Arch Orthop Trauma Surg2013;133(9): 1321–1327

[7] Werner FW, Glisson RR, Murphy DJ, Palmer AK. Force transmission through the distal radioulnar carpal joint: effect of ulnar lengthening and shortening. Handchir Mikrochir Plast Chir 1986;18(5):304–308

[8] Pogue DJ, Viegas SF, Patterson RM, et al. Effects of distal radius fracture malunion on wrist joint mechanics. J Hand Surg Am 1990;15(5):721–727

[9] Kazuki K, Kusunoki M, Shimazu A. Pressure distribution in the radiocarpal joint measured with a densitometer designed for pressure-sensitive film. J Hand Surg Am 1991;16(3):401–408

[10] Martini AK. Secondary arthrosis of the wrist joint in malposition of healed and un-corrected fracture of the distal radius Aktuelle Traumatol 1986;16(4):143–148

[11] Werner FW, Palmer AK, Fortino MD, Short WH. Force transmission through the distal ulna: effect of ulnar variance, lunate fossa angulation, and radial and palmar tilt of the distal radius. J Hand Surg Am 1992;17(3):423–428

[12] Tang JB, Ryu J, Omokawa S, Han J, Kish V. Biomechanical evaluation of wrist motor tendons after fractures of the distal radius. J Hand Surg Am 1999;24(1):121–132

[13] Linscheid RL, Dobyns JH, Beabout JW, Bryan RS. Traumatic instability of the wrist. Diagnosis, classification, and pathomechanics. J Bone Joint Surg Am 1972;54(8):1612–1632

[14] Taleisnik J, Watson HK. Midcarpal instability caused by malunited fractures of the distal radius. J Hand Surg Am 1984;9(3):350–357

[15] Fernandez DL, Geissler WB, Lamey DM. Wrist instability with or following fractures of the distal radius. In: Büchler U, ed. Wrist Instability. London: Martin Dunitz 1996: 181–192

[16] Bade H, Lobeck F. Behavior of the joint surface of the distal radio-ulnar joint in malposition of the distal radius Unfallchirurgie 1991;17(4):213–217

[17] Adams BD. Effects of radial deformity on distal radioulnar joint mechanics. J Hand Surg Am 1993;18(3):492–498

[18] Hagert CG. Distal radius fracture and the distal radioulnar joint—anatomical considerations. Handchir Mikrochir Plast Chir 1994;26(1):22–26

[19] Bronstein AJ, Trumble TE, Tencer AF. The effects of distal radius fracture malalignment on forearm rotation: a cadaveric study. J Hand Surg Am 1997;22(2):258–262

[20] Fellmann J, Kunz C, Sennwald G. Clinical and radiological results 12 years after conservative treatment of distal radius fractures. La Main 1997;2:313–319

[21] McQueen M, Caspers J. Colles' fracture: does the anatomical results affect the final function? J Bone Joint Surg 1988;70B:649–651

[22] Jenkins NH, Mintowt-Czyz WJ. Mal-union and dysfunction in Colles' fracture. J Hand Surg [Br] 1988;13(3):291–293

[23] Cooney WP III, Dobyns JH, Linscheid RL. Complications of Colles' fractures. J Bone Joint Surg Am 1980;62(4):613–619

[24] Aro HT, Koivunen T. Minor axial shortening of the radius affects outcome of Colles' fracture treatment. J Hand Surg Am 1991;16(3): 392–398

[25] Wilhelm A. Denervation of the wrist. Tech Hand Up Extrem Surg 2001;5(1):14–30

[26] Beyermann K, Prommersberger KJ, Krimmer H, Lanz U. Radioscapho-lunate fusion as treatment of posttraumatic radiocarpal arthrosis. Eur J Trauma 2000;26:169–175

[27] Fernandez DL. Radial osteotomy and Bowers arthroplasty for malunited fractures of the distal end of the radius. J Bone Joint Surg Am 1988;70(10):1538–1551

[28] van Schoonhoven J, Fernandez DL, Bowers WH, Herbert TJ. Salvage of failed resection arthroplasties of the distal radioulnar joint using a new ulnar head prosthesis. J Hand Surg Am 2000;25(3):438–446

[29] Prommersberger KJ, van Schoonhoven J. Störungen des distalen Radioulnargelenkes nach distaler Radiusfraktur. Unfallchirurg 2008;111(3):173–184, quiz 185–186

[30] Wada T, Isogai S, Kanaya K, Tsukahara T, Yamashita T. Simultaneous radial closing wedge and ulnar shortening osteotomies for distal radius malunion. J Hand Surg Am 2004;29(2):264–272

[31] Adams BD, Berger RA. An anatomic reconstruction of the distal radioulnar ligaments for posttraumatic distal radioulnar joint instability. J Hand Surg Am 2002;27(2):243–251

[32] Pillukat T, van Schoonhoven J, Prommersberger KJ. Is corrective osteotomy for malunited distal radius fractures also indicated for elderly patients? Handchir Mikrochir Plast Chir 2007;39(1):42–48

[33] Meier R, Prommersberger KJ, van Griensven M, Lanz U. Surgical correction of deformities of the distal radius due to fractures in pediatric patients. Arch Orthop Trauma Surg 2004;124(1):1–9

[34] Jupiter JB, Ring D. A comparison of early and late reconstruction of malunited fractures of the distal end of the radius. J Bone Joint Surg Am 1996;78(5):739–748

[35] Athwal GS, Ellis RE, Small CF, Pichora DR. Computer-assisted distal radius osteotomy. J Hand Surg Am 2003;28(6):951–958

[36] Prommersberger KJ, van Schoonhoven J, Laubach S, Lanz U. Corrective osteotomy for malunited, palmarly displaced fractures of the distal radius. Eur J Trauma 2001;27:16–24

[37] Shea K, Fernandez DL, Jupiter JB, Martin C Jr. Corrective osteotomy for malunited, volarly displaced fractures of the distal end of the radius. J Bone Joint Surg Am 1997;79(12):1816–1826

[38] Fernandez DL. Correction of post-traumatic wrist deformity in adults by osteotomy, bone-grafting, and internal fixation. J Bone Joint Surg Am 1982;64(8):1164–1178

[39] Campbell WC. Malunited Colles' fractures. JAMA 1937;109: 1105–1108

[40] Lanz U, Kron W. Neue Technik zur Korrektur in Fehlstellung verheilter Radiusfrakturen. Handchir Mikrochir Plast Chir 1976;8: 203–206

[41] Viegas SF. A minimally invasive distal radial osteotomy for treatment of distal radius fracture malunion. Tech Hand Up Extrem Surg 1997;1(2):70–76

[42] Melendez EM. Opening-wedge osteotomy, bone graft, and external fixation for correction of radius malunion. J Hand Surg Am 1997;22(5):785–791

[43] Prommersberger KJ, Lanz U. Corrective osteotomy for malunited Colles' fractures. Orthop Traumatol 1998;6:70–76

[44] Prommersberger KJ, Lanz UB. Corrective osteotomy of the distal radius through volar approach. Tech Hand Up Extrem Surg 2004;8(2):70–77

[45] Ring D, Prommersberger K, Jupiter JB. Posttraumatic radial club hand. J Surg Orthop Adv 2004;13(3):161–165

[46] Nagy L. Malunion of the distal end of the radius. In: Fernandez DL, Jupiter JB, eds. Fractures of the Distal Radius. 2nd ed. New York: Springer; 2002:289–344

[47] Ring D, Roberge C, Morgan T, Jupiter JB. Osteotomy for malunited fractures of the distal radius: a comparison of structural and nonstructural autogenous bone grafts. J Hand Surg Am 2002;27(2):216–222

[48] Ozer K, Kiliç A, Sabel A, Ipaktchi K. The role of bone allografts in the treatment of angular malunions of the distal radius. J Hand Surg Am 2011;36(11):1804–1809

[49] Mahmoud M, El Shafie S, Kamal M. Correction of dorsally-malunited extra-articular distal radial fractures using volar locked plates without bone grafting. J Bone Joint Surg Br 2012;94(8):1090–1096

[50] Scheer JH, Adolfsson LE. Non-union in 3 of 15 osteotomies of the distal radius without bone graft. Acta Orthop 2015;86(3):316–320

[51] Pillukat T, Mühldorfer-Fodor M, van Schoonhoven J, Prommersberger KJ. The malunited distal radius fracture—extraarticular correction without bone graft. Handchir Mikrochir Plast Chir 2018;50(3):160–168

[52] Luchetti R. Corrective osteotomy of malunited distal radius fractures using carbonated hydroxyapatite as an alternative to autogenous bone grafting. J Hand Surg Am 2004;29(5):825–834

[53] Yasuda M, Masada K, Iwakiri K, Takeuchi E. Early corrective osteotomy for a malunited Colles' fracture using volar approach and calcium phosphate bone cement: a case report. J Hand Surg Am 2004;29(6):1139–1142

[54] Penning D, Gausepohl T, Mader K. Correction of malunited fractures of the distal radius. Osteosynthese Int 1997;5:143–150

[55] Watson HK, Castle TH Jr. Trapezoidal osteotomy of the distal radius for unacceptable articular angulation after Colles' fracture. J Hand Surg Am 1988;13(6):837–843

[56] Durman DC. An operation for correction of deformities of the wrist following fracture. J Bone Joint Surg 1935;17:1014–1016

[57] Müller LP, Klitscher D, Rudig L, Mehler D, Rommens PM, Prommersberger KJ. Locking plates for corrective osteotomy of malunited dorsally tilted distal radial fractures: a biomechanical study. J Hand Surg [Br] 2006;31(5):556–561

[58] Prommersberger KJ, Van Schoonhoven J, Lanz UB. Outcome after corrective osteotomy for malunited fractures of the distal end of the radius. J Hand Surg [Br] 2002;27(1):55–60

[59] Lozano-Calderón SA, Brouwer KM, Doornberg JN, Goslings JC, Kloen P, Jupiter JB. Long-term outcomes of corrective osteotomy for the treatment of distal radius malunion. J Hand Surg Eur Vol 2010;35(5):370–380

[60] Pillukat T, Gradl G, Mühldorfer-Fodor M, Prommersberger KJ. Malunion of the distal radius—long-term results after extraarticular corrective osteotomy Handchir Mikrochir Plast Chir 2014;46(1):18–25

[61] Bauer DE, Zimmermann S, Aichmair A, et al. Conventional versus computer-assisted corrective osteotomy of the forearm: a retrospective analysis of 56 consecutive cases. J Hand Surg Am 2017;42(6):447–455

[62] Prommersberger KJ, Fernandez DL. Nonunion of distal radius fractures. Clin Orthop Relat Res 2004(419):51–56

22 Arthroscopic-Guided Osteotomy for Intra-articular Malunion

Francisco del Piñal

Abstract

Intra-articular malunion of the radius causes considerable interference with a patient's life: limited and painful range of motion are the norm. Arthroscopic guided osteotomy allows delineation of the original fracture line with minimal additional cartilage injury. The operation enables the surgeon to obtain an anatomic reduction while minimizing the possibility of wrong-site fracture. In the author's experience with intra-articular osteotomies, excellent results can be consistently achieved if one adheres to the described surgical steps. The reader should be warned that the operation ranks among the most difficult arthroscopic procedures a surgeon can be faced with in the wrist. Furthermore, substantial education in classic management of distal radius fractures is required. Otherwise, we risk throwing the patient into a catastrophic situation. The operation with classic arthroscopic technique (wet arthroscopy) is impracticable; thus, familiarity with the dry arthroscopic technique is paramount.

Keywords: distal radius fracture, distal radius malunion, intra-articular osteotomy, arthroscopy, wrist pain

22.1 Introduction

"Arthroscopy is the 'missing link' to achieving a perfect result in distal radius fractures (DRF)." (Piñal in Green 2018).

Intra-articular malunion of the radius causes considerable interference in a patient's life: limited and painful range of motion is the norm (▶Fig. 22.1). Most malunion cases occur because of inappropriate management of the original fracture, and more rarely due to secondary

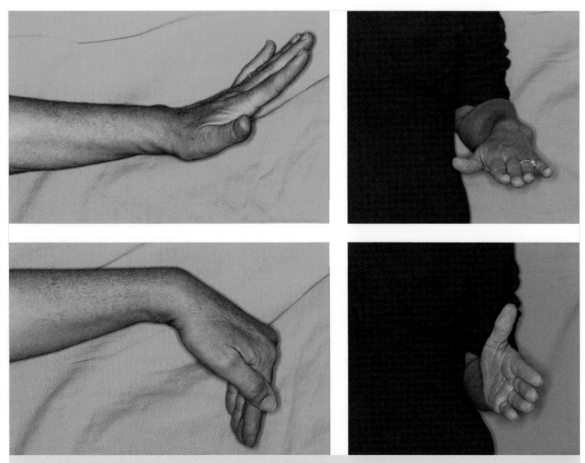

Fig. 22.1 This 50-year-old lady, who works as a cleaner and is also very active at sports, suffered a fracture at work that was treated in a cast. At presentation, 5 months after the injury, she not only had an obvious deformity and pain, but also a limited range of motion. (Copyright © Francisco del Piñal, MD)

subsidence. The former is usually due to not using the arthroscope as the checking tool at the time of fracture management, but the fluoroscope. Indeed, restoring joint anatomy is the main goal when dealing with a DRF. Imaging with a mini fluoroscope is the more common technique for assessing fracture reduction in the operating room. Several papers, however, have demonstrated limitations and poor reliability of this imaging modality for this particular and similar other applications in our field.[1,2,3]

Excellent results have been reported by "outside-in" technique in the treatment of intra-articular malunion.[4,5] However, difficulties were noted with visualization once a reduction was achieved and the procedure relied heavily on fluoroscopy rather than direct visualization, which, as stated, is not a very reliable instrument. We devised a technique under arthroscopy that, under good light and magnification, allowed us to precisely trace the cartilage line of the old fracture with the osteotome. In this way, the possibility of wrong-site fracture during the osteotomy does not exist, thus converting a malunion into an acute fracture.[6,7]

22.2 Indications and Contraindications

Diagnosis of a malunion is often evident from the plain X-ray (▶Fig. 22.2). Nevertheless, a computed tomography (CT) scan with cuts in pure orthogonal planes is invaluable in the decision-making process and for surgeon's orientation at the time of the arthroscopy (▶Fig. 22.3). Besides the standard sagittal, coronal, and axial slices of the CT scan, I have found what I have termed the "articular view" to be extremely useful.[8] This is generated by moving the axis in the coronal and

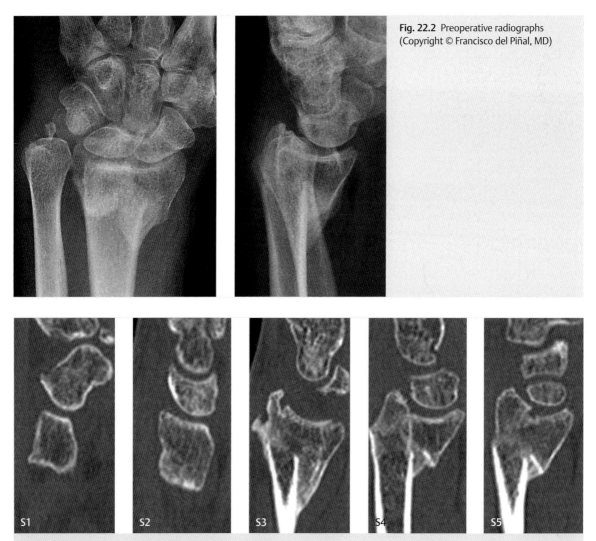

Fig. 22.2 Preoperative radiographs (Copyright © Francisco del Piñal, MD)

S1 S2 S3 S4 S5

Fig. 22.3 On the computed tomography scan, the compound articular and nonarticular deformity can be clearly delineated. The dorsal ulnar fragment that seems to maintain its position relatively well, is also rotated volarly.(Copyright © Francisco del Piñal, MD)

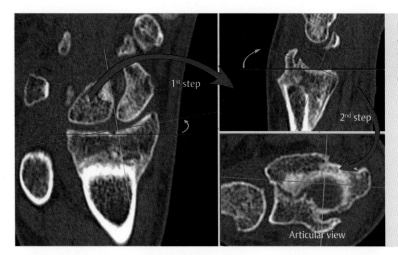

Fig. 22.4 In this "articular view" it can be appreciated that there are anterior-ulnar and scaphoid fossa fragments that are very short but relatively level with each other. (Copyright © Francisco del Piñal, MD)

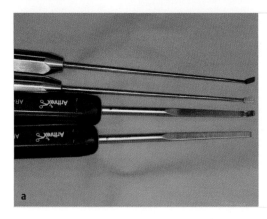
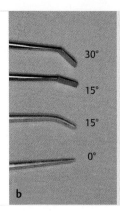

Fig. 22.5 (a, b) Instruments used during the procedure. From *above* to *below*: shoulder periosteal elevator (of 15 and 30° angle) (Arthrex AR-1342–30° and AR-1342–15°, Arthrex, Naples, FL), and straight and curved osteotomes (Arthrex AR-1770 and AR-1771).[8] (Copyright © Francisco del Piñal, MD)

then in the sagittal views, in order to have a tangential scan of the surface of the malunited joint in the axial slice (▶Fig. 22.4).

Traditionally, a 2 mm or greater step-off of the distal radial articular surface was considered an indication for osteotomy. Each patient should be considered on an individual basis. In a young active patient, even 1 mm step-off in the lunate or scaphoid facet should be considered for repair. Alternatively, a low-demand patient with a similar step-off may benefit from a resection arthroplasty, i.e., from levelling the joint—the latter having a much more benign postoperative course.

An additional consideration is the status of the cartilage, which again requires experience to take the appropriate decision. In general, the longer time between the fracture and the visit, and the more the patient has attempted to move the joint, the less cartilage will remain. As a rule, no exact contraindications for the procedure can be given. Factors such as more than 6 months duration after the fracture, very committed patients in rehabilitation, and presence of hardware in the joint all cast a shadow over the possibility of restoration of the joint. By the same token, in order to prevent further damage, when a patient

is seen in the office with a step-off, the physical therapy is to be called off immediately. Furthermore, a splint should be applied to minimize motion while the CT studies are done and surgery is scheduled.

22.3 Surgical Technique

All patients with an intra-articular malunion in the author's practice are managed similarly. First of all, an arthroscopic exploration is performed. Due to the large portals needed to introduce the osteotomes, it is paramount that the surgeon adheres to the dry technique,[8,–10] as otherwise constant loss of vision will occur due to lack of water-tightness. The only special instruments we use are the osteotomes and periosteal elevators borrowed from the shoulder and knee trays. These are 4-mm wide and with different angulations to access the always tight wrist (▶Fig. 22.5).

Under tourniquet, the hand is set in traction from an overhead bow. Traction of 12 to 15 kg is evenly applied to all fingers. Establishing the portals is more difficult than in a standard arthroscopy as the space is collapsed by scar tissue. Once the scar tissue is removed, the cartilage is carefully assessed and a decision is taken as to whether the osteotomy is feasible (▶ Fig. 22.6). Basically, if the cartilage is mostly preserved I will go ahead with the osteotomy. Contrarily, if the cartilage is worn, I prefer to carry out some form of salvage operation: ideally an arthroscopic arthroplasty or a transplant of vascularized cartilage.[11,12,13] If the damage is diffuse and widespread, then the option would be to consider an arthroscopic radioscapholunate fusion.[14,15]

Typically, once the surgeon has opted for an arthroscopy-guided osteotomy, the hand is set on the table and a standard volar-radial approach is carried out exposing the radius. This is needed, above all, to remove the volar callus, but also because there is often hardware to be removed. Furthermore, a volar plate will be used for fixation and has to be preset at this point. Removing the extra-articular callus will weaken the fragment connection.

However, no attempt to release the fragments is made at this stage, as they may break at the wrong spot intra-articularly. The hand is now set in traction, and depending on the type of malunion and the location of the step-off, the so-called straight or tear-line osteotomies are carried out. From a technical standpoint, straight cuts with the straight osteotome are the easiest but only possible when the fracture line is straight and in line with one of the portals (▶ Fig. 22.7). For those malunions not amenable to this simple osteotomy (such as any coronal fracture line), multiple perforations are made with the osteotome creating a sort of "tear line" in the cartilage and subchondral bone for easy breakage when prying with the osteotome (▶ Fig. 22.8). Given the space limitations and the fact that quite commonly the malunions are irregular, one has to be prepared to use any portal, any osteotome, and

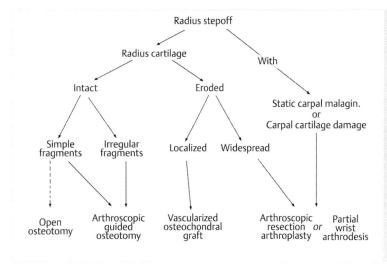

Fig. 22.6 Decision tree for treatment of intra-articular distal radius malunions. While simple configurations could be amenable to open osteotomy, complex ones would require massive exposure and consequently scarring and fragment devascularization. Arthroscopic guided is thus much preferred by the author.[13] (*Source:* Modified from del Piñal et al 2013)

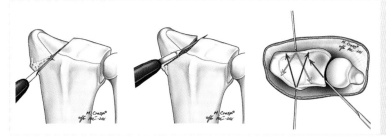

Fig. 22.7 Straight line osteotomy.[8] (Copyright © Francisco del Piñal, MD)

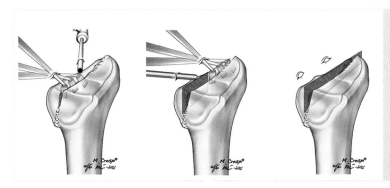

Fig. 22.8 Tear line osteotomy.[8] (Copyright © Francisco del Piñal, MD)

combinations of linear and tear-line osteotomies in order to manage a given malunion.

Once the fragment is mobilized, the redundant callus and fibrous tissue are removed from inside and outside the joint, until easily reducible. Hitherto, the case is managed as for an acute fracture.[8,16,17] The highlights of the surgical management of the case introduced in ▶Fig. 22.1, ▶Fig. 22.2, ▶Fig. 22.3, and ▶Fig. 22.4 are presented in ▶Fig. 22.9, ▶Fig. 22.10, ▶Fig. 22.11, ▶Fig. 22.12, ▶Fig. 22.13, ▶Fig. 22.14, ▶Fig. 22.15, ▶Fig. 22.16, ▶Fig. 22.17, ▶Fig. 22.18, ▶Fig. 22.19, and ▶Fig. 22.20. Most of these patients are discharged 4 months after surgery. However, I warn them that they should keep doing self-directed exercises several times a day, as improvement is expected up to 2 years or more.

In conclusion, the arthroscopy-guided osteotomy allows delineation of the original fracture line with minimal additional cartilage injury. The operation enables the surgeon to obtain an anatomic reduction while minimizing the possibility of wrong-site fracture. In the author's experience with intra-articular osteotomies, excellent results can be consistently achieved if one adheres to the described surgical steps. The reader should be aware that the operation ranks among the most difficult arthroscopic procedures a surgeon can be faced with in the wrist.

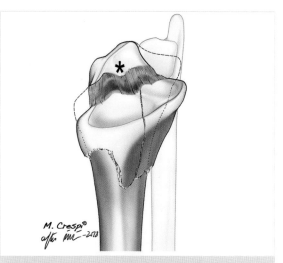

Fig. 22.9 In summary, in the case presented in ▶Fig. 22.1, ▶Fig. 22.2, ▶Fig. 22.3, ▶Fig. 22.4, there is a nonarticular deformity, in which the scaphoid fossa and the volar-ulnar fragment have healed aligned to each other but shortened in relation to the ulna. Furthermore, these two fragments have an articular incongruency with the dorsal-ulnar fragment which itself is also tilted volarly. (The asterisk indicates indicate the volar-radial corner of the posterior-ulnar fragment in all figures of this case). (Copyright © Francisco del Piñal, MD)

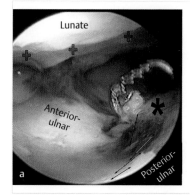
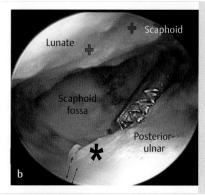

Fig. 22.10 (a, b) First, a radiocarpal arthroscopy was carried out to assess the feasibility of the reconstruction, i.e., the status of the cartilage of the radius and the carpals. The step-off was defined (*arrows*). Typically, after 6 to 8 weeks, step-offs are full of fibrin, making it difficult to gauge the extent of the deformity until such tissue is removed. In this case, an estimate can be inferred from the fact that the shaver is 3 mm in diameter and the dorsal step-off is larger than that. The crosses (+) mark the mirror damage in the lunate. (Copyright © Francisco del Piñal, MD)

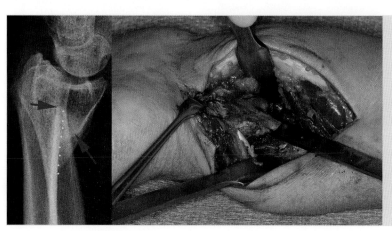

Fig. 22.11 An 8 mm super-thin osteotome is seen sliding on the anterior cortex carefully redefining it and, thus, separating the malunited fragment from the diaphysis (*yellow dots*). No attempt was made to reach the joint with the osteotome. The *arrows* mark the degree of collapse; both *arrows* should eventually meet restoring the length lost at the radius.
(Copyright © Francisco del Piñal, MD)

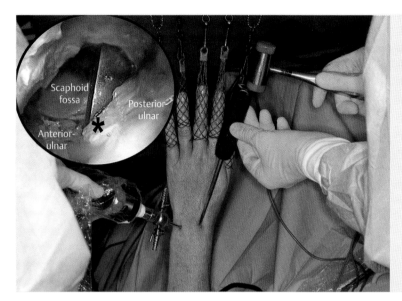

Fig. 22.12 Under arthroscopy the posterior-ulnar and the scaphoid fossa fragments were cut with the osteotome introduced through 3–4 portal. The inset shows the corresponding arthroscopic view. (Copyright © Francisco del Piñal, MD)

Scope in 3-4 / Osteotome in 6R

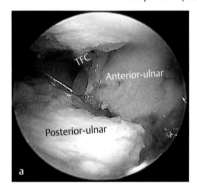
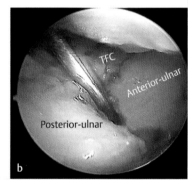

Fig. 22.13 (a, b) Next, the anterior-ulnar fragment was freed from the dorsal-ulnar fragment. The TFC can be seen in the background.
(Copyright © Francisco del Piñal, MD)

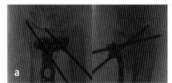
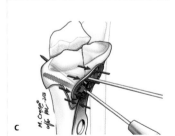
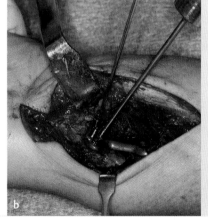

Fig. 22.14 (a–c) Once the anterior-ulnar and the scaphoid fossa fragments were released from the dorsal-ulnar/shaft, a plate was preset (*left*) and then rigidly fixed (*right*) to this component only. This created a stable and manageable "construct" that included the scaphoid fossa/anterior-ulnar fragment and the plate. Great care was taken not to insert locking screws ulnarly so as not to block the reduction that will follow. Note, that at this stage, the extra-articular malalignment was disregarded.
(Copyright © Francisco del Piñal, MD)

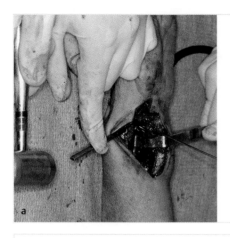
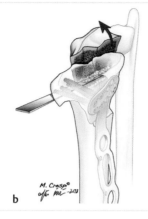

Fig. 22.15 (a, b) Now the malunited dorsal-ulnar fragment was freed from the diaphysis by cutting the dorsal metaphysis with a 4 mm super-thin osteotome introduced from the radial defect.
The fragment was then reduced by rotating it dorsally applying palmar pressure.
(Copyright © Francisco del Piñal, MD)

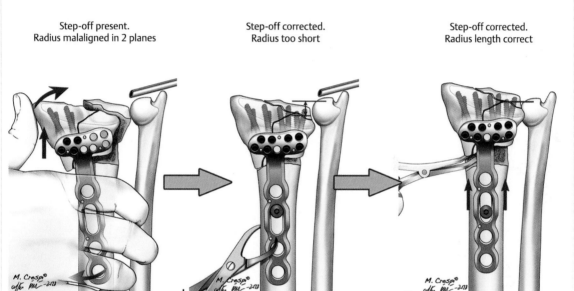

Step-off present.
Radius malaligned in 2 planes

Step-off corrected.
Radius too short

Step-off corrected.
Radius length correct

Fig. 22.16 Summary of the steps to correct the deformity: under arthroscopic control the "construct" was reduced to the dorsal-ulnar fragment **(a)**. Temporary Kirschner wires (K-wires) were replaced by appropriate locking screws, and the stem of the plate was then reduced to the shaft with a bone clamp **(b)**. Finally, by means of a lamina spreader the whole joint-plate unit was distracted until the volar cortex was restored and the variance normalized **(c)**. (Copyright © Francisco del Piñal, MD)

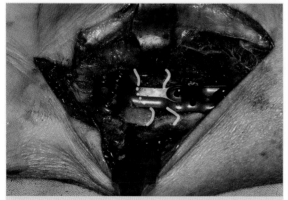

Fig. 22.17 Detail of the lengthening achieved in the volar metaphysis highlighted by lines.
(Copyright © Francisco del Piñal, MD)

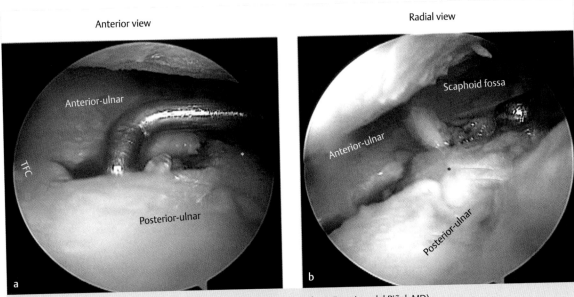

Fig. 22.18 (a, b) Final arthroscopic result with the scope in 6R. (Copyright © Francisco del Piñal, MD)

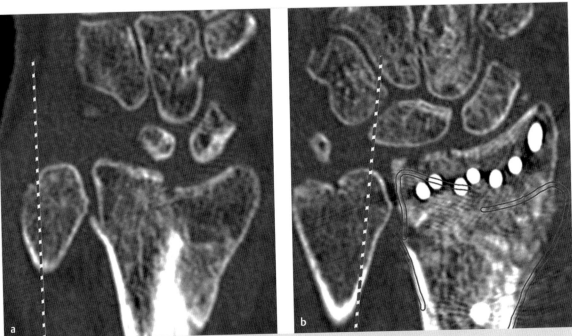

Fig. 22.19 (a, b) Comparative coronal CT scan slices. The outlines of the radius and the axis of the ulna have been marked. Notice the correction of the variance ulnarly but most of all, the collapsed radial column. (Copyright © Francisco del Piñal, MD)

Furthermore, substantial education in classic management of distal radius fractures is required. Otherwise, we risk throwing the patient into a catastrophic situation. The operation with classic arthroscopic technique (wet arthroscopy) is impracticable, thus familiarity with the dry arthroscopic technique is paramount.

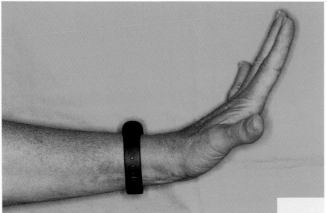
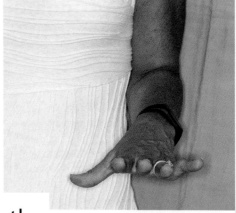

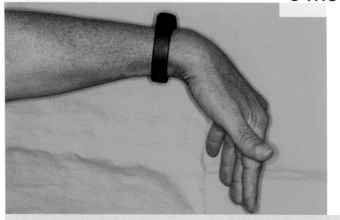
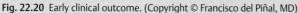
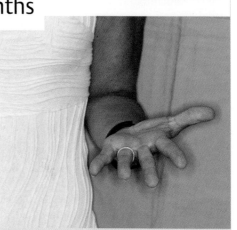

Fig. 22.20 Early clinical outcome. (Copyright © Francisco del Piñal, MD)

References

[1] Edwards CC II, Haraszti CJ, McGillivary GR, Gutow AP. Intra-articular distal radius fractures: arthroscopic assessment of radiographically assisted reduction. J Hand Surg Am 2001;26(6):1036–1041

[2] Lutsky K, Boyer MI, Steffen JA, Goldfarb CA. Arthroscopic assessment of intra-articular distal radius fractures after open reduction and internal fixation from a volar approach. J Hand Surg Am 2008;33(4):476–484

[3] Capo JT, Kinchelow T, Orillaza NS, Rossy W. Accuracy of fluoroscopy in closed reduction and percutaneous fixation of simulated Bennett's fracture. J Hand Surg Am 2009;34(4):637–641

[4] Ring D, Prommersberger KJ, González del Pino J, Capomassi M, Slullitel M, Jupiter JB. Corrective osteotomy for intra-articular malunion of the distal part of the radius. J Bone Joint Surg Am 2005;87(7):1503–1509

[5] Prommersberger KJ, Ring D, González del Pino J, Capomassi M, Slullitel M, Jupiter JB. Corrective osteotomy for intra-articular malunion of the distal part of the radius. Surgical technique. J Bone Joint Surg Am 2006;88(Suppl 1 Pt 2):202–211

[6] del Piñal F, García-Bernal FJ, Delgado J, Sanmartín M, Regalado J, Cerezal L. Correction of malunited intra-articular distal radius fractures with an inside-out osteotomy technique. J Hand Surg Am 2006;31(6):1029–1034

[7] del Piñal F, Cagigal L, García-Bernal FJ, Studer A, Regalado J, Thams C. Arthroscopically guided osteotomy for management of intra-articular distal radius malunions. J Hand Surg Am 2010;35(3):392–397

[8] del Piñal F. Atlas of Distal Radius Fractures. New York: Thieme; 2018

[9] del Piñal F, García-Bernal FJ, Pisani D, Regalado J, Ayala H, Studer A. Dry arthroscopy of the wrist: surgical technique. J Hand Surg Am 2007;32(1):119–123

[10] del Piñal F. Dry arthroscopy and its applications. Hand Clin 2011;27(3):335–345

[11] del Piñal F, Klausmeyer M, Thams C, Moraleda E, Galindo C. Arthroscopic resection arthroplasty for malunited intra-articular distal radius fractures. J Hand Surg Am 2012;37(12):2447–2455

[12] del Piñal F, Garcia-Bernal JF, Delgado J, et al. Reconstruction of the distal radius facet by a free vascularized osteochondral autograft: anatomic study and report of a case. J Hand Surg Am 2005;30A:1200–1210

[13] del Piñal F, Klausmeyer M, Moraleda E, et al. Vascularized graft from the metatarsal base for reconstructing major osteochondral distal radius defects. J Hand Surg Am 2013;38(10):1883–1895

[14] Ho PC. Arthroscopic partial wrist fusion. Tech Hand Up Extrem Surg 2008;12(4):242–265

[15] del Piñal F, Tandioy-Delgado F. (Dry) arthroscopic partial wrist arthrodesis: tips and tricks. Handchir Mikrochir Plast Chir 2014;46(5):300–306

[16] del Piñal F. Technical tips for (dry) arthroscopic reduction and internal fixation of distal radius fractures. J Hand Surg Am 2011;36(10):1694–1705

[17] del Piñal F, Clune J. Arthroscopic management of Intra-articular malunion in fractures of the distal radius. Hand Clin 2017;33(4):669–675

23 Newer Technologies on Managing Distal Radius Fractures

Ladislav Nagy

Abstract

Computer assisted 3D-modelling based on segmentation of CT scans allows for exact assessment of the distal radius morphology in fractures, malunions, and deformities. 3D analysis, virtual planning, and 3D printing enable to plan and accurately perform complex extra- and intra-articular osteotomies, fracture reductions, and osteosyntheses. The clear additional value over the traditional techniques, together with the growing acceptance by the increasingly digital medical community, will eclipse the idle hesitation toward innovation and unfounded misgivings about increased expenses.

Keywords: computer-assisted osteotomy, intraarticular malunion, distal radius malunion, guided osteotomy, virtual planning

23.1 Introduction

The integrity of geometrical shape of the distal radius, due to its two articular surfaces and adjacent joints, has a significant impact on the function of the wrist. Thus, when treating fractures or deformities of the distal radius the prime goal is to restore the original anatomy. However, the radius displays quite a complex three-dimensional (3D) structure, challenging the assessment, the understanding, and the feasibility of repair of the altered structures.

For almost a century, conventional X-rays represented the only method of imaging, evidently a technology that, due to projectional effects, distorts angles and, due to the divergence of the X-ray beams, alters length relationships. This drawback drove several surgeons to use complex mathematical models to compensate for this defect.[1,2,3] But even the most sophisticated calculations were unable to catch up for the limitations of a two-dimensional imaging technique.[2,3,4,5,6] Therefore, conventional radiographs are unable and insufficient to accurately depict a 3D object.[7,8]

With the advent of computed tomography (CT) the radiologists received a powerful tool capable to surmount these problems. However, tied to the traditional way of looking at radiographs, the output of the CT scanners remained hooked to single planes renouncing to extract the totality of the information gathered. It took more than three decades until the manufacturers and radiologists offered rather simplistic measuring and 3D representation options. Still not true 3D images, deprived of the possibility to interact and no attempt to manipulate. Thus, surgeons treating fractures or bone deformities continued to plan their interventions relying mainly on two perpendicular images and only exceptionally took in account rotatory deformities available from clumsy comparison of axial sections.[9]

Although reconstruction of 3D models, 3D analysis, and virtual planning is available since the 1990s, it remained without practical use and spread in orthopaedic surgery. This omission was and still is justified by cost and difficulty. The latter has meanwhile well been resolved—on one hand by the availability of specific software and on the other by the massive intrusion of computer technologies in our daily lives and its inevitable acceptance. The cost indisputably higher than the rule-of-thumb techniques are well in line with other technological advanced treatments, increasingly accepted by providers and patients striving for the best possible result.

Meanwhile thanks to other technical progress, the possibilities have evolved much further; 3D printing allows for manufacturing patient-specific guides and aids in order to transform the virtual plan in the surgical setting.

23.2 Indications

The technique can be used for any fracture or deformity in which a precise preoperative assessment is required, a virtual trial reduction is desired, or intraoperative aids for realizing the planned surgical procedure are needed. The use, therefore, is not dictated by the pathology, but depends solely upon the availability of the software and hardware needed, and the willingness of the surgeon to apply these techniques and tools.

As for the conventional technique, a malunion has to be symptomatic resulting in pain with motion and loading in order to indicate an operative procedure. In extra-articular malunions, pain and reduced function mostly arises on the ulnar side of the wrist presenting as ulnocarpal impaction, incongruity, and/or instability of the distal radioulnar joint. In the radiocarpal joint symptoms result from intra-articular step-off, degenerative arthritis, concomitant ligamentous lesions and, in extra-articular malunions, extrinsic midcarpal instability. There still is not enough data for performing a preventive correction for nonsymptomatic extra-articular malunions, whereas an intra-articular step-off greater than 2 mm might be a more convincing argument being a prearthritic condition.

Nowadays, the minimal first step for a simple 3D analysis is easily available everywhere. Software for segmentation of CT scans can be downloaded for free. With this, at least the virtual radius can be moved in space and observed from any perspective. This permits to assess the orientation of the deformity, the fracture and the fragments in space, especially important and valuable because fracture planes, steps, and gaps are depicted in their true spatial orientation which almost never coincide with the routine projections and therefore tend to be underestimated.

According to the further sophistication of the software available, an increasing number of instruments can be applied: the virtual pathological radius (▶ Fig. 23.1) can be compared with a healthy one (▶ Fig. 23.2) allowing for exact calculation of the deformity, it may be cut in pieces mimicking osteotomies and aligned with the template answering on the feasibility of correction (▶ Fig. 23.3). In fractures, the fragments can be moved until the fracture is reduced.

When these steps in the virtual model finally appear feasible and satisfactory, the preparation of execution of the surgery is done. Appropriate implants are selected and optimally located on the corrected virtual exemplar (▶ Fig. 23.4). Implant site and the trajectories of the screws are implemented in the model (▶ Fig. 23.4). Then the reduction process is reversed returning to the preoperative situation, now however with the afore created

fragments carrying the screw and osteotomy trajectories (▶ Fig. 23.5). Around these and along the bone surface, a mold can be created and prepared to serve as guide for saw cuts,[10] drill holes for the planned plate screws, joysticks for later reduction (▶ Fig. 23.6). For intra-articular osteotomies, which usually do not cross the joint in a straight line, serial close meshed holes are drilled along the desired osteotomy line.[11] Along these perforations, the bone can easily be broken creating a curved osteotomy line (▶ Fig. 23.7). In the cases where locking (fixed angle) plates are used for fracture/osteotomy fixation, the screws inserted in the prepared holes are also used for reduction as their direction is predetermined and not variable. For other types of fixation, reduction guides are necessary. These guides need to be prepared upon the reduced virtual bone in the same manner as the first drill/cutting guide—they accommodate the aforementioned joysticks, now however in the reduced position.

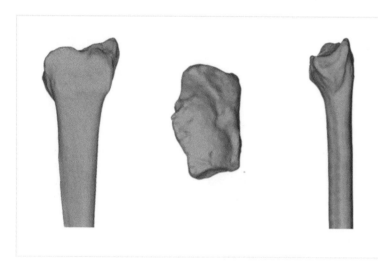

Fig. 23.1 Malunited radius reconstructed from computed tomography.

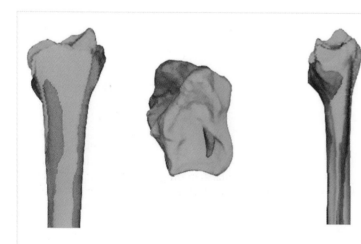

Fig. 23.2 Malunited radius with the opposite healthy radius mirrored and superposed.

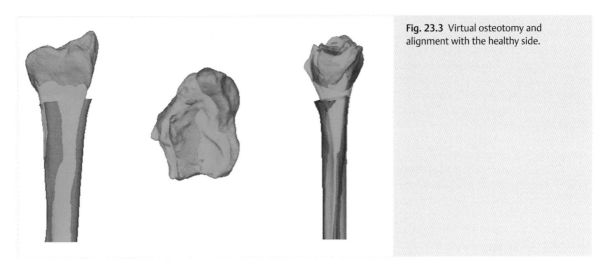

Fig. 23.3 Virtual osteotomy and alignment with the healthy side.

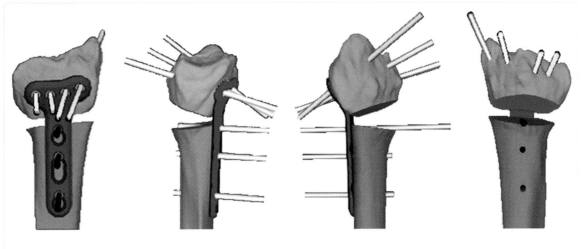

Fig. 23.4 Placement of a T-plate and screw trajectories.

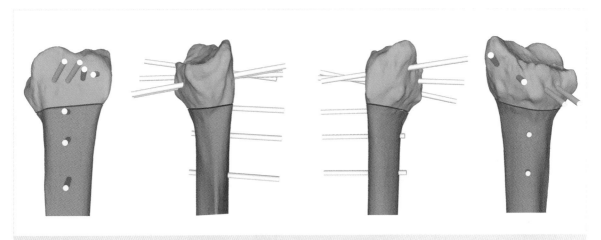

Fig. 23.5 Reversing reduction carrying the screw trajectories on the malunited radius.

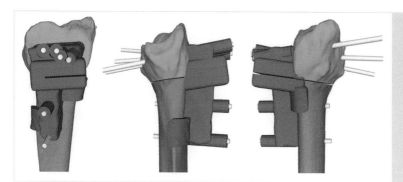

Fig. 23.6 Placing surface mold, drill guides, and saw guide.

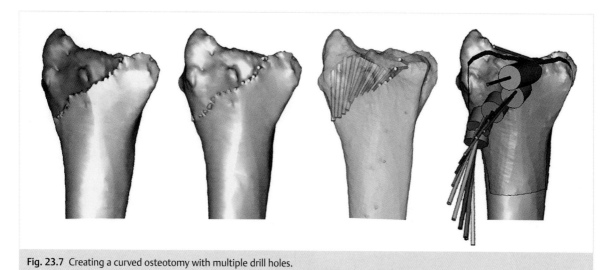

Fig. 23.7 Creating a curved osteotomy with multiple drill holes.

23.3 Surgical Technique

The incision/approach is made according to the site where the position of the gigs and eventually the osteotomy and fixation are planned: palmar, dorsal, radial, or combined. The surface of the bone has to be cleaned meticulously, as (remember!) the gig has been planned with the CT-data, that is, the cortex. Thus, the periosteum and soft tissue has to be locally removed in order to permit an ideal fit of the gigs. Once an undisputed location and perfect fit is found, the gig is pressed on the bone surface and fixed there either by clamps or Kirschner wires (K wires). The holes in the gig are used to correctly place joysticks into the preliminary fragments, drill holes for later screws or for osteotomies, slots allow for perfectly oriented and sized saw cuts. After this the gig is removed, the osteotomies are completed and the fragments are mobilized enough to permit a smooth reduction. The precise reduction is controlled and guaranteed by the reduction guide slid over the prepared joysticks or the fixed-angle plate/screws inserted in one single direction, predefined by the plate/screw-hole geometry.

23.3.1 Extra-articular Malunion

The approach usually is palmar exposing the distal metaphysis of the radius after reflecting the pronator quadratus muscle. The palmar bone surface is flatter and disposes of much less bony landmarks than dorsal, which renders the unmistakable fit of the surface guides more difficult. Therefore, the adaptation of the guides requires the exposure of a larger contact surface or a shape with specs that embrace the radius (▶Fig. 23.8). At the beginning of our experience we used locking plates with a fixed angle of screw insertion.[12] Thus, once the screw trajectories were drilled in the correct predetermined direction the plate positioning was unequivocally determined and the plate acted as a reduction device also. However, the screw placement in the distal fragment could not be adapted to the individual shape especially when this aberrated from the standard anatomy. This adaptation is possible using variable angle locking screws, which have become more and more popular, although at the expense of the virtue of the plate to serve as a reduction device. On the other hand, the predrilling of the holes through the guide that had to be removed before placing and attaching the plate seemed to be a superfluous additional step that is time consuming and fraught with potential error. Thanks to the fact that most extra-articular malunions present a "Colles deformity," the plate can be attached to the distal fragment before completing the osteotomy, provided the shafts of the plate and the radius are oriented diverging in the exact amount and direction of the deformity (▶Fig. 23.9). In order to guarantee this, the space between the plate and the bone shaft has to be determined by the gig. This will present wedge-like therefore we call it a ramp-guide. The undersurface of this wedge-shaped gig fits to the distal radius metaphysis, incorporates a slot for the partial (ulnar sided) osteotomy (▶Fig. 23.10), and drill guides for the plate holes in the shaft. On the upper surface any desired plate can be fastened, which, provided the planning was been correct, fits exactly to the distal fragment (▶Fig. 23.11). Small imperfections of the contact surface can be corrected removing prominences with a rongeur or an osteotome. Then the distal plate is firmly fixed to the distal fragment, the ramp-guide is removed and the partial osteotomy is now completed (▶Fig. 23.12). After mobilization

of the fragments, the plate can be attached to the proximal fragment and the shaft using the prepared screw holes, the osteotomy gap is filled with cancellous bone graft (▶Fig. 23.13). See ▶Fig. 23.14 for a clinical case of extra-articular malunion.

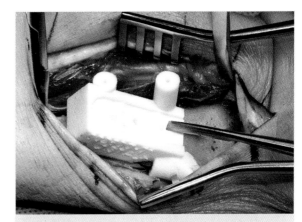

Fig. 23.8 Meticulous fitting of the guide on the palmar bone surface.

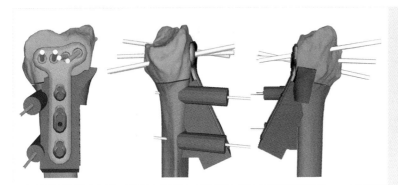

Fig. 23.9 Ramp guide.

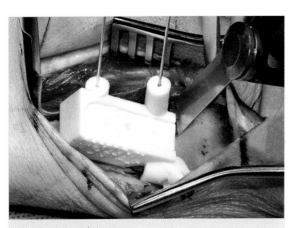

Fig. 23.10 Partial osteotomy.

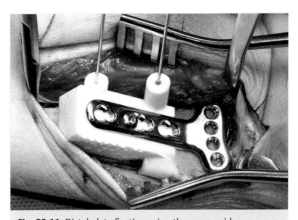

Fig. 23.11 Distal plate fixation using the ramp guide.

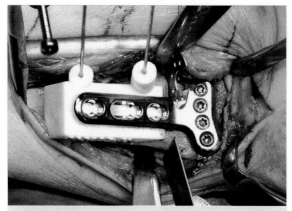

Fig. 23.12 Completion of the osteotomy.

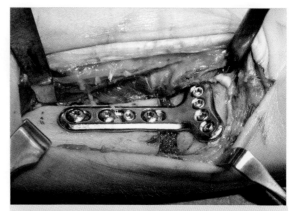

Fig. 23.13 Final presentation after proximal plate fixation and bone grafting.

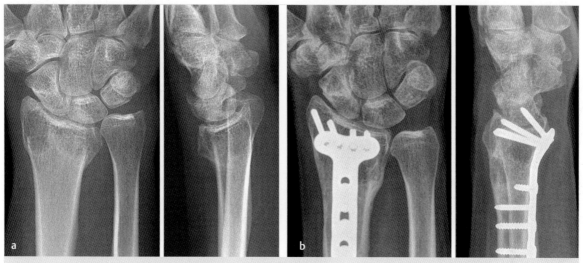

Fig. 23.14 Clinical case. Extra-articular malunion. (a, b) Pre- and postoperative X-rays.

23.3.2 Intra-articular Malunion

In complex, mature intra-articular malunions, 3D analysis and virtual osteotomy planning can already help a lot for deciding whether an osteotomy is possible at all. The joint surface is divided along the lines of the inadmissible step-off, the bone material in the gaps is cut off. Then the fragments are reduced using the contralateral joint image as template (▶Fig. 23.15). Usually one or two displaced fragments are moved onto the best located "main" fragment. In many cases this leads to a symmetrical situation. In other cases, the joint surface, although correctly restored, is not correctly oriented with respect to the shaft, which compels to append a concurrent extra-articular osteotomy in the metaphysis. Guides are prepared for reduction joysticks (▶Fig. 23.16) and for excision of these fragments by close meshed drill holes (▶Fig. 23.17) or saw cuts (▶Fig. 23.18). After osteotomy and mobilization of the fragments (▶Fig. 23.19), the reduction guide is slid over the reduction joysticks (▶Fig. 23.20). This ensures the proper positioning of the fragments, provisional fixation, and finally definitive stabilization with plates or screws (▶Fig. 23.21). Now, with the joint surface reconstructed a concomitant extra-articular deformity can be addressed by a metaphyseal osteotomy as described above. See ▶Fig. 23.22 for a clinical case of intra-articular malunion.

23.3.3 Intra-articular Fractures of the Distal Radius

3D analysis can already be very helpful for fully understanding the fracture pattern. This 3D understanding can further be enhanced if the virtual object is materialized with a printer.[13,14,15,16]

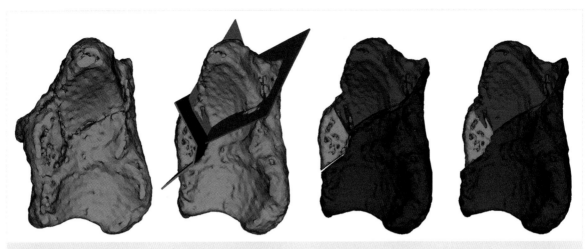

Fig. 23.15 Intra-articular malunion, virtual intra-articular osteotomy, and reduction.

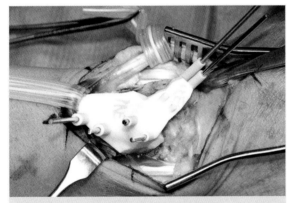

Fig. 23.16 Surface guide for placement of joysticks.

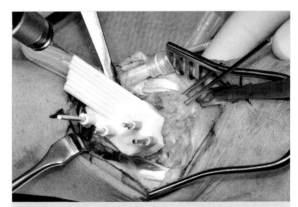

Fig. 23.17 Preparation of osteotomy using multiple drill holes.

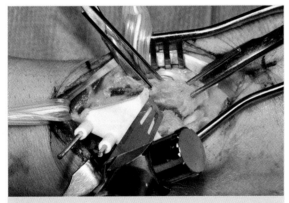

Fig. 23.18 Osteotomy with saw.

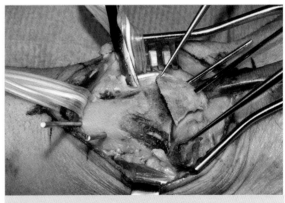

Fig. 23.19 Mobilization of the fragments.

For added steps, a more elaborate software is needed which allows individual manipulation of the separated segmented fragments until anatomical reduction is reached, with or without the help of a template or even haptic devices. It may also include a digital library of fixation devices/plates and tools for fashioning surface-guides

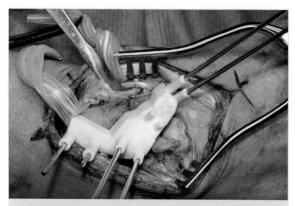

Fig. 23.20 Reduction of the fragments using the guide over the joysticks.

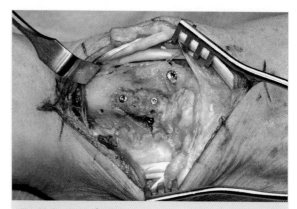

Fig. 23.21 Screw fixation.

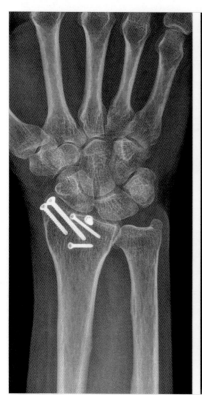
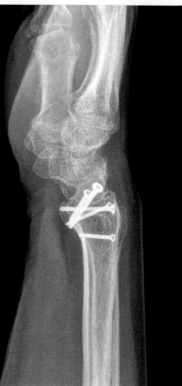

Fig. 23.22 Clinical case. Intra-articular malunion. Postoperative X-rays.

and gigs for preparing appropriate holes for the implant or placement of joysticks. This is especially helpful in fractures where the reduction cannot be sufficiently controlled by direct inspection or intraoperative fluoroscopy (see ▶ Fig. 23.29). This applies for most intra-articular fractures when approached palmarly (▶ Fig. 23.23). The intra-articular fracture line is concealed by the intact palmar capsule and its exact reduction is not possible unless controlled through a second/dorsal approach or wrist arthroscopy.

A precisely fitting surface guide allows for introduction of reduction joysticks into radial styloid (▶ Fig. 23.24) fragment and preparation of drill holes for the plate on the shaft fragment. If dealing with a dorsally tilted teardrop fragment, this is first attached to the plate. In order to fix the plate in the correct angulation,

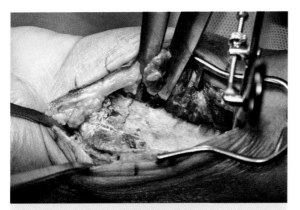

Fig. 23.23 Palmar fracture lines exposed.

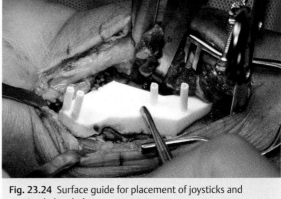

Fig. 23.24 Surface guide for placement of joysticks and proximal plate holes.

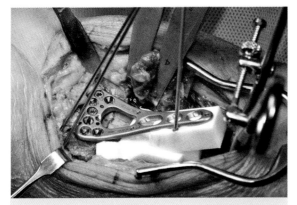

Fig. 23.25 Ramp guide fixed to the teardrop fragment.

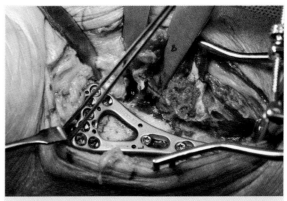

Fig. 23.26 Reduction and fixation of the teardrop fragment with the plate.

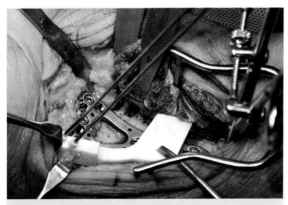

Fig. 23.27 Placement of the reduction guide over the joysticks in the styloid fragment.

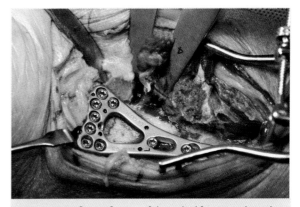

Fig. 23.28 Definitive fixation of the styloid fragment through the plate.

we use a ramp-guide defining the off-standing of the plate and also the location of the plate head and shaft (▶ Fig. 23.25). After removing the ramp-guide, the plate shaft is fixed to the predrilled holes in the proximal main fragment leading to an exact indirect reduction of the palmar-ulnar fragment (▶ Fig. 23.26). Then using the joysticks in the radial styloid fragment and a separate reduction guide, the styloid fragment is moved to the desired position (▶ Fig. 23.27) and stabilized with the additional screws through the plate (▶ Fig. 23.28). See ▶ Fig. 23.29 for a clinical case of intra-articular fracture.

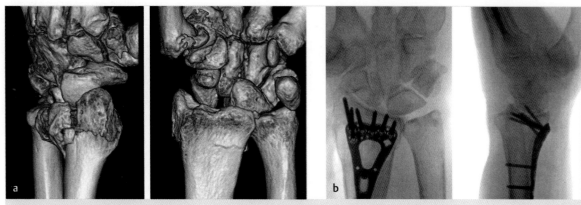

Fig. 23.29 Clinical case. Intra-articular fracture. **(a)** Preoperative 3D CT scan. **(b)** Postoperative X-rays.

So far, the experience with this technique in fresh fractures is limited, mainly due to the time needed to perform the analysis, the planning, and mainly the preparation and printing of the guides. There has been no data on this so far; our experience in a current prospective study has been positive.

23.4 Results

Several authors have reported on computer-assisted extra-articular osteotomies, mostly in case reports or based on small patient cohorts[11,17,18,19,20] which recently prompted a systematic review and meta-analysis including 68 patients from 15 studies.[21] There was a significant and reliable benefit from surgery. Eleven complications were reported, mostly related to the hardware; however, there were no infections or nonunions. A meaningful evaluation with regard to function is not possible due to the low numbers. Few later studies compare relevant patient cohorts[22,23] showing significantly more precise and reliable correction of deformity with the computer-assisted surgery, shorter duration of the operation, less X-ray exposure, and also better clinical results but latter not reaching statistical significance. Evidently, for intra-articular osteotomies no comparison is possible as no suitable reference group is available.

On our patients, we could demonstrate and confirm a very high reliability and precision of the method[24, 25,26,27]: closing wedge and single-cut osteotomies were more accurate than opening wedge osteotomies. Extra-articular osteotomies displayed a residual error of 2 to 4 degrees, intra-articular correction resulted in less than 1 mm residual step-off and 5 degree angulatory deformity. During the last 4 years, 96 extra-articular and 41 intra-articular virtually planned and computer-assisted osteotomies of the distal radius have been sufficiently documented at our institution. Out of these, we had five severe complications: one plate broke, another one bent,

one correction was lost, and there were two cases of complex regional pain syndrome. Only one patient with a painful wrist after intra-articular osteotomy needed a partial arthrodesis of the wrist.

23.5 Pitfalls and Contraindications

As for any osteotomy, the wrist should be free of trophic changes and stiffness. In the presence of degenerative arthritis, the indication for surgery needs to be challenged. Good bone quality is important for the reliable placement of the joysticks and reduction. Long standing significant deformity may have resulted in recalcitrant soft-tissue contracture that will preclude reduction especially gaining length. In these cases, an alternate strategy is preferable: closing wedge or rocking osteotomy of the radius necessitating length adjustment of the ulna by shortening ulna osteotomy when the cartilage in distal radioulnar joint is intact. If this joint presents with post-traumatic or degenerative arthritis, a prosthetic replacement is indicated. This usually allows for adjusting the length according to the corrected radius.

Given that the planning of the surgery and manufacturing of guides was correct, the most important step during the procedure is the perfect fit of the guide(s) on the bone. This entails a meticulous cleaning of the bone surface that is covered by the guide; periosteum and all soft tissue needs to be removed, which is in gross contrast to the lessons learned from soft-tissue sparing, biological surgery.

Substantial attention is needed during drilling and sawing the osteotomy cuts, as the friction of the tool in the guides hampers the perception of depth and resistance. Therefore, the guides should provide a catch adapted to length of the drill/saw blade to be used in order not to penetrate into the joint.

Tips and Tricks

- After exposure of the site of osteotomy, mark the contours of the guide on the bone and compare their location with the preoperative plan with regard to surface landmarks (measure distances).
- Check the length of the drill and saw with respect to the guide in order to avoid penetration into the joint.
- After osteotomy, the fragment needs to be generously mobilized in order to permit unconstrained reduction.
- The osteotomy surfaces should be cleaned and levelled, off-cuts completely removed including the scar tissue located in the intra-articular fracture gaps.

23.6 Conclusion

3D analysis, virtual planning, and computer assistance are powerful tools for improving precision, reliability and, given the time and numbers, also clinical results when performing osteotomies and osteosynthesis of the distal radius. Moreover, it opens new horizons for treating afore unsolvable clinical problems such as complex intra-articular malunion.

With the inevitable spread of easy-to-use software and the responsiveness of the digital generations of surgeons, the hesitation and timidity so far encountered with respect to this kind of surgery are rapidly disappearing; thus, computer assistance no doubt will become standard for correction of deformities and fractures.

References

[1] D'Aubigne RM, Deschamps L. L'osteotomie plane oblique dans la correction des deformations des membres. Bull Mem Arch Chir 1952;8:271–276
[2] Meyer DC, Siebenrock KA, Schiele B, Gerber C. A new methodology for the planning of single-cut corrective osteotomies of mal-aligned long bones. Clin Biomech (Bristol, Avon) 2005;20(2):223–227
[3] Nagy L, Jankauskas L, Dumont CE. Correction of forearm malunion guided by the preoperative complaint. Clin Orthop Relat Res 2008;466(6):1419–1428
[4] Nagy L. Malunion of the distal end of the radius. In: Fernandez DL, Jupiter JB, eds. Fractures of the Distal Radius. New York: Springer; 2002:289–344
[5] Sangeorzan BJ, Sangeorzan BP, Hansen ST Jr, Judd RP. Mathematically directed single-cut osteotomy for correction of tibial malunion. J Orthop Trauma 1989;3(4):267–275
[6] Sangeorzan BP, Judd RP, Sangeorzan BJ. Mathematical analysis of single-cut osteotomy for complex long bone deformity. J Biomech 1989;22(11–12):1271–1278
[7] Christersson A, Nysjö J, Berglund L, et al. Comparison of 2D radiography and a semi-automatic CT-based 3D method for measuring change in dorsal angulation over time in distal radius fractures. Skeletal Radiol 2016;45(6):763–769
[8] Miyake J, Murase T, Yamanaka Y, Moritomo H, Sugamoto K. Comparison of three dimensional and radiographic measurements in the analysis of distal radius malunion. J Hand Surg Am 2012;38E(2):133–143
[9] Bindra RR, Cole RJ, Yamaguchi K, et al. Quantification of the radial torsion angle with computerized tomography in cadaver specimens. J Bone Joint Surg Am 1997;79(6):833–837
[10] Murase T, Oka K, Moritomo H, Goto A, Yoshikawa H, Sugamoto K. Three-dimensional corrective osteotomy of malunited fractures of the upper extremity with use of a computer simulation system. J Bone Joint Surg Am 2008;90(11):2375–2389
[11] Oka K, Moritomo H, Goto A, Sugamoto K, Yoshikawa H, Murase T. Corrective osteotomy for malunited intra-articular fracture of the distal radius using a custom-made surgical guide based on three-dimensional computer simulation: case report. J Hand Surg Am 2008;33(6):835–840
[12] Farshad M, Hess F, Nagy L, Schweizer A. Corrective osteotomy of distal radial deformities: a new method of guided locking fixed screw positioning. J Hand Surg Eur Vol 2013;38(1):29–34
[13] Bizzotto N, Tami I, Santucci A, et al. 3D printed replica of articular fractures for surgical planning and patient consent: a two years multi-centric experience. 3D Print Med 2015;2(1):2
[14] Bizzotto N, Tami I, Tami A, et al. 3D Printed models of distal radius fractures. Injury 2016;47(4):976–978
[15] Chen C, Cai L, Zhang C, Wang J, Guo X, Zhou Y. Treatment of die-punch fractures with 3D printing technology. J Invest Surg 2018;31(5):385–392
[16] Debarre E, Hivart P, Baranski D, Déprez P. Speedy skeletal prototype production to help diagnosis in orthopaedic and trauma surgery. Methodology and examples of clinical applications. Orthop Traumatol Surg Res 2012;98(5):597–602
[17] Athwal GS, Ellis RE, Small CF, Pichora DR. Computer-assisted distal radius osteotomy. J Hand Surg Am 2003;28(6):951–958
[18] Miyake J, Murase T, Moritomo H, Sugamoto K, Yoshikawa H. Distal radius osteotomy with volar locking plates based on computer simulation. Clin Orthop Relat Res 2011;469(6):1766–1773
[19] Schweizer A, Fürnstahl P, Nagy L. Three-dimensional correction of distal radius intra-articular malunions using patient-specific drill guides. J Hand Surg Am 2013;38(12):2339–2347
[20] Zimmermann R, Gabl M, Arora R, Rieger M. Computer-assisted planning and corrective osteotomy in distal radius malunion Handchir Mikrochir Plast Chir 2003;35(5):333–337
[21] de Muinck Keizer RJO, Lechner KM, Mulders MAM, Schep NWL, Eygendaal D, Goslings JC. Three-dimensional virtual planning of corrective osteotomies of distal radius malunions: a systematic review and meta-analysis. Strateg Trauma Limb Reconstr 2017;12(2):77–89
[22] Bauer DE, Zimmermann S, Aichmair A, et al. Conventional versus computer-assisted corrective osteotomy of the forearm: a retrospective analysis of 6 consecutive cases. J Hand Surg Am 2017;42(6):447–455
[23] Buijze GA, Leong NL, Stockmans F, et al. Three-dimensional compared with two-dimensional preoperative planning of corrective osteotomy for extraarticular distal radius malunion. J Bone Joint Surg 2018;100-A:1191–1202
[24] Roner S, Vlachopoulos L, Nagy L, Schweizer A, Fürnstahl P. Accuracy and Early clinical outcome of 3-dimensional planned and guided single-cut osteotomies of malunited forearm bones. J Hand Surg Am 2017;42(12):1031.e1–1031.e8
[25] Stockmans F, Dezillie M, Vanhaecke J. Accuracy of 3D virtual planning of corrective osteotomies of the distal radius. J Wrist Surg 2013;2(4):306–314
[26] Vlachopoulos L, Schweizer A, Graf M, Nagy L, Fürnstahl P. Three-dimensional postoperative accuracy of extra-articular forearm osteotomies using CT-scan based patient-specific surgical guides. BMC Musculoskelet Disord 2015;16:336–344
[27] Yoshii Y, Kusakabe T, Akita K, Tung WL, Ishii T. Reproducibility of three dimensional digital preoperative planning for the osteosynthesis of distal radius fractures. J Orthop Res 2017;35(12):2646–2651

24 Distal Radius in Children and Growth Disturbances

Alexandria L. Case, Joshua M. Abzug

Abstract

Distal radius fractures are the most common fracture in the pediatric population. The vast majority of these injuries can be treated nonoperatively, with or without a closed reduction. In the event that operative intervention is indicated, the majority of fractures can be adequately stabilized with a closed reduction and percutaneous pinning. Plate and screw fixation is rarely necessary and typically reserved for the adolescent population. Complications are fairly uncommon but can occur. A physeal arrest must be monitored for with close follow-up until growth is confirmed. If a physeal arrest occurs, a physeal bar resection, epiphysiodesis of the distal radius and/or ulna, a corrective osteotomy of the radius, and/or an ulna shortening osteotomy may be indicated to optimize outcomes.

Keywords: distal radius, physeal arrest, extraphyseal, Salter–Harris, physeal bar resection, epiphysiodesis, pediatric, adolescent, fracture

24.1 Distal Radius Fractures in Children: Introduction

Distal radius fractures are the most common fractures experienced by children and account for nearly a quarter of all pediatric fractures.[1,2,3] These injuries are classically caused by ground levels falls onto the outstretched upper extremity, particularly in or around the home.[4] Peak frequencies of distal radius fractures are observed around ages 11 to 14 years in male children and ages 8 to 11 years in female children.[5] Epidemiological analyses of distal radius fractures has shown that the prevalence of these injuries in the pediatric population has increased in recent years, likely due to increased sporting participation and changes in typical bone density and body mass index of the population.[5,6]

As the physis is the weakest portion of the musculoskeletal system in the growing child, it is biomechanically prone to fracture before ossified bone of the epiphysis or diaphysis. Within the physis, the zone of provisional calcification is especially susceptible to fracture by mechanical stresses.[7] However, the closer a fracture lies in proximity to the physis, the greater potential for remodeling may be experienced. As such, fractures at or near the physis present unique considerations, which must be considered during the treatment. The most commonly utilized descriptors for distal radius fractures are based on the fracture location, either extraphyseal or physeal fractures.

24.1.1 Extraphyseal Fractures

Extraphyseal distal radius fractures in the pediatric population typically involve the metaphysis of the radius and generally heal without complication. These fractures can be further described with reference to the amount of cortical involvement, either incomplete or complete extraphyseal fractures. More specifically, incomplete extraphyseal fractures are innately stable fractures due to the partially intact cortex remaining outside the fracture line, while complete extraphyseal fractures involve both cortices, thus potentially inducing instability. Incomplete extraphyseal fractures are further subcategorized as either greenstick fractures or torus/buckle fractures. Greenstick fractures are generally caused by a rotational mechanism in which one cortex is entirely disrupted while the other remains intact.[8] Torus/buckle fractures of the distal radius occur when the wrist is axially loaded with mechanical compression.[9] Complete extraphyseal fractures are associated with mechanisms involving excessive rotational or bending forces on the bone.[10]

24.1.2 Physeal Fractures

Distal radius physeal fractures are among the most common physeal fractures observed in growing children.[11] In the distal radius, 75 to 80% of the longitudinal bone growth of the radius originates from the distal radial physis.[12] Therefore, although physeal arrest is a rare complication seen in less than 7% of cases, it is imperative that the treating physician takes all precautions available to preserve growth within the physis to prevent long-term functional and cosmetic deficits.[11,13]

Salter–Harris Classification

Within the broader category of physeal fractures, a subcategorization system proposed by Salter and Harris in 1963 is widely used to further specify the extent of physeal involvement.[14] This classification is based on five primary designations, aptly termed Salter–Harris types I to V (SH I–V). An SH I fracture does not involve any ossified bone, with the fracture line traversing solely through the physis. Type II fractures are the most common type, accounting for nearly three-quarters of all distal radius physeal fractures in children.[14] These fractures are characterized by a fracture line, which extends through the physis and into the metaphysis. An SH III fracture extends from the physis into the epiphysis. Type IV fractures encompass all three of these sections, with a fracture line extending from the epiphysis to the metaphysis, through the physis or vice versa. An SH V fracture is rare and is notably different than the earlier types. These fractures are most often caused by crushing mechanisms or repeated compression and are associated with significantly increased rates of physeal arrest.[14]

24.1.3 Indications and Contraindications

Nondisplaced Fractures

Nondisplaced and minimally displaced fractures do not often require operative intervention. Given the proximity to the physis, particularly for fractures in younger children, distal radius fractures have tremendous potential for remodeling and are often able to be treated conservatively with casting or splinting. In the case of SH types I and II fractures, those that are minimally displaced or nondisplaced can typically be managed conservatively. In particular, fractures with less than 50% displacement and those that limited angulation are often casted and closely followed during the early stages of healing.[15] Current literature describes that fractures with less than 15° of sagittal plane angulation and/or 1 cm of shortening will remodel without substantial functional impairment.[16,17]

Torus/buckle fractures are inherently stable and can typically be treated nonoperatively. However, there is a lack of consensus as to what is truly classified as a buckle/torus fracture.[10] For a stable torus/buckle fracture, immobilization for approximately 3 weeks is recommended in a short-arm cast or splint. For older patients, splints may be utilized for immobilization and weaned as the patient's symptoms improve.

Displaced Fractures

General guidelines indicate that in children under 9 years of age, any amount of displacement and up to 15° of angulation and 45° of malrotation may be treated nonoperatively.[8,16,17] However, some authors recommend that up to 20 to 25° of flexion/extension angulation and 10° of radial/ulnar deviation are acceptable in the younger population.[18] Acceptable amounts of displacement and angulation for nonoperative treatment decrease with age as the remodeling potential diminishes with maturation and closure of the physes. In children 9 years and older, dorsal angulation greater than 20° should be treated with an intervention that improves the alignment.[8] It is important to note that complete fractures and fractures that are not inherently stable should be closely followed with weekly radiographs for up to 3 weeks to ensure maintenance of acceptable alignment.

Additional Indications for Surgical Intervention

Fracture patterns consistent with SH II to IV fractures often require a closed reduction to improve the alignment. Surgical intervention may also be indicated in cases of additional concurrent injuries, open fractures,

floating elbows, suspected neurovascular injury, and/or intra-articular involvement.[19] In these cases, additional preoperative imaging such as computed tomography (CT) or magnetic resonance imaging (MRI) may be ordered to better assess the injury and plan for surgery. Additional surgical indications include complete extraphyseal fractures, which are inherently unstable, an inability to obtain an acceptable reduction with closed means, and the need for correction of a deformity due to insufficient remodeling.

Furthermore, socioeconomic factors need to be considered when evaluating the need for operative intervention, particularly in cases where the angulation, displacement, and/or malrotation are borderline, as the socioeconomic factors may lead to poor compliance regarding the need for close follow-up to monitor for loss of acceptable alignment.

24.1.4 Surgical Technique

Closed Reduction under Anesthesia

Closed reduction under some sort anesthesia is most often the first-line treatment for fractures that are not in acceptable alignment. However, it is important to note that repeated attempts at reduction increase the potential for physeal injury and subsequent growth disturbance, and therefore, we recommend no more than two attempts at reduction in the emergency department followed by no more than two attempts at closed reduction in the operating room. Additionally, late attempts at reduction can also lead to an increase in physeal damage, and therefore, attempts at closed reduction of physeal fractures should be limited to about 2 weeks from the time of injury. If a physeal fracture presents following this time frame, the fracture should be allowed to heal and remodel, even if a malunion develops, as the deformity can be corrected later on if needed without damaging the physis.

The method of anesthesia may vary based on where the closed reduction is taking place (i.e., emergency department vs. operating room) and physician preferences. Commonly, distal radius fractures can be reduced under anesthesia by means of a hematoma or intravenous block, axillary block, self-administered 50/50 nitrous oxide mixture, conscious sedation, general anesthesia, or some combination of these methods.[20,21,22,23,24,25] To perform a closed reduction, traction should initially be applied to unlock the fracture ends. Subsequently, the distal fragment should be translated in the direction opposite the angulation (i.e., volar translation for a dorsally angulated fracture). While maintaining the fracture in a reduced position, the extremity should be immobilized in either a sugar tong splint or long-arm cast. Proper casting technique, including either a three-point or interosseous mold and an optimal cast index, is imperative to optimize the potential to maintain the reduction. Follow-up radiographs over the first 2 to 3 weeks after reduction are imperative to ensure maintenance of acceptable alignment.

Closed Reduction with Percutaneous Pinning (CRPP)

Percutaneous pinning can provide stabilization following a reduction under anesthesia. This procedure is performed in cases of inherently unstable fractures, fractures that have failed prior attempts at closed reduction, and when stabilization of a fracture is needed without the aid of a cast/splint (i.e., open wounds, a floating elbow injury that one does not want to apply a circumferential dressing, or an associated vascular injury that requires close observation). A CRPP procedure minimizes surgical time and invasiveness while providing substantial stability to the fracture.

The procedure is performed utilizing the semisterile technique directly on an inverted large fluoroscopy unit (▶ Fig. 24.1). Alternatively, one can use a hand table or a mini C-arm. Following the closed reduction and confirmation of acceptable alignment in both the coronal and sagittal planes using fluoroscopy, Kirschner wires (K-wires) of appropriate size for the patient's age and size can be inserted either percutaneously or using a small longitudinal incision over the radial styloid. The wire is placed on the radial styloid for physeal fractures or just proximal to the physis for extraphyseal fractures and is driven retrograde, crossing the fracture site in a bicortical manner as confirmed with fluoroscopic imaging. An additional K-wire can be inserted, either in a divergent or crossed manner, if additional stability is thought to be necessary (▶ Fig. 24.2). Once the K-wire(s) have been appropriately placed, they should be bent 90° with the bend approximately 1 cm from the skin surface and then cut such that only about 1 cm of the K-wire persists past the bend. Additional fluoroscopic images should be obtained to ensure there was no loss of alignment during this process. Sterile dressings are then applied followed by application of a well-molded long-arm cast. Follow-up radiographs should be obtained within 1 week following the procedure to ensure that the reduction has been maintained. Additional radiographs are obtained 4 to 6 weeks postoperatively, and if the fracture is healed, the K-wire can be removed in the outpatient setting without any need for anesthesia. Additional follow-up radiographs should be obtained over the course of the next year until either longitudinal growth is confirmed or a physeal bar is apparent.

Open Reduction with Internal Fixation (ORIF)

ORIF is reserved for open fractures, fractures that cannot be closed reduced into acceptable alignment, and late presenting extraphyseal fractures that are substantially angulated. An ORIF of a pediatric or adolescent fracture is analogous to the adult procedure with a few notable differences. First, in younger children that require an ORIF, K-wires can be used as the definitive fixation. Second, for patients that require plate and screw fixation, it is imperative to ensure that the plate remains proximal to the physis if the child is still growing (▶ Fig. 24.3). Third, patients that will be placed in a cast for a prolonged period of time postoperatively may have hardware used that does not completely provide rigid stabilization of the fracture. For example, a smaller size plate and screw construct may be utilized to align the fracture, while a cast or splint immobilizes the extremity for a prolonged period of time to permit fracture healing. Lastly, it is important to note that distal radius fractures that are somewhat proximal in nature may be amenable to treatment with an intramedullary flexible nail.

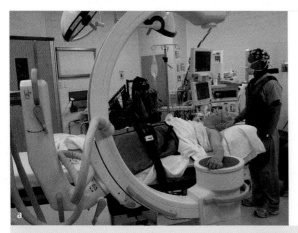
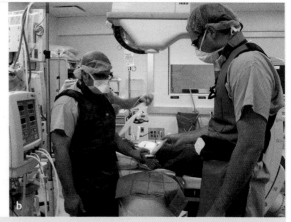

Fig. 24.1 (a) Operating room setup for closed reduction and percutaneous pinning. Note that the standard fluoroscopy unit is inverted and used as the operating room table. (b) Semisterile technique utilized for closed reduction and percutaneous pinning. Note the lack of excessive drapes, gowns, and so forth. (These images are provided courtesy of Joshua M. Abzug, Baltimore, MD.)

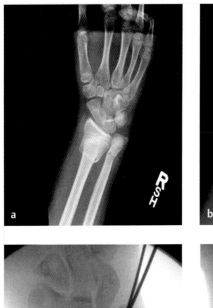

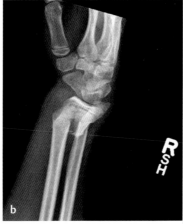

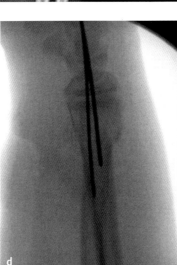

Fig. 24.2 Extraphyseal distal radius fracture with substantial displacement in an 11-year-old female who fell off of a horse. **(a)** Preoperative posteroanterior wrist radiograph. **(b)** Preoperative lateral wrist radiograph. **(c)** Intraoperative posteroanterior fluoroscopic view following CRPP. **(d)** Intraoperative lateral fluoroscopic view following CRPP. (These images are provided courtesy of Joshua M. Abzug, Baltimore, MD.)

Corrective Osteotomies

A corrective osteotomy may be indicated in patients originally treated nonoperatively who experience insufficient remodeling with subsequent loss of functional motion or instability at the distal radioulnar joint (DRUJ).[26] Various osteotomies can be performed, including closing wedge, opening wedge, or dome osteotomies, depending on the deformity present. An ulnar shortening osteotomy, in isolation or in conjunction with the distal radius osteotomy, may also be utilized to address the deformity present. Osteotomies can be stabilized utilizing K-wires or Steinmann pins in young children or with a volar or dorsal plate in older children/adolescents. For patients in need of a lengthening procedure, an external fixator (uniplanar or multiplanar, depending on the correction needed) may be employed or one can achieve the lengthening acutely with the aid of tricortical bone graft. Utilization of ample irrigation during the osteotomy is mandatory to minimize the risk of osteonecrosis. Immobilization for a minimum of 4 weeks is recommended

with an initial follow-up visit 1 week postoperatively to ensure that the osteotomy and subsequent fixation are remaining in proper alignment. At 4 to 6 weeks postoperatively, a thermoplastic splint can be made and the patient can be referred to outpatient therapy.

24.1.5 Results

The proximity of distal radius fractures to the rapidly growing physis in skeletally immature children contributes to the overwhelming rate of excellent outcomes associated with these fractures. Subsequent occupational or physical therapy is rarely required as motion is quickly regained through play and everyday activities. The vast majority of nondisplaced or minimally displaced distal radius fractures are healed without complication. Operative intervention increases the risk of complications, although serious and lasting complications are rarely observed following these injuries in the pediatric and adolescent population.

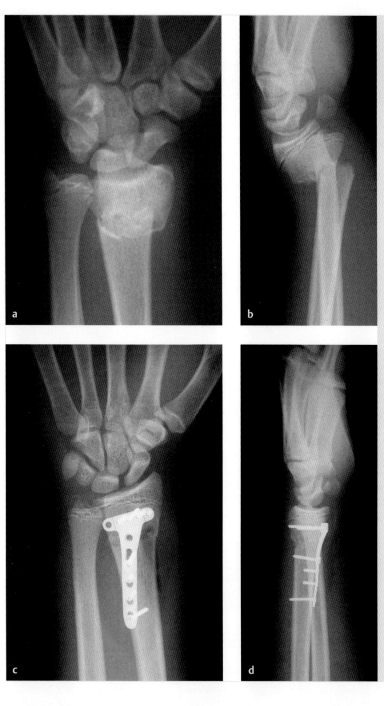

Fig. 24.3 (a) Posteroanterior and **(b)** lateral radiographs of a 15-year-old boy who sustained an extraphyseal distal radius fracture. **(c)** Postoperative posteroanterior and **(d)** lateral radiographs showing the use of the T-plate. Note that the plate is proximal to the physis. (These images are provided courtesy of Shriners Hospital for Children, Philadelphia, PA.)

Complications associated with operative procedures include persistent pain, pin tract infections, scarring, pin migration, physeal damage, and/or tendon irritation. Nonunion is extremely rare but can be present in cases of ORIF due to the amount of trauma incurred during surgery.[27,28] Radioulnar synostosis is another potential complication, which can result fromhigh-energy mechanisms such as motor vehicle or all-terrain vehicle accidents; however, this is exceedingly rare.[8]

24.1.6 Pitfalls

- Failure to have close follow-up to monitor for loss of alignment as this can lead to malunion and long-term functional deficits.
- Poor casting technique can contribute to loss of alignment.
- Failure to continue follow-up after initial treatment to ensure no growth arrest occurred can lead to delayed diagnosis and ulnar abutment syndrome.

- Failure to recognize concomitant injuries in the upper extremity may lead to functional impairment and poor outcomes.

24.2 Growth Disturbances Following Distal Radius Fractures: Introduction

Despite the low reported incidence, 1 to 7%, of physeal arrest associated with distal radius fractures, this complication is recognized as one of the most detrimental consequences of these injuries.[11,13] The ossification of the distal radius epiphysis begins at about 8 months of age with physeal closure occurring around the age of 14 to 15 years in females and 16 to 17 years in males. A variety of factors, both known and unknown, may contribute to the premature closure of the physis. One known factor is direct damage to the proliferative and/or reserve zones of the physis. Additional factors include late attempts at reduction (greater than 14 days postinjury), multiple attempts at reduction, substantial physeal trauma during operative intervention, extensive trauma to the physis at the time of injury, and/or repetitive stresses across the physis such as during activities like gymnastics.[29,30]

Acute distal radius fractures should be monitored following the healing of the acute fracture with radiographs at approximately 3-month intervals to monitor for physeal arrest. The radiographs should be continued until definitive longitudinal growth is present or a physeal injury is confirmed. An increase in the ulnar variance is concerning for physeal arrest and should be further investigated, utilizing advanced imaging to assess the

distal radius physis.[31] CT and/or MRI (▶ Fig. 24.4) can accurately diagnose and locate a physeal bar as well as assess the specific size and location of the area of early ossification.[32,33]

A partial or complete physeal arrest of the distal radial physis may occur following a fracture but is also observed in skeletally immature athletes who endure repetitive stress on the physis through repeated movement such as those introduced throughout gymnastics. For this reason, gymnasts often utilize splints, which prevent hyperextension of the wrist in an attempt to limit the amount of force that is directly applied to the physis.

Physeal arrests are classified as either complete or partial, depending upon the amount of the physis, which has begun to, or is already, ossified. In the case of a partial physeal arrest, the term *physeal bar* is often used to describe the portion of the physis, which has early ossification secondary to trauma. The most commonly observed type of partial physeal arrest is a central growth arrest, in which the portion of early ossification is located centrally within the physis, while the medial and lateral aspects of the physis attempt to continue to propagate new bone growth. These types of physeal arrests are often treated by physeal bar resections with interposition, assuming the physeal bar accounts for less than 50% of the physis. Peripheral physeal arrests are those in which the physeal bar is located either medially or laterally. These physeal arrests have substantially greater impacts on the observable deformity of the wrist. Given the location of these physeal bars, an epiphysiodesis is often considered if the patient is close enough to skeletal maturity to prevent a substantial limb-length discrepancy. In the case of SH III and SH IV fractures, linear

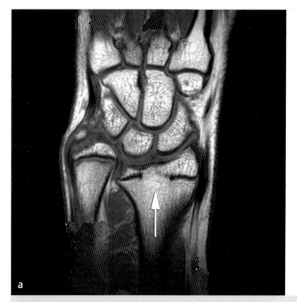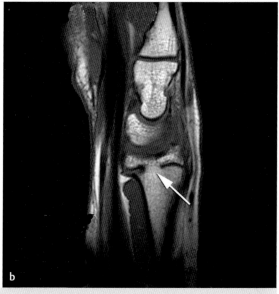

Fig. 24.4 (a) Coronal and **(b)** sagittal T1-weighted magnetic resonance images of the wrist showing a central bar (*arrows*) traversing the distal radius physis. (These images are provided courtesy of Shriners Hospital for Children, Philadelphia, PA.)

physeal arrests may be observed to follow the path of the former fracture line. As the physeal bar associated with these fractures may be quite small, continued growth of the physis on either side of this physeal bar may lead to the breakage of the bar, permitting continued growth of the radius. Alternatively, a transverse physeal bar may develop along the course of the intraphyseal fracture line.[31]

If close follow-up does not occur following an acute fracture, a physeal arrest is often not identified until it becomes symptomatic years after the initial injury. A study by Waters et al reported that the average time from initial injury to corrective surgery for physeal arrest was 38 months (range: 6–120 months).[34]

24.2.1 Indications and Contraindications

The treatment of a physeal arrest is dependent upon a number of factors, including patient age/gender, remaining growth potential, and familial history of late growth spurts. In the case of female patients, the onset of menarche plays an important role during the treatment discussion, as this is indicative of cessation of growth within 2 years in the majority of patients. The location and size of the physeal arrest are also key determinants when discussing the treatment strategy.

A partial physeal arrest may be treated with a physeal bar resection with interposition grafting. This procedure is ideally performed when the physeal bar is centrally located and makes up less than 50% of the physis. However, it should be noted that this procedure is less reliable than the other options subsequently listed. If the radial physis has completely ossified but the ulnar physis is still actively contributing to the length of the ulna, ultimately ulna abutment syndrome will develop. Therefore, it is prudent to perform a procedure to stop longitudinal growth of the ulna or a procedure to lengthen the radius, thus minimizing the potential for ulna abutment syndrome, bowing of the forearm, decreased forearm rotation, and/or a cosmetic deformity. A discussion between the surgeon, the patient, and the family should occur to discuss the available surgical procedures and their outcomes. If the ulnar physis is closing and the radial physis has already arrested, it may be ideal to manage the patient conservatively. However, if any true growth is remaining, the most reliable treatment in older children and adolescents is a completion ulna epiphysiodesis. It is important to note that this will lead to a limb-length discrepancy and the patient and the parents must be made aware of that. In young children, a radial lengthening may be optimal; however, the parents must understand the high complication rate associated with this procedure as well as the fact that multiple lengthenings may be needed during the growing years. Ultimately, the decision to operate or not to operate as well as which procedure to perform

should be a shared decision-making process between the surgeon, the patient, and the family.

24.2.2 Surgical Techniques

Physeal Bar Resection

In cases of central physeal bar formation, a physeal bar resection may be performed to remove the ossified portion of the physis to allow for continuation of growth along the remaining, functioning portions of the physis. This procedure is ideal in cases of early identification and can minimize the impact of a physeal arrest. The treating surgeon will need to remove the entire physeal bar to ensure that the physis is not tethered in any way. In the distal radius, this procedure is commonly performed through a longitudinal dorsal incision over the distal radius. Following exposure of the physis, a burr is used to remove the ossified area of the physis. The normal surrounding physis has a bluish hinge and should remain intact. Fluoroscopy should be utilized judiciously during the procedure to ensure that the bar has been removed in its entirety but the damage to the surrounding intact physis is minimal. It is imperative that the portion of resected physis is replaced by a filler material, or "plug," to prevent recurrence of the physeal bar. The interposed material may vary between surgeons but can include fat interposition, sourced from the surrounding soft tissue during the resection, or substances such as methyl methacrylate or silicone rubber.[7,35,36,37] The patient must be followed long-term until skeletal maturity to ensure that the physis continues to grow and no new physeal bar develops. Occasionally, the remaining intact physis just "peters out" and stops growing before the normal uninjured ulna, and this must be monitored for.

Epiphysiodesis

Epiphysiodesis procedures involve the removal of the normal healthy growth plate and can be utilized in cases of either partial or complete physeal arrest. This procedure is commonly performed in older children and adolescents who have limited growth potential remaining at the radius and/or ulna. In cases of complete physeal arrest of the radius, epiphysiodesis procedures may be performed bilaterally to prevent a limb-length discrepancy from occurring. Although the techniques for these procedures may vary amongst surgeons, an epiphysiodesis is a relatively efficient and reliable procedure that can be performed through a small incision. Following the incision, blunt dissection is carried down to the bone. Subsequently, a guidewire for a cannulated drill is placed into the physis under fluoroscopic guidance. The drill is then placed over the guidewire to create a tract and the guidewire is removed. The drill is reintroduced and used to ablate the physis. Care should be taken during this process to ensure that the drill is appropriately aligned

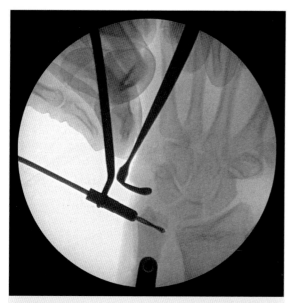

Fig. 24.5 Intraoperative fluoroscopic image of the wrist demonstrating the use of a cannulated drill to perform an ulnar epiphysiodesis. (The image is provided courtesy of Joshua M. Abzug, Baltimore, MD.)

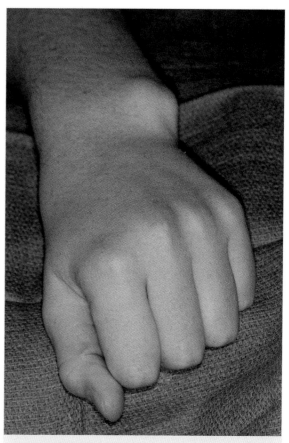

Fig. 24.6 Clinical photograph of the hand and wrist demonstrating a prominent ulnar head following physeal arrest of the distal radius. (The image is provided courtesy of Shriners Hospital for Children, Philadelphia, PA.)

with the physis and is placed at the appropriate depth (▶ Fig. 24.5). Additionally, a curette or burr can be placed in the tract to remove any remaining physeal cartilage. Patients are subsequently immobilized for approximately 2 weeks, after which they should be followed with radiographs taken 3 to 6 months postoperatively to monitor the effect of the procedure and ensure that bone growth has ceased.

Corrective Osteotomies

Dependent upon the location, severity, and time of diagnosis of the physeal arrest, a corrective osteotomy may be warranted. An osteotomy can be indicated when the physeal arrest is diagnosed after growth has ceased, when the substantial deformity is present or when the ulna is substantially longer than the radius (▶ Fig. 24.6). Often, these scenarios occur in cases in which the physeal arrest occurs outside the period of typical fracture follow-up and is not observed until it becomes symptomatic or an additional injury requiring radiographs is obtained. Radial osteotomies are indicated for partial growth arrests that result in angular deformities at the wrist, which can be painful at presentation, and also create the potential for long-term complications such as arthritis and degenerative changes at the wrist due to malalignment between the radius and ulna and the carpal bones. These procedures are specifically beneficial in correcting malalignment in the coronal and sagittal planes. Additionally, one can correct the deformity and simultaneously lengthen the radius acutely. The use of tricortical

bone graft is ideal when performing an acute lengthening of the radius (▶ Fig. 24.7). Close follow-up should be continued until the bony union is observed on radiographs.

If a patient begins experiencing ulnar abutment syndrome, a condition that is hallmarked by pain from excessive impaction between the ulna and carpal bones (▶ Fig. 24.8), an ulnar shortening osteotomy may be indicated. By shortening the ulna, pain caused by ulnar impaction into the lunate or triquetrum can be alleviated. A shortening osteotomy of the ulna may be successful in restoring stability and alignment at the DRUJ to normalize biomechanics at the wrist without requiring additional procedures or treatment. In patients with bone growth remaining, a distal ulnar epiphysiodesis may be recommended to prevent the need for a repeat ulnar shortening osteotomy. Ulnar shortening osteotomies are most effective when the discrepancy between the radial and ulnar lengths is less than 12 to 15 mm, as larger osteotomies can present technical challenges and increase the risk of complications such as nonunion. When performing an ulnar osteotomy, the cut should be made as distal as possible while ensuring there is

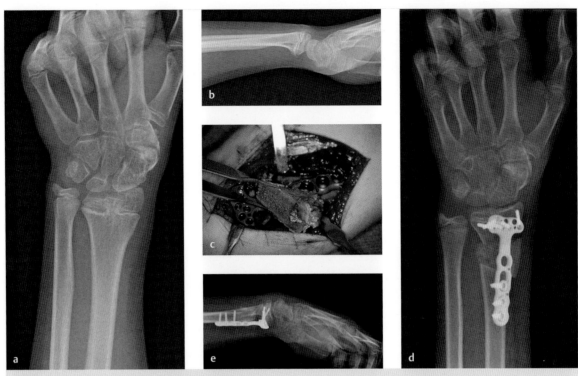

Fig. 24.7 **(a)** Preoperative posteroanterior and **(b)** lateral radiographs of the distal radius demonstrating physeal arrest in an 11-year-old boy following a fracture. **(c)** Intraoperative fluoroscopic image showing a corticocancellous iliac crest autograft used to perform an acute radius lengthening. **(d)** Postoperative posteroanterior and **(e)** lateral radiographs demonstrating the plate and screw construct. (These images are provided courtesy of Shriners Hospital for Children, Philadelphia, PA.)

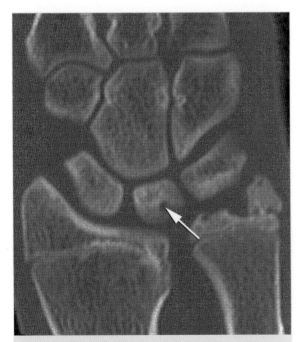

Fig. 24.8 Coronal computed tomography (CT) scan of the wrist demonstrating physeal arrest of the ulnar half of the distal radius. Note the early arthritic changes demonstrated by the cystic lesion (*arrow*) on the lunate caused by ulnar abutment. (The image is provided courtesy of Joshua M. Abzug, Baltimore, MD.)

enough space for adequate fixation distally. To minimize the potential disruption of the blood supply, the amount of periosteum disrupted should be minimal, ideally only disrupting the periosteum at the level of the planned osteotomy. A wedge of bone equal to the desired amount of shortening should be removed, and the hardware is placed to compress the bone at the osteotomy site. Several commercially available systems exist that permit the osteotomy to occur with malrotation of the fragments. Placement of the plate on the volar aspect of the ulna can reduce irritation caused by hardware and decrease the potential for hardware removal (▶Fig. 24.9). Close follow-up is necessary to monitor the osteotomy site until the union is confirmed.

Distraction Osteogenesis

Distraction osteogenesis is an alternative to an acute lengthening or corrective osteotomy, particularly in cases with a limb-length discrepancy of 5 mm or greater.[38] These procedures effectively address length discrepancies without requiring permanent hardware. A circular external fixator is used over an extended period of time to address both length and angular deformities. However, such procedures introduce risk for increased complications and unplanned returns to the operating room. Complications may include pin tract infections, skin tenting,

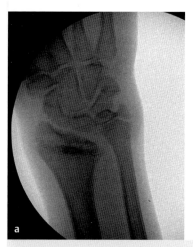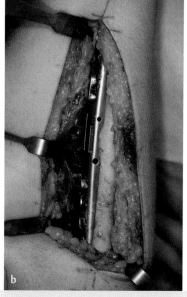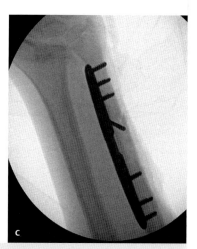

Fig. 24.9 (a) Preoperative fluoroscopic image of the distal radius demonstrating physeal growth arrest and ulnar abutment. **(b)** Intraoperative photograph showing the volar placement of the ulnar shortening osteotomy plate. **(c)** Postoperative fluoroscopic image of the radius and ulna demonstrating placement of the osteotomy plate following an ulnar shortening of 15 mm. Note the oblique cut and placement of the lag screw. (These images are provided courtesy of Joshua M. Abzug, Baltimore, MD.)

dermatitis, and ulnar subluxation.[38] The primary advantage of such procedures is to allow for correction of angular deformities that cannot be optimally managed with wedge osteotomies. Additionally, the extended period of time in which the external fixator is in place allows for gradual manipulation as the healing progresses.[38,39] Uniplanar devices can be used if no deformity correction is needed. The parents and child must be educated regarding the prolonged time the child will be in the frame as well as the potential complications associated with this treatment option.

24.2.3 Results

Operative procedures following physeal arrest of the distal radius physis are focused on alleviating pain and minimizing long-term functional impairment caused by uneven growth between the radius and ulna or from substantial limb-length discrepancies. Current literature assessing the long-term follow-up of the procedures utilized to treatment distal radius physeal arrests is limited but suggests that the aforementioned procedures may successfully restore anatomic alignment of the wrist and reduce symptoms induced by the physeal arrest.

24.2.4 Pitfalls

- Failure to monitor for physeal arrest following an acute fracture is the number one pitfall associated with distal radius physeal arrest, as early diagnosis

permits less invasive management and minimization of long-term functional deficits.
- Failure to ablate the entire physis during an epiphysiodesis may result in further, and potentially worsened, deformities and functional impairment. Use of intraoperative fluoroscopy is recommended to reduce the risk of such complications.
- Improper wedge approximation during a corrective osteotomy may result in an unplanned return to the operating room. This can be avoided utilizing thorough preoperative planning and radiographic assessment.

Tips and Tricks

Acute distal radius fracture evaluation:
- Ensure the entire upper extremity is assessed to rule out concomitant injuries.
- Ensure true anteroposterior and lateral views are obtained so that adequate assessment of angulation can occur.
- Fractures treated with closed means, with or without a closed reduction, should be followed weekly for at least 2–3 wk to monitor for loss of alignment.
- Closed reduction and percutaneous pinning procedures can be performed utilizing the semisterile technique, thus limited healthcare costs and waste.
- All physeal fractures must be followed until longitudinal growth in the distal radius is confirmed or one identifies a physeal arrest.

Distal radial physeal arrest treatment:
- Early recognition of a physeal arrest in an older child/ adolescent is most reliably treated with a completion epiphysiodesis of the distal radius combined with a distal ulna epiphysiodesis.

24.3 Conclusion

Distal radius fractures are extremely common injuries in the pediatric population and typically result in successful healing and return to preinjury function. Nonoperative treatment with casting or splinting is often sufficient for nondisplaced or minimally displaced fractures. In the case of a fracture with substantial displacement or angulation, closed reduction and casting are typically sufficient to yield an excellent outcome. Operative intervention is reserved for fractures that failed closed treatment and those in which acceptable alignment was not able to be obtained with closed methods. Although the rate of physeal arrest following a fracture of the distal radius in children is low, appropriate caution should be taken during the initial treatment to minimize the risk. This includes the utilization of adequate anesthesia during reduction attempts, avoiding multiple reduction attempts, and avoiding late reduction attempts. If a physeal arrest does develop, procedures including physeal bar resection, epiphysiodesis, wedge osteotomies, ulnar shortening osteotomy, and/or distraction osteogenesis may be performed to prevent or correct limb-length discrepancies, forearm deformities, and/or functional impairment at the wrist/forearm.

References

[1] Landin LA. Fracture patterns in children. Analysis of 8,682 fractures with special reference to incidence, etiology and secular changes in a Swedish urban population 1950–1979. Acta Orthop Scand Suppl 1983;202:1–109

[2] Cheng JC, Shen WY. Limb fracture pattern in different pediatric age groups: a study of 3,350 children. J Orthop Trauma 1993;7(1):15–22

[3] Landin LA. Epidemiology of children's fractures. J Pediatr Orthop B 1997;6(2):79–83

[4] Rodríguez-Merchán EC. Pediatric fractures of the forearm. Clin Orthop Relat Res 2005;(432):65–72

[5] Skaggs DL, Loro ML, Pitukcheewanont P, Tolo V, Gilsanz V. Increased body weight and decreased radial cross-sectional dimensions in girls with forearm fractures. J Bone Miner Res 2001;16(7):1337–1342

[6] Khosla S, Melton LJ III, Dekutoski MB, Achenbach SJ, Oberg AL, Riggs BL. Incidence of childhood distal forearm fractures over 30 years: a population-based study. JAMA 2003;290(11):1479–1485

[7] Bright RW. Operative correction of partial epiphyseal plate closure by osseous-bridge resection and silicone-rubber implant. An experimental study in dogs. J Bone Joint Surg Am 1974;56(4):655–664

[8] Noonan KJ, Price CT. Forearm and distal radius fractures in children. J Am Acad Orthop Surg 1998;6(3):146–156

[9] Bae DS, Howard AW. Distal radius fractures: what is the evidence? J Pediatr Orthop 2012;32(Suppl 2):S128–S130

[10] Dua K, Abzug JM, Sesko Bauer A, Cornwall R, Wyrick TO. Pediatric Distal Radius Fractures. Instr Course Lect 2017;66:447–460

[11] Lee BS, Esterhai JL Jr, Das M. Fracture of the distal radial epiphysis. Characteristics and surgical treatment of premature, post-traumatic epiphyseal closure. Clin Orthop Relat Res 1984;(185):90–96

[12] Digby KH. The measurement of diaphysial growth in proximal and distal directions. J Anat Physiol 1916;50(Pt 2):187–188

[13] Buterbaugh GA, Palmer AK. Fractures and dislocations of the distal radioulnar joint. Hand Clin 1988;4(3):361–375

[14] Salter R, Harris WR. Injuries involving the epiphyseal plate: AAOS instructional course lecture. J Bone Joint Surg Am 1963;45:587–622

[15] Egol KA, Koval KJ, Zuckerman JD. Handbook of Fractures. 4th ed. Philadelphia, PA: Lippincott Williams & Wilkins; 2010

[16] Do TT, Strub WM, Foad SL, Mehlman CT, Crawford AH. Reduction versus remodeling in pediatric distal forearm fractures: a preliminary cost analysis. J Pediatr Orthop B 2003;12(2):109–115

[17] Roy DR. Completely displaced distal radius fractures with intact ulnas in children. Orthopedics 1989;12(8):1089–1092

[18] Bae DS. Pediatric distal radius and forearm fractures. J Hand Surg Am 2008;33(10):1911–1923

[19] Bae DS, Waters PM. Pediatric distal radius fractures and triangular fibrocartilage complex injuries. Hand Clin 2006;22(1):43–53

[20] Price CT, Choy JY. Current practice of sedation and pain management in the reduction of pediatric forearm fractures: A survey. Orthop Trans 1995;19:42

[21] Juliano PJ, Mazur JM, Cummings RJ, McCluskey WP. Low-dose lidocaine intravenous regional anesthesia for forearm fractures in children. J Pediatr Orthop 1992;12(5):633–635

[22] Wedel DJ, Krohn JS, Hall JA. Brachial plexus anesthesia in pediatric patients. Mayo Clin Proc 1991;66(6):583–588

[23] Varela CD, Lorfing KC, Schmidt TL. Intravenous sedation for the closed reduction of fractures in children. J Bone Joint Surg Am 1995;77(3):340–345

[24] Evans JK, Buckley SL, Alexander AH, Gilpin AT. Analgesia for the reduction of fractures in children: a comparison of nitrous oxide with intramuscular sedation. J Pediatr Orthop 1995;15(1):73–77

[25] Hennrikus WL, Shin AY, Klingelberger CE. Self-administered nitrous oxide and a hematoma block for analgesia in the outpatient reduction of fractures in children. J Bone Joint Surg Am 1995;77(3):335–339

[26] Miller A, Lightdale-Miric N, Eismann E, Carr P, Little KJ. Outcomes of isolated radial osteotomy for volar distal radioulnar joint instability following radial malunion in children. J Hand Surg Am 2018;43(1):81.e1–81.e8

[27] Lewallen RP, Peterson HA. Nonunion of long bone fractures in children: a review of 30 cases. J Pediatr Orthop 1985;5(2):135–142

[28] Fernandez FF, Eberhardt O, Langendörfer M, Wirth T. Nonunion of forearm shaft fractures in children after intramedullary nailing. J Pediatr Orthop B 2009;18(6):289–295

[29] Abzug JM, Zlotolow DA. Pediatric Hand and Wrist Fractures. Curr Orthop Pract 2012;23:327–330

[30] Valverde JA, Albiñana J, Certucha JA. Early posttraumatic physeal arrest in distal radius after a compression injury. J Pediatr Orthop B 1996;5(1):57–60

[31] Abzug JM, Little K, Kozin SH. Physeal arrest of the distal radius. J Am Acad Orthop Surg 2014;22(6):381–389

[32] Young JW, Bright RW, Whitley NO. Computed tomography in the evaluation of partial growth plate arrest in children. Skeletal Radiol 1986;15(7):530–535

[33] Sailhan F, Chotel F, Guibal AL, et al. Three-dimensional MR imaging in the assessment of physeal growth arrest. Eur Radiol 2004;14(9):1600–1608

[34] Waters PM, Bae DS, Montgomery KD. Surgical management of posttraumatic distal radial growth arrest in adolescents. J Pediatr Orthop 2002;22(6):717–724

[35] Langenskiöld A. Partial closure of the epiphyseal plate. Principles of treatment. 1978. Clin Orthop Relat Res 1993;(297):4–6

[36] Peterson HA, Madhok R, Benson JT, Ilstrup DM, Melton LJ III. Physeal fractures: Part 1. Epidemiology in Olmsted County, Minnesota, 1979–1988. J Pediatr Orthop 1994;14(4):423–430

[37] Lonjon G, Barthel PY, Ilharreborde B, Journeau P, Lascombes P, Fitoussi F. Bone bridge resection for correction of distal radial deformities after partial growth plate arrest: two cases and surgical technique. J Hand Surg Eur Vol 2012;37(2):170–175

[38] Page WT, Szabo RM. Distraction osteogenesis for correction of distal radius deformity after physeal arrest. J Hand Surg Am 2009;34(4):617–626

[39] Gündeş H, Buluç L, Sahin M, Alici T. Deformity correction by Ilizarov distraction osteogenesis after distal radius physeal arrest. Acta Orthop Traumatol Turc 2011;45(6):406–411

25 Open Surgery for Chronic Scapholunate Injury

Dirck Ananos, Marc Garcia-Elias

Abstract

A wrist is unstable when it gives way under physiologic loads. Injury to the scapholunate (SL) ligament tends to cause wrist instability particularly when the so-called helical antipronation ligaments (HAPLs) cannot send proper proprioceptive information to the intracarpal supinator muscles, the ultimate SL joint stabilizers. Several HAPL reconstructions using local tendons have been proposed. Those tendon grafts, however, do not contain active mechanoreceptors. Furthermore, it is not known whether a properly vascularized and innervated environment will help new receptors to grow into the graft and reinitiate the process of joint stabilization. This chapter will explain commonly used SL reconstructions, with the understanding that these need to be still regarded as experimental at this point in time.

Keywords: Carpal bones, ECRL tendon, FCR tendon, ligamentoplasty, misalignment, spiral tenodesis, three-ligament tenodesis, wrist instability

25.1 Introduction

This chapter should not start without first clarifying some carelessly used terminology. Particularly problematic are the concepts of wrist misalignment and carpal instability. There are two meanings for the term "stability": one derives from the verb "to stand," that is, to be capable of resisting loads; the other, rather different, comes from the verb "to stay," that is, to remain permanently unaltered. If we believe that both meanings are complementary descriptions of one single condition, we are creating the basis for misleading expressions such as "static instability." The problem is not only semantic. If all malalignments were to be considered permanently unstable, all should be surgically intervened, and this, obviously, would be dangerously wrong. Reality is less dramatic, fortunately. Most carpal instabilities deteriorate with time. After carpal collapse, most capsules and allied soft tissues undergo a process of contraction, all empty spaces fill up with fibrosis, and the wrist becomes osteoarthritic. In fact, down the line, most misaligned wrists become stiff and, in many instances, asymptomatic. (▶Fig. 25.1). Certainly, clarifying what is unstable and what is not becomes a practical necessity.[1]

25.1.1 Terminology

- *Instability* is defined as the inability of a load-bearing structure to resist normal amount of loads without collapsing. A wrist is stable when it is capable of bearing physiologic loads without yielding. If it gives way when loaded, a wrist is unstable. If an alteration of forces induces the carpus to collapse, that wrist is by definition unstable, despite being well aligned.
- *Misalignment* refers to an improper position of one of many elements of a load-bearing structure in the three-dimensional space. A misaligned wrist may become evident by the presence of a widened SL gap or by increased angulation of an SL angle. However, it is important to understand that "instability" and "misalignment" are not synonyms. Instability is a dynamic term that cannot be measured in static terms (millimeter of a gap or degrees of an SL angle). Only carpal misalignment may be quantified this way. Therefore, the wrist with an SL injury may be both misaligned and unstable, either or neither.

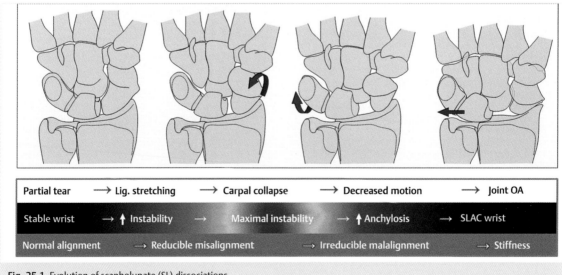

Partial tear	→ Lig. stretching	→ Carpal collapse	→ Decreased motion	→ Joint OA
Stable wrist	→ ↑ Instability	→ Maximal instability	→ ↑ Anchylosis	→ SLAC wrist
Normal alignment	→ Reducible misalignment	→ Irreducible malalignment	→ Stiffness

Fig. 25.1 Evolution of scapholunate (SL) dissociations.

- *Stiffness* is a clinical sign experienced by a patient whose wrist has had an abnormal reduction in the range of motion. Hence, stiffness and instability are mutually exclusive wrist dysfunctions. A joint may be unstable or stiff but not both.
- *Clinical symptoms* are usually the reason why patients seek attention. In other joints, symptoms are directly proportional to the severity of the case. This, however, cannot be always said if we assess carpal dysfunctions. The symptoms of pain and instability may not exist even in the presence of severe misalignment. Indeed, the rate of asymptomatic osteoarthritic wrists is unknown but certainly more common than usually assumed. For this reason, we propose including clinical symptoms as another variable to consider for the assessment and treatment of carpal dysfunctions.

25.1.2 Ligaments Involved in Scapholunate Instability

Ligaments are not merely static cables binding bones together, but complex arrangements of dense collagen fibers that contain sensorial elements (mechanoreceptors) able to detect changes in carpal bone position, and transmit this information to the sensorimotor system for centralized control of neuromuscular joint stabilization.[1,2,3,4] Depending upon the direction of their fascicles, some carpal ligaments are naturally aligned to detect one particular type of intracarpal displacement, while others are ready for a different type of torque. The so-called helical antipronation ligaments (HAPLs) are specialized in preventing carpal collapse when the distal row is torqued into pronation.[5] While the dorsal and volar ligaments are considered primary SL stabilizers, the HAPLs have a secondary, yet very important role in wrist stabilization (▶ Fig. 25.2, ▶ Fig. 25.3).

25.2 Indications

For an SL-dissociated wrist to be a good candidate for carpal realignment using neighboring tendon,
- The dissociation must be complete and nonrepairable.
- Carpal misalignment must be easily reducible.
- The periscaphoid cartilages must be normal.
- The injury must be the only cause of unpleasant symptoms such as pain, weakness, and/or a giving way sensation.

When all the above coexist in a wrist with normal radiolunate relationship (no ulnar translocation and no excessive rotation of the lunate), the so-called three-ligament tenodesis extensor carpi radialis longus (3LT-ECRL) tendon ligamentoplasty is indicated.[6,7]

When the lunate exhibits an abnormal coronal and/or sagittal misalignment, indicating the presence of an unstable SL dissociation plus a radiocarpal derangement, the so-called spiral ECRL technique will be preferred.[8]

An SL gap is not an indication for surgery without clinical findings.

Treatment during early stages of the condition, in which alignment is maintained by secondary stabilizers, should be directed at restoration of neuromuscular control of SL joint stability.[4] In these cases, surgery is not indicated.

25.3 Surgical Technique

The technique outlined here was developed following on the previously described concept of HAPL.[5] This group is composed of the long radiolunate, the volar component of the lunotriquetral, scaphotriquetral (or dorsal intercarpal), dorsal scapholunate, scaphocapitate and radioscaphocapitate ligaments and their function is to prevent excessive pronation of the distal carpal row. When there

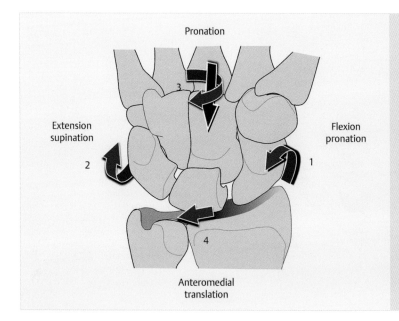

Pronation

Extension supination

Flexion pronation

Anteromedial translation

Fig. 25.2 Movement of carpal bones when subjected to an axial load.

is an injury to the SL ligament and its secondary stabilizers, the scaphoid flexes and pronates out of its fossa. The ECRL tenodesis aims to realign the scaphoid back to its anatomical position by restoring this group of ligaments instead of solely addressing the dorsal SL ligament.[7] Two versions of the procedure exist as described below: ECRL-3LT (▶Fig. 25.4) and ECRL spiral tenodesis (▶Fig. 25.5).

A dorsal wrist incision is made while identifying and protecting sensory branches of the ulnar and radial nerves. Access is gained through the third extensor compartment. Extensor retinacular flaps are raised from second to fifth compartments. Resection of the posterior interosseous nerve (PIN) may be performed, depending on the nerve status. If the aforementioned nerve is identified with normal features, a PIN-sparing proximally based capsulotomy is performed[9] and the diagnosis of SL instability is assessed and confirmed.

At this stage, it is essential to determine if the scaphoid and lunate are easily reducible. Any soft-tissue reconstruction will fail if they are not. This is determined by traction to the index and middle fingers. This maneuver should reduce the proximal carpal row without excessive force.

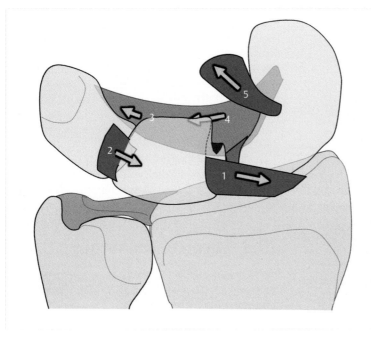

Fig. 25.3 Helical antipronation ligaments (HAPLs). For full description refer to text.
1. Long radiolunate
2. Volar lunotriquetral
3. Dorsal scaphotriquetral
4. Dorsal scapholunate
5. Scaphocapitate

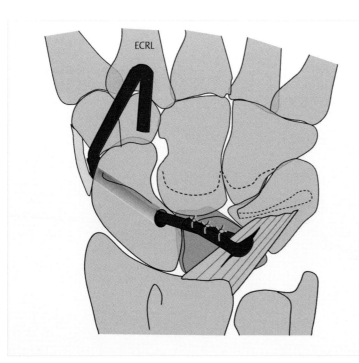

Fig. 25.4 Extensor carpi radialis longus three-ligament tenodesis (ECRL-3LT).

In addition, the wrist should be visually explored to search for signs of damaged cartilage. This is also a contraindication to continue.

A 2-cm transverse incision is made on the dorsoradial surface of the forearm, just proximal to the oblique contour of the abductor pollicis longus (APL) muscle belly. A distally based strip of ECRL tendon (3-mm diameter) is harvested with the aid of a tendon passer. We believe that the ECRL tendon has better control of the tendency of the scaphoid to flex and pronate because of its anatomical position and its vector of pull (▶ Fig. 25.6). A volar wrist tendon would not have the mechanical advantage of this

tendon to induce as much extension and supination on the scaphoid.[4]

The harvested tendon is brought from dorsal to palmar around the radial side of the distal scaphoid, through the triangular space formed by the inner aspect of the scaphotrapeziotrapezoidal (STT) ligament, the radial surface of the distal scaphoid, and the proximolateral corner of the trapezium. To achieve this, a blunt mosquito is passed from dorsal to volar and used to tent the volar wrist skin. A small skin incision is made onto the tented skin and a tendon passer is used to transfer the ECRL graft from dorsal to volar.

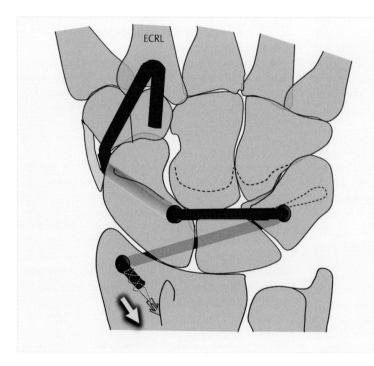

Fig. 25.5 Extensor carpi radialis longus (ECRL) spiral tenodesis.

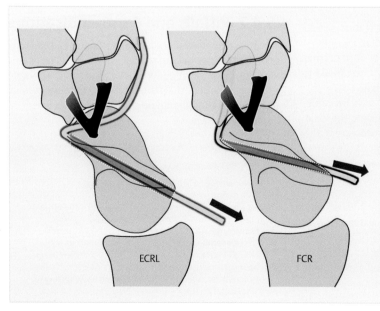

Fig. 25.6 Vector of pull of extensor carpi radialis longus (ECRL) versus flexor carpi radialis (FCR).

A Kirschner wire (K-wire) and a 2.7-mm cannulated drill are then used to make a tunnel through the scaphoid, connecting the distal/radial corner of the scaphoid tuberosity and a point on the dorsal/ulnar surface of the scaphoid where the dorsal SL ligament had originally inserted. Using a tendon passer, the ECRL tendon graft is then passed through this tunnel from volar to dorsal.

Traction on the tendon as it passes through the tunnel should reduce the scaphoid onto extension and supination. An interference screw is used now to secure the tendon onto the scaphoid.

To recreate an SL ligament, the dorsal surface of the lunate is decorticated until bleeding cancellous bone is encountered. An anchor is placed onto this surface and the sutures are used to tie down the ECRL tendon onto the lunate.

If the radiocarpal joint is stable (i.e., the lunate does not displace ulnarly), the procedure ends by securing the end of the tendon onto the radiotriquetrum ligament and thereby indirectly onto the triquetrum. This procedure receives the name of *ECRL-3LT*.

If the scaphoid still feels unstable, further stability can be obtained by placing two 1.2-mm K-wires to hold the scaphoid in reduction. One across the SL interval and a second one from the scaphoid to the capitate to prevent rotation of the scaphoid. Tension must be exerted on the ECRL tendon during K-wire placement. However, in most cases, K-wires should not be necessary.

Alternatively, if the radiocarpal joint is unstable with ulnar translocation of the lunate, the procedure can be continued with a full *ECRL spiral tenodesis* as described below.

The wrist is now turned around again and surgery is continued on the volar aspect. The carpal tunnel is opened through an extended approach and the pisotriquetral joint is identified via palpation. A K-wire is placed through the triquetrum avoiding this joint. A tunnel is created around the wire with a 2.7-mm cannulated drill from volar to dorsal and the tendon is thus passed through the triquetrum from dorsal to volar and subsequently from ulnar to radial along the floor of the carpal tunnel deep to its soft-tissue contents (flexor tendons and median nerve) in an extra-articular plane.

If the volar component of the SL joint feels unstable, anchors may be used to secure the tendon onto the volar surface of the lunate and scaphoid to reconstruct the volar SL ligament. Otherwise, the tendon graft is secured onto the radial styloid either with a transosseous suture or via a suture anchor. The excess graft is trimmed and the wound is closed in layers.

The wrist is placed in a plaster splint for 2 weeks and immobilization is continued with a removable orthosis until removal of K-wires at 8 to 10 weeks (if they were placed). Physiotherapy should emphasize on strengthening scaphoid supinators: ECRL, APL, and flexor carpi radialis (FCR) while minimizing extensor carpi ulnaris activation (scaphoid pronator).[10]

25.4 Results, Pearls, and Tips

25.4.1 Case Example

SL ligament reconstruction with an ECRL tendon is a relatively new technique with good initial results.[11] A 43-year-old male patient sustained a low-energy trauma after he fell off his bike onto an outstretched arm. Examination revealed a tender SL interval with a positive scaphoid shift test. Wrist range of motion was impaired (flexion to extension: 0–40°) and the grip strength was 14% of the unaffected side (8 vs. 58 kg). X-rays and magnetic resonance imaging confirmed a misaligned proximal row of the carpus.

He attended our department 6 weeks after injury and at this stage, it was deemed that the SL ligament was not suitable for a direct repair. We decided to proceed with an ECRL tenodesis as outlined above.

Standard postoperative rehabilitation as previously described was instated. He returned to full work duties as a fireman 5 months postoperatively. Disabilities of the arm, shoulder, and hand score at 17 months after surgery was 14, revealing full satisfaction. Grip strength on the affected side increased to 45 kg (76% of the contralateral side).

As with any new procedure, caution must be exerted. We believe that this technique is a marked biomechanical improvement to previous ligament reconstructions. The use of a dorsal wrist tendon allows for more effective control of the flexion and pronation tendency of the scaphoid. It is also an improvement to the previous 3LT technique with a more accurate reconstruction of the dorsal SL ligament and the ability to control the ulnar translocation of the carpus. It also allows for a possible volar SL ligament reconstruction.

This is a relatively new technique and only short-term results are available. We will continue to assess our results and long-term follow-up will be published when available.

25.4.2 Pitfalls and Contraindications

As emphasized above, carpal ligamentoplasties using tendon grafts are *not* recommended when carpal misalignment cannot be easily reduced, the local joint cartilages are damaged, and/or the patient is not symptomatic. Joint salvage procedures should be considered in the presence of cartilage damage.

> **Tips and Tricks**
>
> - Avoid damage to the branches of the superficial radial nerve during harvest of the ECRL tendon.
> - Passage of ECRL from dorsal to volar via an intracapsular approach will avoid entrapment of the radial artery.
> - Choosing the most radial wrist extensor (ECRL over extensor carpis radialis brevis) will avoid graft incarceration in the STT joint.
> - The surgeon must be aware of the potential for scaphoid or triquetrum avascular necrosis secondary to drilling of these carpal bones.

25.5 Conclusion

Adequate function of the so-called HAPLs is the key to avoid complications when treating chronic injury to the SL ligaments. This novel way of interpreting SL carpal dyskinetics has evolved into the design of several open or arthroscopy-guided techniques. In this chapter, the so-called ECRL-3LT and the ECRL spiral tenodeses are analyzed and the results of these experimental surgical techniques are discussed.

The SL ligament reconstruction presented in this chapter is the result of an evolution from our previous technique (3LT),[6] which described the use of a volar wrist graft (FCR) to stabilize the radial column of the carpus.

The distal end was used to reinforce the radiotriquetral ligament. With this new technique, we not only reconstruct the dorsal SL ligament but it is also possible to address the secondary stabilizers in a full spiral that recreates the HAPL complex.[10]

We now use a dorsal wrist tendon for the tenodesis as this offers a better mechanical advantage to counteract the pathological flexion and pronation of the scaphoid after SL ligament injuries (▶Fig. 25.7). In addition, it is preferable to preserve FCR as it is an important scaphoid stabilizer.

It is important to reiterate that the general concepts described at the beginning of this chapter should be fully understood to provide the correct treatment to the patient.

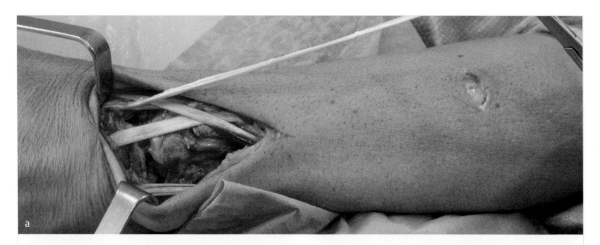

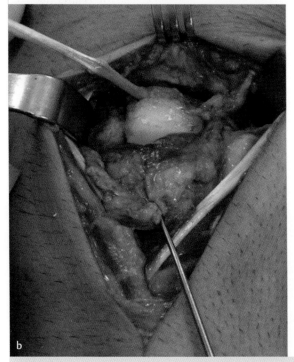
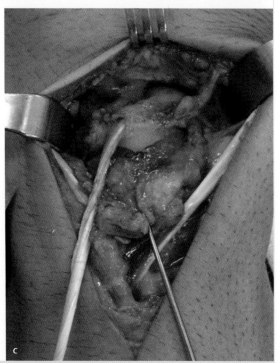

Fig. 25.7 (a–c) Scaphoid reduction (supination and extension) upon traction of extensor carpi radialis longus (ECRL).

References

[1] Garcia-Elias M, Lluch AL. Wrist instabilities, misalignments and dislocations. In: Wolfe S, Pederson W, Hotchkiss R, et al, eds. Green's operative hand surgery. 7th ed. Atlanta (GA): Elsevier Health Science; 2016:418–478

[2] Hagert E, Garcia-Elias M, Forsgren S, Ljung BO. Immunohistochemical analysis of wrist ligament innervation in relation to their structural composition. J Hand Surg Am 2007;32(1):30–36

[3] Hagert E. Proprioception of the wrist joint: a review of current concepts and possible implications on the rehabilitation of the wrist. J Hand Ther 2010;23(1):2–17

[4] Esplugas M, Garcia-Elias M, Lluch A, Llusá Pérez M. Role of muscles in the stabilization of ligament-deficient wrists. J Hand Ther 2016;29(2):166–174

[5] Garcia-Elias M, Puig de la Bellacasa I, Schouten C. Carpal Ligaments: A Functional Classification. Hand Clin 2017; 33(3):511–520

[6] Garcia-Elias M, Lluch AL, Stanley JK. Three-ligament tenodesis for the treatment of scapholunate dissociation: indications and surgical technique. J Hand Surg Am 2006;31(1):125–134

[7] Kakar S, Greene RM, Garcia-Elias M. Carpal Realignment Using a Strip of Extensor Carpi Radialis Longus Tendon. J Hand Surg Am 2017;42(8):667.e1–667.e8

[8] Chee KG, Chin AY, Chew EM, Garcia-Elias M. Antipronation spiral tenodesis—a surgical technique for the treatment of perilunate instability. J Hand Surg Am 2012;37(12):2611–2618

[9] Hagert E, Ferreres A, Garcia-Elias M. Nerve-sparing dorsal and volar approaches to the radiocarpal joint. J Hand Surg Am 2010; 35(7):1070–1074

[10] Holmes M, Taylor S, Miller C, et al. Early outcomes of "The Birmingham Wrist Instability Programme": A pragmatic intervention for stage one scapholunate instability. Hand Ther 2017;22(3): 90–100

[11] Garcia-Elias M, Ortega Hernandez D. Tendon Reconstruction of the Unstable Scapholunate Dissociation. A Systematic Review. In: Giddins G, Leblebicioğlu G, eds. Evidence Based Data in Hand Surgery and Therapy. Federation of European Societies for Surgery of the Hand Instructional Courses 2017. Ankara, Turkey: Iris Publications; 2017:355–368

26 Arthroscopic Scapholunate Repair

Max Haerle, Christophe Mathoulin

Abstract

The treatment of lesions of the scapholunate ligament of the wrist has always been a challenge for surgeons. Stability was possibly obtained by conventional open surgical methods, but at the cost of severe stiffness in flexion. This impeded the possibility of recovery in high-level athletes, for example. Since the development of wrist arthroscopy in general and the creation of EWAS in particular, the understanding and treatment of these lesions has been reversed. In recent years, we have developed precise, efficient, and reproducible techniques that allow the stability and preservation of normal wrist movements. In this article we present the indications, techniques, and outcomes of arthroscopic repair of scapholunate ligament.

Keywords: scapholunate ligament, wrist arthroscopy, capsulodesis

26.1 Introduction

The scapholunate (SL) complex consists of the intrinsic and extrinsic ligaments. The intrinsic portion of the scapholunate interosseous ligament (SLIL) has three segments: dorsal, volar, and proximal. The dorsal segment is biomechanically the most important. It is made up of very thick transverse fibers that resist rotation. The volar segment of the SLIL consists of long, oblique fibers that allow sagittal rotation. The proximal segment consists of nonvascularized fibrocartilage that is often perforated secondary to degeneration in the elderly. The main extrinsic ligaments of the SL complex are the radioscaphocapitate ligament, the long and short radiolunate ligaments, and the dorsal radiocarpal and dorsal intercarpal ligaments. The impact of these ligaments also being damaged on SL instability is not fully understood.

We should remember that an isolated acute SL ligament injury without instability will heal by simple immobilization in slight extension for 6 weeks.

Not correctly treated, isolated SL ligament injuries may not lead to SL dissociation on radiographs even when instability is present. On the other hand, slight weakening of the SL ligament that is not visible on X-rays can lead to pain. Typically, both the intrinsic and extrinsic systems must be damaged for complete SL diastasis to be visible on X-rays. In most cases, radiological abnormalities are not visible immediately after SL ligament injury, but appear over time because of gradual destruction of the entire ligament system. A period of "dynamic" instability, one that is visible only under certain loading conditions (e.g., tight fist), can be differentiated from "static" instability, one in which significant bone shifts are often found too late to be repaired if they cannot be reduced. This explains why this pathology is often diagnosed too late.

The concept of the interosseous ligament itself should be limited to the proximal portion, which is the only nonvascularized fibrocartilaginous portion, and therefore not repairable. Conversely, the volar and dorsal portions of the SL ligament are completely integrated into the extrasynovial volar and dorsal extrinsic ligament systems and have well-developed vascularity.

The more elastic volar and dorsal extrinsic carpal ligaments allow the distal parts of the scaphoid, lunate, and triquetral to shift slightly in the sagittal plane and control torsion of the scaphoid–lunate–triquetral chain. Reconstruction of only the dorsal capsule ligament complex seems to be sufficient to represent a solution for SL stabilization and minimizes stiffness as long as the bones are satisfactorily reduced.

The treatment approach for SL dissociation has evolved in recent years due to the development of wrist arthroscopy, which was a significant technological revolution in the 1990s just like microsurgery was in the 1970s.

Salvà-Coll, Garcia-Elias et al in 2011[1] showed the importance of distal scaphoid stabilization, particularly the role of the flexor carpi radialis. Meade et al,[2] Short et al,[3] and Berger et al[4] showed that the SLIL actually consisted of three parts, with the dorsal part being the main stabilizer of the SL joint. Mataliotakis et al[5] and Hagert[6] emphasized the importance of innervation to proprioception, which allows the entire peripheral musculotendinous system to respond and protect the SL gap. They suggested that proprioception plays an important role in protecting the SL dissociation, and that it is important to protect both the anterior and posterior interosseous nerves.

Elsaidi et al[7] carried out a cadaver study in which they sequentially cut the various ligament components (volar, interosseous, and dorsal) and then loaded the wrist. They found that dorsal tipping of the lunate with scaphoid horizontalization, such as in cases of severe SL instability, occurs only when the dorsal attachments of the dorsal intercarpal ligament are cut.

We have observed cases of arthroscopically obvious midcarpal SL instability where the SLIL (dorsal, proximal, and volar) was intact. It was only during the systematic exploration of the dorsal capsule that we discovered isolated tears in the dorsal capsule, which was detached from the dorsal portion of the SL ligament, with easy access to the midcarpal joint from the radiocarpal joint.[8]

In a cadaver laboratory, we used radiographs and arthroscopy to evaluate loaded and unloaded wrists after progressively sectioning the stabilizers. This work revealed worsening of the SL dissociation in all cases in which the attachment between the dorsal capsule and SL ligament was cut.[9]

An additional cadaver study was carried out to demonstrate the presence of this anatomical structure (DCSS, the dorsal capsuloligamentous scapholunate septum), which was found in all the specimens. It consists of two transverse arches assembled into a third arch, which is larger than the other two. This capsule–ligament structure joins the dorsal portion of the SL ligament with the dorsal capsule.[10] This forms an extremely solid dorsal complex consisting of the dorsal portion of the SL ligament—a true dorsal SL ligament—the DCSS and the dorsal intercarpal, particularly the sacrotuberous ligament, and the proximal portion of the dorsal intercarpal. These three structures are closely interlinked and appear to be the key to SL stability. Therefore, arthroscopic repair aims to reconstruct the DCSS.[11,12]

26.2 Indications

This technique is recommended in all cases of SL instabilities lower than Geissler grade 4. It is very suitable for fresh cases as for older cases because aggressive shaving recreates a fresh lesion. An acute ligament injury with no dissociation may heal by immobilization.

For more unstable cases the success rate was lower, which means that other techniques may help in the future or to be a secondary option or to be then the primary choice.

26.3 Surgical Technique

A diagnostic arthroscopy is of best value in SL lesions. The scope is inserted through the 3–4 radiocarpal portal to visualize the SLIL. However, the dorsal portion of SLIL can be best seen with the scope in the 6R portal. A probe is used to assess the nature of the SL ligament injury.

In case the ligament is ruptured in the center, with two ligament stumps remaining attached to the scaphoid and lunate, the original *Mathoulin SL suture technique* to suture the ligament arthroscopically is performed.

An absorbable monofilament suture (3–0 or 4–0) is passed through a needle. This needle is inserted through the 3–4 portal, and then shifted slightly distally so as to cross the joint capsule. The needle is localized inside the joint through the scope and then pushed through the SLIL stump on the scaphoid side. The needle is then oriented dorsal to volar and angled proximal to distal, allowing it to enter the midcarpal joint. A second needle and suture are then inserted parallel to the first into the SLIL stump attached to the lunate (▶ Fig. 26.1). The scope is returned to the midcarpal ulnar portal. The two tips of the needles are now found inside the midcarpal joint, after they have passed between the scaphoid and lunate. The two sutures can be caught through the midcarpal radial portal (▶ Fig. 26.2).

The needles are removed and both sutures are pulled outside. A knot is tied between the two sutures. Traction is applied to both sutures through portal 3–4 to pull the first distal knot into the medio-carpal joint. This knot is going to be positioned between the scaphoid and the lunate (▶ Fig. 26.3) just volar to the remaining dorsal portions of the SLIL. The degree of reduction in the SL gap is determined by maintaining tension on the sutures after releasing wrist traction. If reduction is satisfactory, the ligament is sutured to the dorsal capsule by the last knot, which is tied subcutaneously (▶ Fig. 26.4).

If reduction is insufficient, Kirschner wires (K-wires) will need to be added to stabilize the SL joint and potentially the scaphocapite joint. The wrist is immobilized

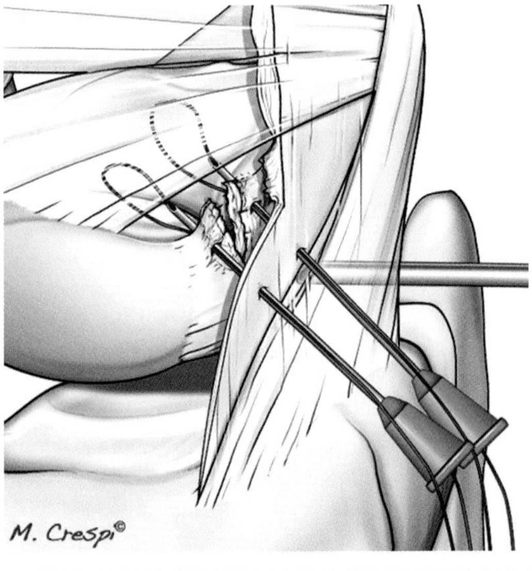

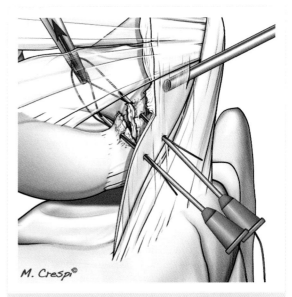

Fig. 26.1 Arthroscopic view of the needles passing through the capsule and dorsal portions of the SLIL. The needle is angled dorsal to volar and proximal to distal so it can penetrate into the midcarpal joint. (*Source:* Reproduced from Mathoulin C. Wrist Arthroscopy Techniques, 2nd Edition; © 2019 Thieme Publishers.)

Fig. 26.2 Drawing of sutures retrieval using a hemostat introduced through the MCR portal. (*Source:* Reproduced from Mathoulin C. Wrist Arthroscopy Techniques, 2nd Edition; © 2019 Thieme Publishers.)

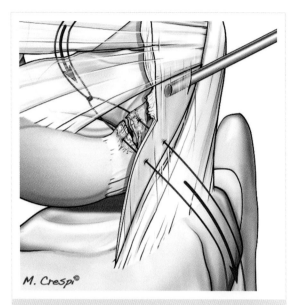

Fig. 26.3 Drawing of traction placed on the proximal suture ends to bring the knot back into the joint. (*Source:* Reproduced from Mathoulin C. Wrist Arthroscopy Techniques, 2nd Edition; © 2019 Thieme Publishers.)

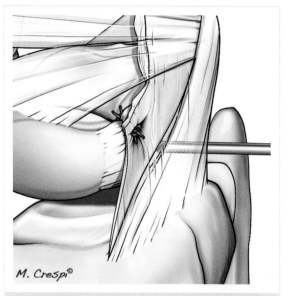

Fig. 26.4 Drawing of the suturing between the SL and dorsal capsule with one intra-articular knot located in front of the dorsal portion of SLIL and one extra-articular subcutaneous dorsal knot located behind the dorsal capsule.
(*Source:* Reproduced from Mathoulin C. Wrist Arthroscopy Techniques, 2nd Edition; © 2019 Thieme Publishers.)

in extension (45–60 degrees) with an anterior splint for 6 weeks in cases of suture repair only, and for 8 weeks in cases of associated K-wire fixation.

It is true that in many cases the ligament is avulsed from the lunate or from the scaphoid. Therefore, Haerle hypothesized that the effect of Mathoulin technique lays more in a capsulodesis effect rather than in suturing the SLIL, which has low healing potential anyway. For these cases, he developed the *Haerle capsulodesis technique* by arthroscopy.

The stability of the SL is usually assessed from midcarpal portals, by inserting a probe into the palmar, central, and dorsal portions of the SL joint. Then, the grade of instability is assessed according to Geissler or the European Wrist Arthroscopy Society (EWAS) for every portion of the interosseous ligament.[13]

The first most important step of the technique is to shave the radiocarpal and midcarpal dorsal capsular segments adjacent to the SL space aggressively. Hereby we recreate a fresh lesion of those ligaments and capsular segments.

The skin incision to the 3–4 portal is slightly enlarged and the extensor tendons of the third–fourth compartment are gently kept aside. Thereafter, under arthroscopic control (6R portal) the first needle is inserted into the radiocarpal compartment ulnar to the 3–4 portal. This needle is slightly retracted and then passed on the dorsal horn of the scaphoid with slight radial divergence into the midcarpal compartment, transpiercing the radial septum portion (see ▶ Fig. 26.5; ▶ Fig. 26.6). The second needle is now inserted into the radiocarpal compartment ulnarly to the 3–4 portal, slightly retracted and passed dorsally to the lunate with slight radial divergence into the midcarpal compartment, transpiercing the ulnar portion of the dorsal septum (see ▶ Fig. 26.7).

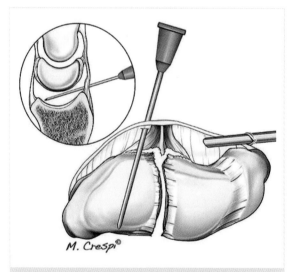

Fig. 26.5 Needles are first introduced at the radiocarpal joint under arthroscopic control with the optic in 6R.
(*Source:* From Haerle M., Del Gaudio T. Arthroscopic dorsal capsulodesis in SL instability. In: Atzei A, Coert JH, Haugstvedt J-R, eds. Arthroscopic Management of Radial-Sided Wrist Pain. Springer; In Press.)

Basically, it is a very similar technique to Mathoulin until this point. The difference lies in fact that Mathoulin tries to catch the remnants of the ligament stumps by a convergent direction of the needles, while Haerle tries to catch the most possible amount of capsule that remains inserted to the scaphoid and lunate by diverging the needles.

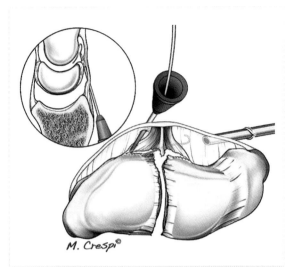

Fig. 26.6 First needle is passed dorsally to the lunate in the midcarpal joint. The second needle is passed dorsally to the scaphoid in midcarpal joint. (*Source:* From Haerle M., Del Gaudio T. Arthroscopic dorsal capsulodesis in SL instability. In: Atzei A, Coert JH, Haugstvedt J-R, eds. Arthroscopic Management of Radial-Sided Wrist Pain. Springer; In Press.)

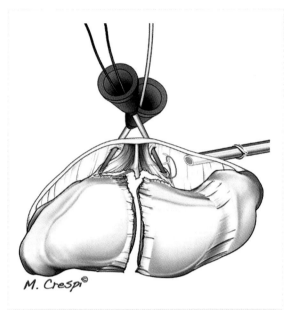

Fig. 26.7 The direction of the needles is divergent in order to catch as much as possible of the DCSS. The optic is then moved in MCU portal and the two sutures are picked out through MCR. Then a loop technique is applied. (*Source:* From Haerle M., Del Gaudio T. Arthroscopic dorsal capsulodesis in SL instability. In: Atzei A, Coert JH, Haugstvedt J-R, eds. Arthroscopic Management of Radial-Sided Wrist Pain. Springer; In Press.)

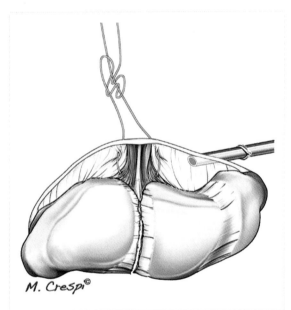

Fig. 26.8 The loop pulls out the 20 suture and the knot will be closed after removing traction and slight dorsiflexion. (*Source:* From Haerle M., Del Gaudio T. Arthroscopic dorsal capsulodesis in SL instability. In: Atzei A, Coert JH, Haugstvedt J-R, eds. Arthroscopic Management of Radial-Sided Wrist Pain. Springer; In Press.)

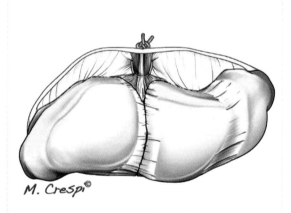

Fig. 26.9 The closed knot will approximate the lunate and the scaphoid in their physiologic position and the capsule adheres to the two bones. (*Source:* From Haerle M., Del Gaudio T. Arthroscopic dorsal capsulodesis in SL instability. In: Atzei A, Coert JH, Haugstvedt J-R, eds. Arthroscopic Management of Radial-Sided Wrist Pain. Springer; In Press.)

The first needle carries a 2–0 multistranded polyethylene suture, and the second needle a looped suture thread. The polyethylene suture is pulled out through the looped suture thread and exteriorized (see ▶Fig. 26.8). Traction is released and a knot is tied on the top of the dorsal capsule on the floor of the fourth extensor sheet (see ▶Fig. 26.9).

Repositioning and stability of the suture are evaluated by arthroscopy.

Postoperatively, the wrist is immobilized in a forearm cast for 8 weeks. K-wires are needed only in singular cases. No physiotherapy is applied to improve wrist flexion for up to 3 months postoperative to give the ligaments the time to heal without being stretched out.

26.4 Results

In *Mathoulin series*, there were 139 males and 82 females with a mean age of 38.11 ± 11.33 years (range: 17–63 years). The mean time since injury was 7.13 ± 1.33 months (range: 3–26 months) and the mean follow-up was 39.43 ± 7.05 months (range: 12–83 months). The mean range of motion improved in all directions. The mean difference between the preoperative and postoperative extension was 14.03 degrees (standard error of the mean, SEM = 1.27 degrees; $p < 0.001$), while the mean difference between the preoperative and postoperative flexion was 11.14 degrees (SEM = 1.3 degrees; $p < 0.0001$). The mean difference in the visual analogue scale (VAS) score was −5.46 (SEM = 0.19; $p < 0.0001$). The mean postoperative grip strength on the affected side was 38.42 ± 10.27 kg (range: 20–60 kg) as compared with mean preoperative grip strength of 24.07 ± 10.51 kg (range: 8–40 kg; $p < 0.0001$). The mean postoperative grip strength of the operated side was 93.4% of that on the unaffected side. In 19% of cases, the dorsal intercalated segment instability (DISI) was uncorrected on postoperative radiographs. The mean difference between the preoperative and postoperative SL angles was −9.45 degrees (SEM = 1.37 degrees; $p < 0.0001$). The mean postoperative disabilities of the arm, shoulder, and hand (DASH) score was 9.4 ± 6.71 as compared with mean preoperative DASH score of 47.04 ± 17.23 ($p < 0.0001$). There was a negative correlation between the overall DASH score and the postoperative correction of the DISI deformity with a lower DASH score associated with increasing SL angles (▶ Fig. 26.7).

All patients returned to work in an average of 9 weeks (range: 1–12 weeks) and the all professional athletes resumed their sporting activities at their preinjury levels. Two hundred and fifteen patients (95.7%) were very satisfied or satisfied with their result. Five patients had a fair result and one was unsatisfied, mainly due to postoperative wrist stiffness and nonreduction of the SL gap. All failures were cases of Garcia-Elias stage 5 dissociation (5/7).

The *study of Haerle was* set out as a bicenter study with Orthopädie Rosenberg in St. Gallen, Switzerland (Dr. med. Nicole Schmelzer-Schmied). The study collective comprised 63 patients with a mean follow-up of 2 years. The collective comprised 25 acute and 38 chronic SL lesions; 47 patients presented dynamic and 13 a static SL instability.

The patients were stratified according to Messina-EWAS classification.[13] Here, 33 patients (52%) showed proximal and posterior scapholunate interosseous ligament (SLIOL) tears and were classified stage 3b, followed by 22 (35%) patients with complete SLIOL lesions and wide detachment of the dorsal capsular structures, which were classified stage 3c. The remaining eight patients showed high-grade instabilities with arthroscopic drive-through sign from medio- to radiocarpal; six were classified as stage 4, and two were classified as stage 5.

Mean postoperative VAS at rest decreased about 90% (from 2.0 pre- to 0.2 postoperative), and mean postoperative VAS under load about 70% (from 5.3 pre- to 1.6 postoperative).

Initially, wrist flexion was decreased. On long term mean range of motion (ROM) was not relevantly decreased. When compared to contralateral ROM we found a slight overall decrease of 9.5 degrees.

While positive preoperative Watson test was found in 30 patients, postoperative positive Watson test persisted in nine patients. Of those, two patients were classified stage 5, followed by four stage 4 patients and three stage 3c patients according to Messina-EWAS classification. Looking through the records of these patients, we found that the majority of them intraoperatively presented with a high-grade SL instability, accompanied by static SL dissociation on radiographies. Three out of those nine were complete failures, which needed wrist salvage procedures in the further course. SL dissociation was significantly reducible by arthroscopy in these patients.

Regarding grip strength, no significant postoperative impairment was found, when compared to contralateral side. Mean postoperative Mayo wrist score was 83, and mean DASH score of 12.7.

Pre- and postoperative SL gap among acute and chronic lesions was assessed separately. Analyses revealed a significant postoperative reduction of the SL gap among both acute and chronic lesions in posteroanterior and clenched fist views, ranging from 0.1 to 0.3 mm.

SL gap in pre- and postoperative posteroanterior and clenched fist views was analyzed among dynamic and static SL instabilities. Dynamic instabilities ($n = 47$) revealed a statistically high significant mean postoperative gap reduction from 2.2 to 2.0 mm ($p < 0.001$) in posteroanterior and from 2.9 to 2.6 mm ($p < 0.001$) in clenched fist views, respectively. Static instabilities ($n = 13$), however, showed a statistically not significant tendency of gap reduction in posteroanterior views, namely from 3.6 to 3.3 mm, while we noticed a statistically not significant increase from 3.9 to 4.0 mm in clenched fist views. Statistical significance was probably not reached because of the small number in this subgroup analysis.

26.5 Pitfalls and Contraindications

Some of our cases with high-grade injuries were clear failures. This type of capsuloligamentous suture is insufficient if a lunotriquetral instability is associated. In both techniques, this seems to be connected to the complete detachment of the dorsal capsule to the proximal row. In these cases, the capsulodesis effect is lost and the biological healing is not effective. Therefore, we do not currently recommend this technique in cases of Geissler stage 4 or in association with lunotriquetral instabilities. Fixed dissociations need other solutions as well.

26.6 Conclusion

The results of this study reinforces our view that arthroscopic stabilization of the SL joint is a reality.[12] The underlying principle is to return the damaged structures to the correct anatomical position, to allow our body's innate repair ability to take over.

This is why this technique is very successful in the early instabilities. In older cases lower than Geissler grade 4, these instabilities are treated as fresh ones after aggressive shaving. In Geissler 4 or even more unstable cases the rate of failures raises. Other techniques such as transosseous anchorage of the capsule or neoligaments must probably be used in the future for cases of greater instability.

When performing wrist arthroscopy to remove the K-wires in the second month, we were surprised to find that the dorsal portion was very well healed but the proximal portion of SLIL was not healed at all. The proximal nonvascularized portion of the SLIL likely does not act as a stabilizer of the SL joint. Probably its avascularity leads to a very low healing potential.

Proprioception is likely underestimated, as it plays an important role in stabilizing the SL gap. The musculotendinous response to trauma (i.e., stretching) of the dorsal and volar portions of the SL ligament provides a protective countereffect. Thus, it seems crucial to preserve the innervated areas. As such, arthroscopic techniques cause less denervation than open surgical SL ligament repair methods do.

In summary, recent data and clinical findings lead us to think that the proximal, nonvascularized portion of the SLIL does not contribute to SL stability. Repairing it is now unrealistic. Proprioception must be taken into account and thus significant innervation must be preserved. The concept of scaphotrapeziotrapezoid ligament damage in rotary subluxation of the scaphoid should be revisited, even if we cannot forget the role of extrinsic ligaments in maintaining carpal stability. The dorsal intrinsic and extrinsic ligament system, particularly the DCSS, is a key component of SL stability. The concept of a SL complex is a reality that requires a more systematic analysis in regards to the extent of ligament damage, which may be repaired by the presented techniques. Arthroscopic techniques cause less damage and less denervation in this type of injury.

Therefore, we currently adopt Mathoulin technique of SL ligament suture or Haerle technique of capsulodesis, depending on the presence or not of ligament stumps. Both techniques have shown stable results in all cases excluding the major instabilities or fixed dissociations. Here, future technical developments and long-term studies will show more evidence and alternative solutions.

References

[1] Salvà-Coll G, Garcia-Elias M, Llusá-Pérez M, Rodríguez-Baeza A. The role of the flexor carpi radialis muscle in scapholunate instability. J Hand Surg Am 2011;36(1):31–36

[2] Meade TD, Schneider LH, Cherry K. Radiographic analysis of selective ligament sectioning at the carpal scaphoid: a cadaver study. J Hand Surg Am 1990;15(6):855–862

[3] Short WH, Werner FW, Sutton LG. Dynamic biomechanical evaluation of the dorsal intercarpal ligament repair for scapholunate instability. J Hand Surg Am 2009;34(4):652–659

[4] Berger RA, Imeada T, Berglund L, An KN. Constraint and material properties of the subregions of the scapholunate interosseous ligament. J Hand Surg Am 1999;24(5):953–962

[5] Mataliotakis G, Doukas M, Kostas I, Lykissas M, Batistatou A, Beris A. Sensory innervation of the subregions of the scapholunate interosseous ligament in relation to their structural composition. J Hand Surg Am 2009;34(8):1413–1421

[6] Hagert E, Persson JK, Werner M, Ljung BO. Evidence of wrist proprioceptive reflexes elicited after stimulation of the scapholunate interosseous ligament. J Hand Surg Am 2009;34(4):642–651

[7] Elsaidi GA, Ruch DS, Kuzma GR, Smith BP. Dorsal wrist ligament insertions stabilize the scapholunate interval: cadaver study. Clin Orthop Relat Res 2004;(425):152–157

[8] Binder AC, Kerfant N, Wahegaonkar AL, Tandara AA, Mathoulin CL. Dorsal wrist capsular tears in association with scapholunate instability: results of an arthroscopic dorsal capsuloplasty. J Wrist Surg 2013;2(2):160–167

[9] Overstraeten LV, Camus EJ, Wahegaonkar A, et al. Anatomical description of the dorsal capsulo scapholunate septum (DCSS)—anatomical staging of scapholunate instability after DCSS sectioning. J Wrist Surg 2013;2(2):149–154

[10] Tommasini Carrara de Sambuy M, Burgess TM, Cambon-Binder A, Mathoulin CL. The anatomy of the dorsal capsulo-scapholunate septum: a cadaveric study. J Wrist Surg 2017;6(3):244–247

[11] Mathoulin CL, Dauphin N, Wahegaonkar AL. Arthroscopic dorsal capsuloligamentous repair in chronic scapholunate ligament tears. Hand Clin 2011;27(4):563–572, xi

[12] Wahegaonkar AL, Mathoulin CL. Arthroscopic dorsal capsuloligamentous repair in the treatment of chronic scapho-lunate ligament tears. J Wrist Surg 2013;2(2):141–148

[13] Messina JC, Van Overstraeten L, Luchetti R, Fairplay T, Mathoulin CL. The EWAS classification of scapholunate tears: an anatomical arthroscopic study. J Wrist Surg 2013;2(2):105–109

27 Treatment of Lunotriquetral Injuries

Benjamin F. Plucknette, Haroon M. Hussain, Lee Osterman

Abstract

Lunotriquetral (LT) injuries are rare and challenging to diagnose both clinically and radiographically. If initial nonoperative interventions fail, a number of operative options are described. Initially, wrist arthroscopy (including the midcarpal joint) should be performed to confirm the diagnosis, identify concomitant injuries, and guide the treatment. When LT instability is present without arthrosis or volar intercalated segment instability (VISI), ligament debridement and capsular shrinkage is effective. Repair or reconstruction is required in the presence of correctable VISI. For chronic LT injuries without arthrosis or VISI in the setting of ulnar positive or neutral variance, ulnar shortening osteotomy is the most appropriate treatment. Finally, in the presence of LT arthrosis or fixed VISI, partial wrist denervation may be offered to maintain motion and grip strength; however, long-term studies for this procedure are lacking, and LT arthrodesis or other salvage options may eventually be required for definitive management.

Keywords: lunotriquetral instability, lunotriquetral tear, volar intercalated segment instability, lunotriquetral repair, lunotriquetral reconstruction, lunotriquetral arthrodesis, ulnar shortening osteotomy, partial wrist denervation, wrist arthroscopy

27.1 Anatomy

While this chapter focuses on the treatment of lunotriquetral (LT) injuries, some attention must also be given to the anatomy, diagnosis, and classification, as the injury pattern guides the treatment.

Like the scapholunate (SL) interosseous ligament, the LT is composed of three subregions: dorsal, membranous,

and volar. The volar region is the strongest and considered to be the major stabilizer of the lunate–triquetrum interval. The volar and dorsal subregions merge with their respective extrinsic ligaments to further constrain LT motion (▶Fig. 27.1).

Mechanically, the triquetrum links the proximal and distal carpal row motion through its contact with the hamate. During ulnar deviation, the extensor carpi ulnaris (EUC) with its attachment at the base of the fifth metacarpal forces the hamate to corkscrew and engage the triquetrum pushing it into extension. The triquetrum by its interosseous attachment to the lunate brings the lunate into extension, which helps guide the scaphoid into its horizontal position. The reverse happens in radial deviation.

27.2 Diagnosis and Classification

Various classifications of LT injury have been described but the authors prefer the simple outline presented in ▶Table 27.1. Any classification begins with a thorough

Table 27.1 Classifications of lunotriquetral injury

Traumatic	Degenerative
Acute isolated tear • Membranous • Complete	Attritional lesion with ulnar impaction syndrome
Acute perilunate dislocation	
VISI • Chronic > 3 mo	

Abbreviation: VISI, volar intercalated segment instability.

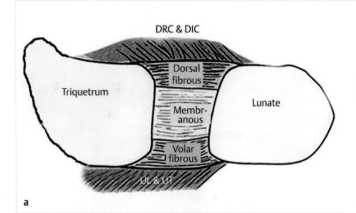
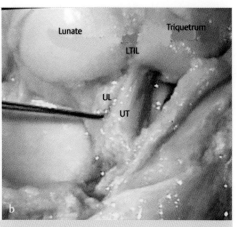

Fig. 27.1 (a, b) The lunotriquetral (LT) ligament is tripartite with a dorsal and fibrous section and a central membranous component. The volar and dorsal fibrous components merge with the extrinsic ligaments that are major contributors to LT overall stability. Ulnar extrinsic ligaments merging with fibrous component of LTIL. DRC, dorsal radiocarpal ligament; DIC, dorsal intercarpal ligament; UL, ulnolunate ligament; UT, ulnotriquetral ligament; LTIL, lunotriquetral interosseous ligament.

history and physical examination, which lead the surgeon to suspect LT involvement. It is important to note that LT injuries present on a spectrum based on the degree of injury. Horii performed a kinematic study of the intact wrist followed by serial sectioning of the LT ligaments followed by the dorsal radiocarpal ligament (DRC)/dorsal intercarpal (DIC) ligaments.[1] The pathognomonic volar intercalated segment instability (VISI), increase in LT motion, and catch-up-clunk associated with ulnar deviation only appeared after additional sectioning of the DRC/DIC (▶Fig. 27.2). The authors asserted that the subtle changes to LT kinematics that accompanied LT

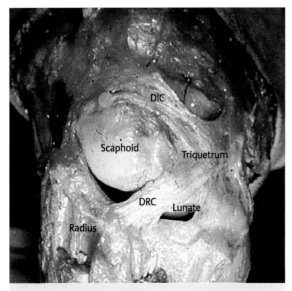

Fig. 27.2 The triquetrum is a stronghold of ligament attachments. Volar intercalated segment instability (VISI) requires more than an isolated lunotriquetral (LT) ligament tear. DRC, dorsal radiocarpal ligament; DIC, dorasl intercarpal ligament.

ligament injuries in the absence of DRC/DIC injury would be difficult to detect clinically or radiographically but sufficient to generate synovitis, altered joint mechanics, and increased ligamentous tension. Therefore, patients with a complete LT injury but intact DRC/DIC can present without obvious radiographic findings and only subtle examination findings including some negativespecial tests.

In the history of ulnar wrist pain, an understanding of the timing of symptomology is critical because it may directly affect the treatment options. Patients with acute injuries often describe a fall on an outstretched hand or, less frequently, a rotary mechanism.[2] Generally, acute tears are associated with the history of a known traumatic event and a firm timeline regarding the pain history, whereas chronic tears are often insidious or may be incited by a trivial trauma (acute on chronic).[3] Patients complain of weakness with ulnar-sided wrist pain, and carefully delineating the exact site of pain also aids in the diagnosis.

Patients with LT injuries will complain of pain directly over the dorsal LT joint, which is more distal and a subtly different location than those complaining of triangular fibrocartilage complex (TFCC) tears, ECU, pisotriquetral arthritis, or distal radioulnar joint pathology.[1]

Examination consists of range of motion (ROM) measurements, grip testing, palpation, and special tests. Reagan studied 35 patients with LT sprains and found that examination universally produced tenderness over the dorsal LT, restricted wrist ROM, and weakened grip.[2] Linscheid is credited with the description of a click when transitioning from radial to ulnar deviation in the presence of an LT ligament tear.[2,4,5] The diagnosis is further supported by special tests such as the LT ballottement (or Reagan shuck) test, the LT compression test (▶Fig. 27.3), the ulnocarpal stress test, the presence of a fovea sign, the derby test, and the shear (or Kleinman) test. The LT ballottement test is performed by fixing the lunate with the thumb and the index finger of one hand while, with

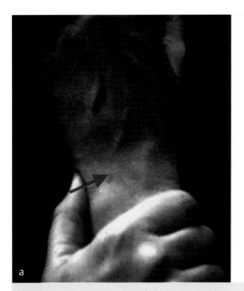
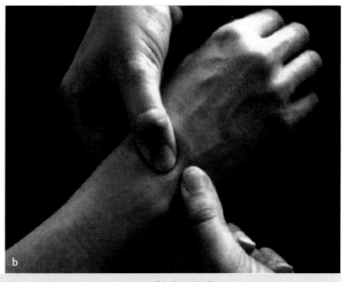

Fig. 27.3 Stress tests to identify lunotriquetral (LT) pathology. **(a)** The LT compression test. **(b)** The LT ballottement test.

the other hand, displacing the triquetrum and pisiform first dorsally and then palmarly. A positive result elicits pain, crepitus, and excessive laxity.[2] The Reagan test has a reported sensitivity of 64% and specificity of 44%.[5,6] The compression test is abnormal when pain is elicited as the triquetrum is radially compressed into a stabilized lunate. With the ulnocarpal stress test, pain is created when the wrist is fully ulnarly deviated, followed by wrist pronosupination.

The fovea sign is present when the patient's pain is recreated with deep palpation of the ulnar fovea.[5] While the fovea sign does not directly detect LT ligament tears, it can identify injury to the secondary stabilizers of the LT joint—mainly the ulnar extrinsic ligaments. The fovea sign is more closely associated with TFCC tears, but there is a reported sensitivity of 74% and specificity of 97% for ulnar extrinsic pathology.[5,7] The Derby test is a complex, three-part examination maneuver that takes the patient's subjective feelings of instability into account. The examination is well represented by Rhee et al both pictorially and in video form.[5] The Derby test has a reported sensitivity of 77% and specificity of 89%.[5,8]

Following clinical diagnosis, plain radiographs are obtained to evaluate the carpal alignment. Standard anteroposterior, lateral, and oblique views of the wrist should be obtained at a minimum. Grip views should also be obtained to evaluate ulnar variance. When obtaining grip views, it is important to standardize the positioning to wrist neutral pronosupination (requiring the film to be performed with the shoulder abducted to 90 degrees), as ulnar variance is altered with different degrees of pronosupination. Including the contralateral wrist is valuable for comparison. Next, critical evaluation of Gilula arcs is performed to evaluate the congruity of the carpal rows.[9]

With LT injury, radiographs can be normal or Gilula arcs I and II may be disrupted and accompanied by LT overlap.[9] (▶ Fig. 27.4) Although common in SL ligament injury, gapping is infrequent with LT injuries.[10] In acute patterns, the LT injury may be only one component of a larger injury pattern, as is the case with perilunate injuries. To support this concept, Lichtman et al suggested that some LT injuries are probably "forme fruste" perilunate patterns.[4] With a diagnosis of perilunate injury, the associated LT injury is often obvious on plain radiographs based on interruption of Gilula arcs (▶ Fig. 27.4). The lateral radiograph is scrutinized for the presence of VISI. The normal SL angle is 47 degrees while VISI is diagnosed with an SL angle of less than 30 degrees. The normal LT angle is 14 degrees, but this angle decreases to a negative value in the presence of VISI.[2] Since VISI is only noted after disruption of secondary stabilizers (DRC/DIC ligaments and scaphotrapeziotrapezoid ligament), it will only be appreciated in more severe injuries or in chronic injury patterns with ligamentous attenuation.[1]

Advanced imaging is debated. Gilula argued that the word "tear" should not be used when referring to LT lesions noted on arthrography due to the high incidence of degenerative perforations, which may result in false positives in the setting of acute injury.[11] Historically, arthrographic tears based on dye extravasation between joints has fallen out of favor due to the aforementioned frequency of degenerative perforations and the 13% rate of communication between the midcarpal and radiocarpal joints in normal individuals.[10,12] Furthermore, Cantor demonstrated a 59% rate of LT tear in the asymptomatic wrist of those with a contralateral symptomatic LT tear.[13] Viegas performed dissections on 100 cadavers and noted no attritional tears in specimen under the age of 45 but a 27.6% rate of perforations in the LT ligament in those older than 60 years.[14] The article concluded that there is a significant rate of perforation of the LT ligament in the general population.

Wrist MRI is considered a diagnostic help, although even the newer 3T magnets have only 25 to 75% sensitivity for diagnosing LT tears (▶ Fig. 27.5).[15] The

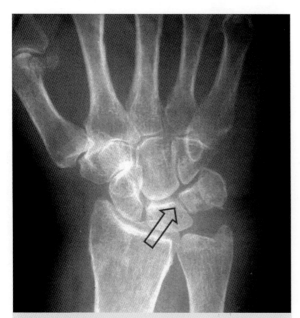

Fig. 27.4 Plain radiograph of acute lunotriquetral (LT) tear with disruption of Gillula arcs (*arrow*).

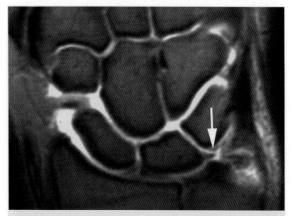

Fig. 27.5 Gadolinium MRI showing a lunotriquetral (LT) ligament tear.

Table 27.2 Arthroscopic staging of lunotriquetral lesions

LT tear	X-ray	MRI	Radiocarpal	Midcarpal
Partial	nl	Variable Arthroscopic perforation	Membranous tear No synovitis	nl
Grade 1	nl	Variable Artho perforation	Complete tear Mild synovitis	Straight probe insertion Hamate nl
Grade 2	nl	abnl	Complete tear Synovitis	Twisted probe insertion Hamate erosions
Grade 3	Variable Gilula arc	abnl	Complete tear Synovitis	Trocar insertion Hamate erosions
Ulnar Impaction With LT tear	+ ulnar variance	+ TFC + LT tear =/- lunate Chondral lesion	Tears TFC and LT Lunate erosion Synovitis	Findings like stages 1, 2, or 3

Abbreviations: abnl, abnormal; LT, lunotriquetral; nl, normal; TFC, triangular fibrocartilage.

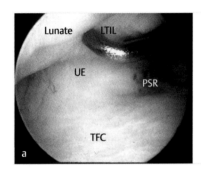

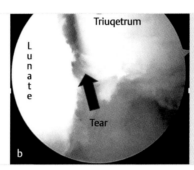

Fig. 27.6 (a, b) Arthroscopic 6R portal view. **(a)** Normal lunotriquetral (LT) interval. LTIL, lunotriquetral interosseous ligament; UE, ulnar extrinsic ligaments; TFC, triangular fibrocartilage; PSR, prestyloid recess.

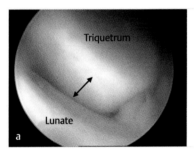

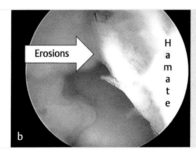

Fig. 27.7 (a) Grade 2 lunotriquetral (LT) tear, radial midcarpal view. Note: 3 mm offset in LT alignment. Gap will admit a twisted probe. **(b)** Hamate erosions in a grade 2 LT tear (the HALT [Hamete arthrosis lunotriquetral] lesion).

significance of the tear requires clinical correlation. Some authors continue to use bone scans, which will demonstrate increased uptake in the LT joint, but this test is nonspecific.[16,17]

Wrist arthroscopy remains the gold standard for diagnosis of ligamentous injury in the wrist and offers an approach to staging LT lesions (▶Table 27.2). Given the wide curvature of the radiocarpal joint, the best visualization of the LT interval is from an ulnar portal either 4–5 or 6R. The use of a probe to assess ligament integrity is important (▶Fig. 27.6a, b). Unlike a torn SL, there is never a drive-through opening. Midcarpal arthroscopy is essential to evaluate the degree of instability and the joint reaction to that instability. In the midcarpal joint, one can assess the congruency of the concave LT interface and the degree of the step off. Instability can be dynamically evaluated using the probe and trocar (▶Fig. 27.7a). Normally it will barely admit a probe. In grade 1 it will admit a standard arthroscopic probe, in grade 2 the probe can be twisted, and in grade 3 the 2.9 mm trocar can be inserted. Furthermore, the degree of instability relates to the reaction at the hamate interface. Palmer described the

HALT (Hamete arthrosis lunotriquetral) lesion (hamate impaction secondary to LT instability).[3,18] The greater the hamate erosion, the greater the instability (▶Fig. 27.7b). These findings are incorporated in the arthroscopic staging of the LT lesions. Hofmeister et al found that midcarpal arthroscopy confirmed the radiocarpal diagnosis 21% of the time and added to the radiocarpal diagnosis 82% of the time.[19] We have previously demonstrated the frequency of additional injuries associated with LT tears (synovitis 85%, LT chondromalacia 40%, TFCC tears 40%, triquetrohamate chrondromalacia 30%, and ulnar extrinsic ligament tears 30%).[20] Treatment is then based on patient pain and impairment, acuity and arthroscopic staging.

27.3 Treatment of Acute LT Injuries

Acute injuries present on a spectrum from membranous tear to a perilunate injury. Perilunate injuries are beyond the scope of this chapter, and injuries discussed herein are limited to instances when the LT injury is the primary diagnosis. Our initial management of any isolated LT injury is nonoperative. When symptoms are recalcitrant to nonoperative management, operative management is carried out.

27.3.1 Nonoperative Management

Patients are referred to occupational therapy (OT) for the fabrication of a custom molded thermoplast splint, which is contoured to support the pisiform. In addition, formal OT is conducted with an emphasis on ECU proprioception and strengthening. Kobayashi et al demonstrated that LT ligament injury results in altered carpal kinematics, with the proximal carpal row migrating into flexion and supination.[21] Leon-Lopez at al built on the work of Kobayashi by sectioning the LT ligament and then testing each forearm muscle to determine the effect on LT kinematics.[22] They demonstrated that the ECU can affect a countering force via pronation, and the ECU was determined to be the only muscle that exerts a pronation force on the proximal carpal row. A trial of nonoperative management should consist of at least a 6- to 12-week course. Splinting can be supplemented with nonsteroidal anti-inflammatory drugs and corticosteroid injections as needed.

Reagan et al demonstrated good results with nonoperative treatment in six of seven acute tears, but only one of four chronic tears.[2]

27.3.2 Operative Management

When patients continue to be symptomatic after appropriate nonoperative management, surgical management is indicated. Arthroscopy allows for confirmation of the diagnosis and grading of the tear severity, as well as documentation of the presence or absence of degenerative changes. All of these factors contribute to the selection of the ultimate surgical technique directed at the LT injury. As in most injuries the final treatment decision depends on the circumstances of the patient, the preference of the surgeon, and the acuteness and grade of the injury. There are no validated best scientific algorithms and only level 4 evidence for any particular treatment paradigm.

Acute grade 1 and 2 lesions are frequently treated with debridement and capsular shrinkage. Ruch et al demonstrated 93% patient satisfaction, 100% relief of mechanical symptoms, and no degenerative changes at an average follow-up of 34 months after LT debridement alone.[23] Weiss et al reported complete resolution of symptoms or only occasional symptoms in seven of nine patients with a complete LT tear treated with debridement alone.[24] They also noted 100% complete resolution or only occasional symptoms in patients with partial LT tears treated with debridement despite these patients returning to heavy labor. Lee et al performed debridement with capsular shrinkage on partial LT tears and noted significant pain improvement with an excellent or good outcome for the entire cohort (11 excellent; 3 good).[25] It is important to note that associated pathology diagnosed on arthroscopy should also be addressed concomitantly with the LT pathology. We have previously reported our results on debridement, joint reduction, and pinning of LT injuries while simultaneously addressing associated pathology, with 80% good to excellent results at an average follow-up of 20 months.[22]

When gross instability, usually grade 3, is noted, open treatment with LT repair is considered. There is a paucity of literature to support open repair of the LT ligament, which we postulate is secondary to the low frequency in which the diagnosis is made acutely; however, repair maybe attempted if the adequate residual LT tissue remains, regardless of chronicity. Stabilization with LT pinning or screws is used for 8 weeks (▶Fig. 27.8), followed by a dart throwers rehabilitation

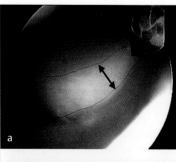
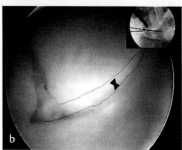
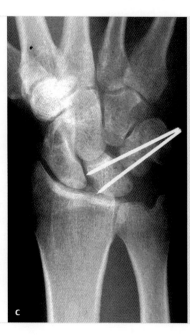

Fig. 27.8 **(a)** Grade 2 lunotriquetral (LT) tear with unreduced stepoff in midcarpal joint. **(b)** Arthroscopic view of grade 2 LT tear reduced. **(c)** Radiograph of pinned LT joint following reduction and heat capsulodesis. The pins are buried and kept in place for 8 weeks.

program and return to full functional use on average around 4 months. Reagan reported good patient satisfaction in six of seven repairs with an average follow-up of 44 months.[2]

27.4 Treatment of Chronic Lunotriquetral Injuries

Chronic grades 1 and 2 tears are effectively managed with debridement and capsular shrinkage in a similar fashion to acute tears. When there is a high-grade tear of chronic nature with instability or VISI, there are several treatment options including the following: LT ligament repair, LT ligament reconstruction, partial wrist denervation (PWD), LT arthrodesis, and ulnar shortening osteotomy (USO) (▶Table 27.3). Shin et al retrospectively compared the outcomes of 57 patients that underwent LT repair, LT reconstruction, or LT arthrodesis.[26] While disabilities of the arm, shoulder, and hand (DASH) scores did not differ between the groups, they found a significantly higher rate of remaining symptom free in the reconstruction group (69% reconstruction, 14% repair, and < 1% arthrodesis). They also noted a lower rate of reoperation at 5 years in the reconstruction group (31% reconstruction, 77% repair, and 78% arthrodesis). Reconstruction should be considered in the presence of correctable VISI without arthrosis. There are a number of reconstructive options described. Reagan et al were the first to describe the use of a distally based strip of ECU passed through drill holes in the triquetrum to reconstruct the ligament.[2] They reported a good outcome in the one patient they treated by this method. Shin et al modified the technique by drilling a common volar point in the LT joint with pins directed ulnarly through the lunate and radially through the triquetrum.[17] These pin tracks are enlarged to an appropriate size to allow for the passage of a strip of ECU. The ECU is passed radially through both bone tunnels before being drawn ulnarly across the LT surface to reconstruct the dorsal ligament and sutured to itself. Shahane described a technique of ECU tenodesis involving drill holes in the triquetrum only.[27] The distally based strip of ECU is passed radially through the tunnel, passed through the dorsal radioulnar ligament, and sutured to itself. They described their outcomes on 46 patients at an average of 39 months as 41% excellent, 22% good, 24% satisfactory, and 13% poor. Eighty-seven percent of their cohort stated they would have the surgery again if they had a similar problem. Omokawa et al described the use of the DRC with Kirschner wires (K-wire) immobilization as a capsulodesis in 11 patients.[28] They demonstrated mixed outcomes with 7 good or excellent and 4 fair or poor at an average follow-up of 31 months. Antti-Poika et al described a transverse split in the extensor retinaculum.[29] The radially based distal limb of the split retinaculum is anchored to both the dorsal lunate and triquetrum

Table 27.3 Treatment options for high-grade tear of chronic nature with instability

- Open repair grade 3
  - Dorsal transverse in line with fifth extensor compartment
  - Ligament sparing approach
  - Freshen ligament and lunate edges
  - Trans-osseous drill holes through triquetrum
  - Reduce triquetrolunate posture
  - Capsular closure
  - K-wires or screw for 8 weeks
  - May augment with Swivel locks and labral tape
- Reconstruction with tendon graft
  - Dorsal ligament sparing incision
  - Distally based extensor carpi ulnaris tendon strip
  - Opposing transosseous tunnels
  - K-wires: 8 weeks

Or

  - Tendon graft
  - Circumferential through lunate and triquetrum
  - Extracapsular, capture ulnar extrinsic
  - Two incisions, volar and dorsal
  - Avoid pisiform and ulnar nerve
  - K-wires: 8 weeks

Abbreviation: K-wire, Kirschner wires.

with bone anchors after reduction. They reported on 26 patients at an average follow-up of 39 months and noted good or excellent results in 88%, fair results in 12%, and no poor results.

Lastly we have been using a variation of the combined volar and dorsal "box" reconstruction advocated by Ho for chronic SL instability.[30] In this technique a tendon graft is passed extracapsular from dorsal to volar through the lunate. Using a volar incision and avoiding the pisiform and ulnar nerve, the graft is passed from volar to dorsal through the triquetrum. The graft is then cinched extracapsularly and dorsally. Early results have been promising.

USO is authors' preferred option that has only recently begun to be studied with regard to LT pathology. USO is classically considered when there is evidence of ulnar abutment and ulnar positive variance without the presence of VISI. The theoretical mechanism of efficacy for USO is tightening of the ulnar extrinsic ligaments (ulnotriquetral and ulnolunate), and thereby stabilizing the LT joint. Gupta and Osterman performed a biomechanical study that demonstrated diminished LT motion with increased tension of the ulnar extrinsic ligaments.[31] Given this experimental data, the authors will use it as their go to procedure even when there is neutral or slight negative variance and an LT instability. It is also their choice when primary repair has failed. Mirza et al retrospectively reviewed 53 patients after USO for arthroscopically confirmed isolated LT tears at an average follow-up of 12 months.[16] The authors shortened the ulna 2.5 mm regardless of ulnar variance (including some that started with ulnar negative variance), with the intent of tightening the ulnar extrinsic ligaments (▶ Fig. 27.9).

They noted good or excellent outcomes in 83% and argued that USO has a similar increase in grip strength and similar complication rate to intracarpal procedures. Iwatsuki et al performed a second look arthroscopy at the time of plate removal in 50 patients that underwent USO.[32] At the time of initial arthroscopy, 50% of the patients had LT ligament degeneration. Patients had similar outcomes after USO regardless of the presence or severity of LT ligament involvement. The second look arthroscopy was performed at an average follow-up of 39 months. The

authors found that, in those previously diagnosed with LT degeneration, the Geissler class improved in 11, remained the same in 9, and worsened in 2.

When significant LT arthrosis or fixed VISI is present, salvage options are considered. Many of the salvage options sacrifice ROM and grip strength to achieve pain relief. One early, nondefinitive salvage option that maintains ROM and grip strength is PWD.

Hofmeister et al described their results of anterior interosseous nerve and posterior interosseous nerve neurectomies through a single dorsal incision for the treatment of carpal instability, and this is the only study regarding the procedure specifically for this pathology.[33] In their prospective study, 48 patients were followed up for an average of 28 months and noted to have significant improvement in pain and DASH scores. However, the authors emphasize that 16 wrists required additional surgery and that the procedure should be offered

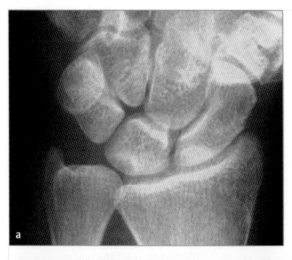
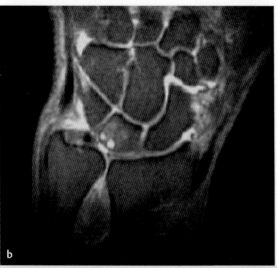
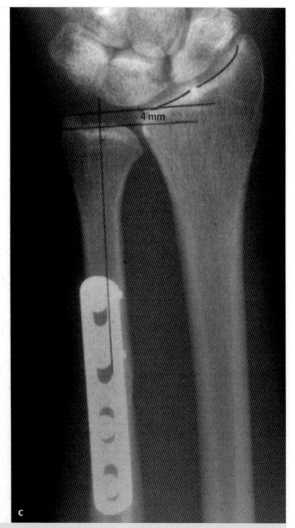

Fig. 27.9 (a) Radiograph of ulnar impaction with proven arthroscopic triangular fibrocartilage and lunotriquetral (LT) tears. **(b)** MRI of the same case. **(c)** Definitive treatment with ulnar shortening osteotomy.

with the understanding that it may only delay the need for a more definitive procedure. The denervation procedure was noted to have a low morbidity, and it did not complicate the definitive procedure, when required. Weinstein et al performed a similar procedure for chronic wrist pain in 19 patients with an average follow-up of 2.5 years.[34] Eighty-five percent of patients were satisfied, and 90% of patients stated they would choose the same surgery again. The authors noted failure in three patients within the follow-up period and found that failure typically occurred within 1 year of the procedure. While robust support in the literature and long-term outcomes are lacking, the procedure appears to offer at least short-term pain relief without evidence of sacrificing proprioception.[35]

LT arthrodesis has fallen out of favor secondary to a high reported rate of nonunion. A meta-analysis by Larsen et al demonstrated that the current body of literature is limited to small studies, with the largest cohort reported on 26 patients.[36,37] Nonunion rates ranged from 0 to 50% between studies and a combined rate of 27%. Despite the risk of nonunion, LT arthrodesis remains the option of choice when treating an unstable LT joint/ fixed VISI with associated degenerative changes. Fixed VISI is not adequately treated with soft-tissue LT reassociation procedures.[38] The method of fixation and length of immobilization may directly impact the union rate. Nelson et al described their cohort of patients that underwent LT arthrodesis and noted 100% fusion rate in those whose fixation included a headless compression screw combined with more than 6 weeks of immobilization.[39] In comparison, their fusion rate was only 50% in those whose fixation included k-wires only combined with less than 6 weeks of immobilization. Guidera et al reported on the largest cohort of 26 patients and demonstrated 100% union.[37] The authors used two parallel k-wires for fixation and emphasized that maintaining the preoperative bony dimensions with precise preparation and bone grafting is more essential than the fixation method. A number of authors have noted that patient function and satisfaction are high when union is achieved, also highlighting that patients with a congenital LT coalition are often asymptomatic.[37]

In summary, LT injuries can be difficult to diagnose and subtle on examination/radiographs. Initial management should consist of nonoperative modalities. When operative management is undertaken, wrist arthroscopy (including the midcarpal joint) should be performed to confirm the diagnosis, identify concomitant injuries, and guide the treatment. In both acute and chronic stage 1/2 injuries without arthrosis or instability, ligament debridement and capsular shrinkage is effective. Similar treatment may be carried out for stage 3/4 injuries without arthrosis or VISI, but repair or reconstruction is required in the presence of correctable VISI. It should be noted that ligament reconstruction has better outcomes

than repair. For chronic LT injuries without arthrosis or VISI in the setting of ulnar positive or neutral variance, ulnar shortening osteotomy is the most appropriate treatment. Finally, in the presence of LT arthrosis or fixed VISI, PWD may be offered to maintain motion and grip strength. However, long-term studies for this procedure are lacking, and LT arthrodesis or other salvage options may eventually be required.

References

[1] Horii E, Garcia-Elias M, An KN, et al. A kinematic study of lunotriquetral dissociations. J Hand Surg Am 1991;16(2):355–362

[2] Reagan DS, Linscheid RL, Dobyns JH. Lunotriquetral sprains. J Hand Surg Am 1984;9(4):502–514

[3] Slutsky DJ, Trevare J. Scapholunate and lunotriquetral injuries: arthroscopic and open management. Sports Med Arthrosc Rev 2014;22(1):12–21

[4] Lichtman DM, Noble WH III, Alexander CE. Dynamic triquetrolunate instability: case report. J Hand Surg Am 1984;9(2):185–188

[5] Rhee PC, Sauvé PS, Lindau T, Shin AY. Examination of the wrist: ulnar-sided wrist pain due to ligamentous injury. J Hand Surg Am 2014;39(9):1859–1862

[6] LaStayo P, Howell J. Clinical provocative tests used in evaluating wrist pain: a descriptive study. J Hand Ther 1995;8(1):10–17

[7] Tay SC, Tomita K, Berger RA. The "ulnar fovea sign" for defining ulnar wrist pain: an analysis of sensitivity and specificity. J Hand Surg Am 2007;32(4):438–444

[8] Christodoulou L, Bainbridge LC. Clinical diagnosis of triquetrolunate ligament injuries. J Hand Surg [Br] 1999;24(5):598–600

[9] Gilula LA, Weeks PM. Post-traumatic ligamentous instabilities of the wrist. Radiology 1978;129(3):641–651

[10] Nicoson MC, Moran SL. Diagnosis and treatment of acute lunotriquetral ligament injuries. Hand Clin 2015;31(3):467–476

[11] Gilula LA, Palmer AK. Is it possible to call a "tear" on arthrograms or magnetic resonance imaging scans? J Hand Surg Am 1993;18(3):547

[12] Kessler I, Silberman Z. An experimental study of the radiocarpal joint by arthrography. Surg Gynecol Obstet 1961;112:33–40

[13] Cantor RM, Stern PJ, Wyrick JD, Michaels SE. The relevance of ligament tears or perforations in the diagnosis of wrist pain: an arthrographic study. J Hand Surg Am 1994;19(6):945–953

[14] Viegas SF, Ballantyne G. Attritional lesions of the wrist joint. J Hand Surg Am 1987;12(6):1025–1029

[15] Anderson ML, Skinner JA, Felmlee JP, Berger RA, Amrami KK. Diagnostic comparison of 1.5 Tesla and 3.0 Tesla preoperative MRI of the wrist in patients with ulnar-sided wrist pain. J Hand Surg Am 2008;33(7):1153–1159

[16] Mirza A, Mirza JB, Shin AY, Lorenzana DJ, Lee BK, Izzo B. Isolated lunotriquetral ligament tears treated with ulnar shortening osteotomy. J Hand Surg Am 2013;38(8):1492–1497

[17] Shin AY, Bishop AT. Treatment options for lunotriquetral dissociation. Tech Hand Up Extrem Surg 1998;2(1):2–17

[18] Harley BJ, Werner FW, Boles SD, Palmer AK. Arthroscopic resection of arthrosis of the proximal hamate: a clinical and biomechanical study. J Hand Surg Am 2004;29(4):661–667

[19] Hofmeister EP, Dao KD, Glowacki KA, Shin AY. The role of midcarpal arthroscopy in the diagnosis of disorders of the wrist. J Hand Surg Am 2001;26(3):407–414

[20] Osterman AL, Seidman GD. The role of arthroscopy in the treatment of lunatotriquetral ligament injuries. Hand Clin 1995;11(1):41–50

[21] Kobayashi M, Garcia-Elias M, Nagy L, et al. Axial loading induces rotation of the proximal carpal row bones around unique screw-displacement axes. J Biomech 1997;30(11–12):1165–1167

[22] León-Lopez MM, Salvà-Coll G, Garcia-Elias M, Lluch-Bergadà A, Llusá-Pérez M. Role of the extensor carpi ulnaris in the

stabilization of the lunotriquetral joint. An experimental study. J Hand Ther 2013;26(4):312–317, quiz 317

[23] Ruch DS, Poehling GG. Arthroscopic management of partial scapholunate and lunotriquetral injuries of the wrist. J Hand Surg Am 1996;21(3):412–417

[24] Weiss AP, Sachar K, Glowacki KA. Arthroscopic debridement alone for intercarpal ligament tears. J Hand Surg Am 1997;22(2):344–349

[25] Lee JI, Nha KW, Lee GY, Kim BH, Kim JW, Park JW. Long-term outcomes of arthroscopic debridement and thermal shrinkage for isolated partial intercarpal ligament tears. Orthopedics 2012;35(8):e1204–e1209

[26] Shin AY, Weinstein LP, Berger RA, Bishop AT. Treatment of isolated injuries of the lunotriquetral ligament. A comparison of arthrodesis, ligament reconstruction and ligament repair. J Bone Joint Surg Br 2001;83(7):1023–1028

[27] Shahane SA, Trail IA, Takwale VJ, Stilwell JH, Stanley JK. Tenodesis of the extensor carpi ulnaris for chronic, post-traumatic lunotriquetral instability. J Bone Joint Surg Br 2005;87(11):1512–1515

[28] Omokawa S, Fujitani R, Inada Y. Dorsal radiocarpal ligament capsulodesis for chronic dynamic lunotriquetral instability. J Hand Surg Am 2009;34(2):237–243

[29] Antti-Poika I, Hyrkäs J, Virkki LM, Ogino D, Konttinen YT. Correction of chronic lunotriquetral instability using extensor retinacular split: a retrospective study of 26 patients. Acta Orthop Belg 2007;73(4):451–457

[30] Ho PC, Wong CW, Tse W. Arthroscopic-assisted combined volar and dorsal reconstruction with tendon graft for chronic SL instability. J Wrist Surg 2015;4:252–263

[31] Gupta R, Bingenheimer E, Fornalski S, McGarry MH, Osterman AL, Lee TQ. The effect of ulnar shortening on lunate and triquetrum motion—a cadaveric study. Clin Biomech (Bristol, Avon) 2005;20(8):839–845

[32] Iwatsuki K, Tatebe M, Yamamoto M, Shinohara T, Nakamura R, Hirata H. Ulnar impaction syndrome: incidence of lunotriquetral ligament degeneration and outcome of ulnar-shortening osteotomy. J Hand Surg Am 2014;39(6):1108–1113

[33] Hofmeister EP, Moran SL, Shin AY. Anterior and posterior interosseous neurectomy for the treatment of chronic dynamic instability of the wrist. Hand (N Y) 2006;1(2):63–70

[34] Weinstein LP, Berger RA. Analgesic benefit, functional outcome, and patient satisfaction after partial wrist denervation. J Hand Surg Am 2002;27(5):833–839

[35] Milone MT, Klifto CS, Catalano LW III. Partial wrist denervation: the evidence behind a small fix for big problems. J Hand Surg Am 2018;43(3):272–277

[36] Larsen CF, Jacoby RA, McCabe SJ. Nonunion rates of limited carpal arthrodesis: a meta-analysis of the literature. J Hand Surg Am 1997;22(1):66–73

[37] Guidera PM, Watson HK, Dwyer TA, Orlando G, Zeppieri J, Yasuda M. Lunotriquetral arthrodesis using cancellous bone graft. J Hand Surg Am 2001;26(3):422–427

[38] Sachar K. Ulnar-sided wrist pain: evaluation and treatment of triangular fibrocartilage complex tears, ulnocarpal impaction syndrome, and lunotriquetral ligament tears. J Hand Surg Am 2012;37(7):1489–1500

[39] Nelson DL, Manske PR, Pruitt DL, Gilula LA, Martin RA. Lunotriquetral arthrodesis. J Hand Surg Am 1993;18(6):1113–1120

28 Arthroscopic Management of Perilunate Dislocation and Fracture Dislocation

Jae Woo Shim, Jong-Pil Kim, Min Jong Park

Abstract

Perilunate injuries are highly unstable carpal dissociations and their management remains challenging and controversial. The key to successful treatment of perilunate injuries is the restoration of normal alignment of the carpal bones, followed by stable maintenance until healing. Recent arthroscopic techniques as minimally invasive treatment have emerged with results similar to or better than those of open approach, as well as having less post-traumatic arthrosis.

Arthroscopic reduction was attempted in case of manual reduction failure. In those cases, the lunate, which had volarly dislocated, was effectively reduced by pulling it dorsally with use of a probe. Once the dislocation has been reduced, arthroscopic restoration of the carpal bones and percutaneous fixation are possible. After evaluation of the radiocarpal joint, debridement were performed to facilitate reduction of the proximal intercarpal joint. Kirschner wires were inserted percutaneously into the scaphoid and triquetrum. When the anatomic reduction was restored, the wires were then driven across the intercarpal intervals into the lunate. For trans-scaphoid type injuries, wires driven across fracture line and percutaneous scaphoid fixation using a cannulated headless auto compression screw was performed.

Arthroscopic reduction with percutaneous fixation is a reliable minimally invasive surgical method for acute perilunate injuries in that it provides proper restoration and stable fixation of carpal alignment and results in satisfactory functional and radiological outcomes on a midterm basis.

Keywords: wrist, arthroscopy, lunate, scaphoid, dislocation, fracture, reduction

28.1 Introduction

Perilunate injuries are highly unstable carpal dissociations, characterized by a complete loss of contact between the lunate and surrounding carpal bones. Perilunate injuries are referred to as lesser arc injuries when ligaments around the lunate are involved only, whereas dislocations associated with fractures (perilunate fracture dislocations) are referred to as greater arc injuries (▶Fig. 28.1).[1] Greater arc injuries most commonly involve fractures through the scaphoid (trans-scaphoid perilunate fracture dislocation), accounting for approximately 95% of perilunate fracture dislocations (▶Fig. 28.2).[2]

Perilunate injuries are caused by high-energy impact, such as falling from a height, motor vehicle accidents, or play injury from contact sports. The mechanism of these injuries includes forceful hyperextension, ulnar deviation, and intercarpal supination of the wrist along with axial load. The force is applied to the scaphoid (causing a trans-scaphoid fracture) or to the scapholunate ligament (causing a scapholunate dissociation). The force then progresses through the scaphocapitate and capitolunate joint or capitate, finally reaching the lunotriquetral ligament or triquetrum. Based on these pathomechanics, Mayfield et al[1] described a spectrum of injuries characterized by four distinct stages (▶Fig. 28.3).

In Stage 1 injuries, the scapholunate ligament and the radioscapholunate ligament are torn. In case of Stage 2 injuries, the force is transmitted to the lunocapitate articulation where the capitate dislocates; the radioscaphocapitate ligament, dorsal intercarpal ligament, and radial collateral ligament are injured. In Stage 3 injuries, energy propagates into the lunotriquetral joint, resulting in the lunotriquetral ligament tear and a triquetral dislocation. In Stage 4 injuries, the lunate dislocates volarly and no longer remains within the lunate fossa as a result of ulnotriquetral and dorsal radiocarpal ligament tears.

The key to successful treatment of perilunate injuries is the restoration of normal alignment of the carpal bones, followed by stable maintenance until healing.[4,5] Although it is usually possible to grossly reduce the dislocation by closed manipulation, restoration of anatomic alignment of all injured structures cannot be achieved by closed means.[6] Complete restoration of proximal carpal bones

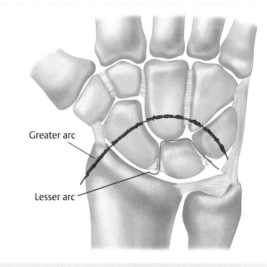

Fig. 28.1 Patterns of greater arc and lesser arc injuries. Greater arc injuries involve a fracture of any bone in the sequence of the radial styloid, scaphoid, capitate, hamate, or triquetrum, whereas lesser arc injuries involve pure ligaments around the lunate. (*Source:* Reproduced with permission from Park MJ. Hand and Upper Extremity Surgery: The Wrist and Elbow. Seoul: Panmun; 2017.[3])

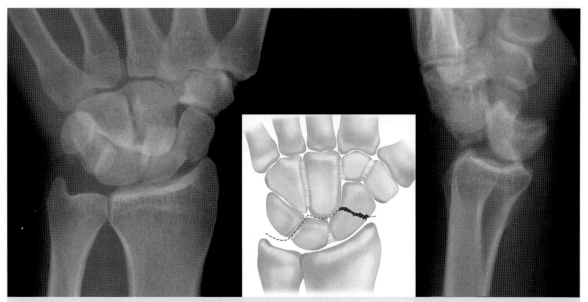

Fig. 28.2 The most common form of perilunate injuries is trans-scaphoid perilunate fracture dislocation, which is the combination of greater arc and lesser arc injuries. (*Source:* Reproduced with permission from Park MJ. Hand and Upper Extremity Surgery: The Wrist and Elbow. Seoul: Panmun; 2017.[3])

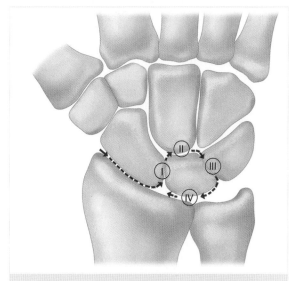

Fig. 28.3 Mechanism of perilunate injuries described by Mayfield et al. The separation progress from radial side of the lunate to ulnar side. It shows a spectrum in that the separation progresses according to the degree of external force. (*Source:* Reproduced with permission from Park MJ. Hand and Upper Extremity Surgery: The Wrist and Elbow. Seoul: Panmun; 2017.[3])

makes good results and prevents sequelae such as nonunion, chronic instability, and arthritis.[7,8] The generally accepted treatment has been open primary repair or reconstruction of the ligaments with open reduction and internal fixation of the fractures.[4,9,10,11]

Arthroscopic treatment allows anatomic reduction of intercarpal articulations and proper reestablishment of carpal stability.[11,12,13] Recent arthroscopic techniques as a minimal invasive treatment have

emerged with results similar to or better than those of open approach, as well as having less posttraumatic arthrosis.[13,14,15,16,17,18]

28.2 Indications

Acute dislocation failing to manual reduction and chronic dislocation without reduction necessarily require open surgery, but once the dislocation has been reduced, arthroscopic restoration of the carpal bones and percutaneous fixation are possible. The perilunate injuries are combined injury of interosseous ligaments and carpal bones fracture. Arthroscopic approach is possible for each, so that the perilunate injuries can be successfully treated with arthroscopy.[15,19] The most common form of perilunate injuries is the trans-scaphoid perilunate fracture dislocation, which is a good indication of arthroscopy surgery because the scapholunate ligament is intact.[5,20]

The feasibility of arthroscopic technique in presence of median nerve dysfunction and whether intercarpal ligaments can achieve reliable healing that is sufficient enough to maintain carpal stability without a direct repair are uncertain and debatable.

28.3 Surgical Technique

Before arthroscopy was performed, a closed reduction had been attempted. When the gross reduction was not amenable to initial closed reduction, this maneuver was not repeated in order to prevent further cartilage or soft-tissue damage. Arthroscopic reduction was attempted in case of manual reduction failure.

Wrist arthroscopy was performed under brachial plexus block or general anesthesia. The hand was suspended using a traction tower with 10 to 15 lb of traction. The forearm was wrapped with a compressive elastic bandage, and continuous saline irrigation was instilled by gravity infusion from an elevated bag to minimize fluid extravasation. After clot and debris were removed through the 3–4 and 4–5 portals, the palmar capsular ligaments, scapholunate and lunotriquetral ligaments, and triangular fibrocartilage complex were carefully evaluated. Arthroscopic findings of patients who had failed to achieve a gross reduction by a closed manipulation revealed that palmar capsular ligaments were torn and interposed between the lunate and capitate. In those cases, the lunate, which had volarly dislocated with or without proximal fragment of the scaphoid, was effectively reduced by pulling it dorsally with use of a probe. Extensive injury to the radioscaphocapitate ligament with relatively intact long and short radiolunate ligaments was the consistent finding, which can be explained anatomically based on the pathology of perilunate injury.

After evaluation of the radiocarpal joint, our attention was directed toward the midcarpal joint, in which the main disruption had occurred. The midcarpal space was entered at the midcarpal radial and midcarpal ulnar portals. Bone or cartilage fragments and frayed edges of torn palmar capsular ligaments were thoroughly debrided or removed to facilitate reduction of the proximal intercarpal joint. Probing the intercarpal joint of the proximal carpal row showed gross instability of both the scapholunate and lunotriquetral articulations in perilunate dislocations and the lunotriquetral joint in trans-scaphoid perilunate fracture dislocations from the complete tear (▶ Fig. 28.4a, b).

Once the injury pattern was identified, Kirschner wires (K-wires) were inserted percutaneously into the scaphoid and triquetrum and an additional K-wire placed dorsally into the lunate under a fluoroscope (▶ Fig. 28.4c). After longitudinal traction was released, the scapholunate and lunotriquetral intervals were reduced by manipulating the K-wires as joysticks, as viewed directly in the midcarpal portals. When the anatomic reduction was restored, the wires were then driven across the intercarpal intervals into the lunate (▶ Fig. 28.4d, e). For trans-scaphoid type injuries, the reduction of the scaphoid fragments was attempted by manipulating provisional K-wires driven into the distal fragment and not across the fracture site, and an additional K-wire was placed on the dorsum of the proximal pole of the scaphoid. These wires were used as joysticks to reduce the fracture further anatomically, while viewing the articular surface from the midcarpal portal. K-wires in the distal pole of the scaphoid were advanced across the fracture site into the proximal fragment after a congruous articular surface was obtained (▶ Fig. 28.4d, e).

Percutaneous scaphoid fixation using a cannulated headless auto compression screw (Acutrak; Acumed, Beaverton, OR, United States) was attempted in patients who did not have comminution in the scaphoid.

The Acutrak screw was introduced after a guidewire was properly advanced from dorsal to volar along the central axis of the scaphoid under fluoroscopic control, as described by Slade et al.21 The patients who had combined intercarpal ligamentous injuries had additional 1.2-mm K-wire fixation into the intercarpal joint under arthroscopic assistance. Finally, the wires were bent, cut, and buried underneath the skin (▶ Fig. 28.4f, g).

After the operation, the wrist was immobilized in a short-arm thumb spica cast. In pure ligamentous injuries, the K-wires were removed at 10 weeks. In patients with a scaphoid fracture that had been fixed with K-wires, the K-wires were removed when there was radiographic evidence of a union. Intensive physiotherapy was started.

28.4 Results

28.4.1 Clinical Results

Kim et al[15] reported results of arthroscopic management in 20 patients with perilunate injuries at a mean follow-up of 31.2 months. Five patients were perilunate dislocations, 12 trans-scaphoid perilunate fracture dislocations, and 3 trans-scaphoid trans-triquetral perilunate fracture dislocations. The mean flexion was 51 degrees (range: 25–70 degrees), which was 79% compared with the contralateral wrist. The mean extension was 53 degrees (range: 30–70 degrees), which was 80% of the contralateral wrist. The mean grip strength was 78% (range: 62–94%) of the contralateral wrist at the final evaluation. The overall functional outcomes according to the Mayo wrist score (MWS) were rated as excellent in 3 patients, good in 8, fair in 7, and poor in 2.

Liu et al[17] reported results of arthroscopic management in 24 patients with perilunate dislocation also. The range of flexion–extension motion of the injured wrist averaged 86% of the values for the contralateral wrist. The grip strength of the injured wrist averaged 83% of the values for the contralateral wrists. According to MWS, overall functional outcomes were rated as excellent in 13 patients (54%), good in 6 (25%), fair in 4 (17%), and poor in 1 (4%).

Oh et al[18] compared the results of arthroscopic and open techniques for trans-scaphoid perilunate fracture dislocations. Twenty patients were included in the study, 11 were operated by arthroscopy, and 9 were operated by open technique. The mean flexion–extension arc was significantly greater in arthroscopy group (125.0 degrees) than in open group (105.6 degrees). The mean MWS was 85.5 in arthroscopy group and 79.4 in open group.

28.4.2 Radiological Results

Although the results showed a tendency toward a gradual loss of reduction with time, this would not indicate the loss of stability based on the facts that a small change in parameters was observed and the final radiological values were within normal ranges in most patients.

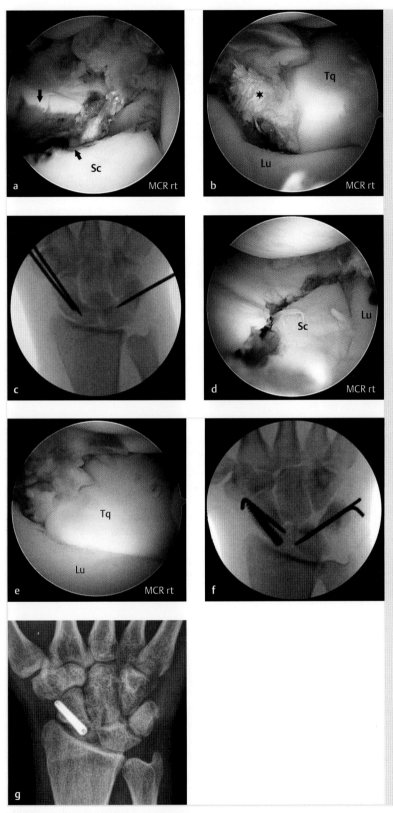

Fig. 28.4 A 19-year-old man with transscaphoid perilunate fracture dislocation on his right side wrist underwent arthroscopic reduction and percutaneous fixations. Findings at the midcarpal portal showing scaphoid fracture (**a**, *arrow* showing displaced scaphoid fracture) and dissociation of lunotriquetral joint (**b**, *star* showing torn lunotriquetral ligament). Kirschner wires were inserted percutaneously into the distal scaphoid and triquetrum (**c**). After arthroscopic assisted reduction and percutaneous fixation, accurate articular reductions of the scaphoid (**d**) and triquetrum. (**e**) can be obtained. Postoperative radiographs showing well-established carpal alignment with anatomic reduction of the scaphoid fracture (**f**). Ten month follow-up radiographs showing union of fractures and normal carpal alignment without evidence of arthritis (**g**). MCR Rt, midcarpal radial portal right; Sc, scaphoid; Lu, lunate; Tq, triquetrum. *(Source:* Reproduced with permission from Park MJ. Hand and Upper Extremity Surgery: The Wrist and Elbow. Seoul: Panmun; 2017.[3])

In Kim et al's study,[15] the mean scapholunate gap during the follow-up period had increased by 0.3 mm (range: 0–0.9 mm). The mean scapholunate angle had increased by 3 degrees (range: 0–8 degrees), and the mean carpal height ratio had decreased by 0.02 (range: 0–0.04). At the final follow-up, 15 patients had a normal scapholunate angle (normal range: 30–60 degrees) and 16 patients had a normal carpal height ratio (normal range: 0.51–0.57). No patients had radiographic evidence of arthritis of either the radiocarpal or midcarpal joint.

In Oh et al's comparative study,[18] the mean scapholunate angle was 47.2 degrees, radiolunate angle was 1.7 degrees, and lunotriquetral distance was 2.0 mm in arthroscopy group. There was no difference between the two groups. Four patients exhibited midcarpal arthritis on radiographs at the last follow-up.

28.5 Complications

In Kim et al's study,[15] among the 15 trans-scaphoid perilunate injuries, nonunion of the scaphoid developed in 2, 1 patient underwent a scaphoid excision, and four-corner fusion was subsequently performed.

In Liu et al's study[17] scaphoid nonunion developed in 1 of 24 patients. In Oh et al's study,[18] there was no nonunion in arthroscopy group, but 1 of 9 patients in open group had nonunion at final follow-up.

28.6 Pitfalls and Contraindications

- Although it is important to place the screw as close as possible to the central axis of the scaphoid, surgeons should attempt to place the screw slightly dorsal because trans-scaphoid perilunate injuries are commonly comminuted. Otherwise, it may compress the fracture back into volarly flexed angulation (i.e., humpback deformity).
- We prefer buried K-wire fixation of the lunotriquetral and triquetrocapitate intervals because restoration of intercarpal integrity has been shown to be a key determinant of the outcome.[9]

Tips and Tricks

- In trans-scaphoid perilunate injuries, scaphoid fracture is commonly comminuted and interposed by palmar capsular ligament, making it difficult to obtain anatomical reduction. Thorough debridement of interposed ligament and removal of small fracture fragments should be performed prior to reduction of scaphoid fracture and intercarpal joints.
- If the fracture is proximal in the scaphoid, it is highly unstable. We prefer to introduce an additional K-wire on the dorsum of the proximal fragment to use as a joystick with two K-wires driven into the distal fragment. After obtaining precise articular reduction, distal K-wires are advanced into the proximal fragment through the fracture site. One of two distal pins can be used as anti-rotation pin while a headless screw is placed in the scaphoid.
- We reduce the lunotriquetral joint using provisional K-wires introduced into the triquetrum and a probe, viewing through the 4–5 portal, which provide a better repositioning of torn intercarpal ligaments in our experience.

28.7 Conclusion

Arthroscopic reduction with percutaneous fixation is a reliable minimally invasive surgical method for acute perilunate injuries in that it provides proper restoration and stable fixation of carpal alignment and results in satisfactory functional and radiological outcomes on a midterm basis.

References

[1] Mayfield JK, Johnson RP, Kilcoyne RK. Carpal dislocations: pathomechanics and progressive perilunar instability. J Hand Surg Am 1980;5(3):226–241

[2] Herzberg G, Comtet JJ, Linscheid RL, Amadio PC, Cooney WP, Stalder J. Perilunate dislocations and fracture-dislocations: a multicenter study. J Hand Surg Am 1993;18(5):768–779

[3] Park MJ. Hand and Upper Extremity Surgery: The Wrist and Elbow. Seoul: Panmun; 2017

[4] Herzberg G, Forissier D. Acute dorsal trans-scaphoid perilunate fracture-dislocations: medium-term results. J Hand Surg [Br] 2002;27(6):498–502

[5] Kozin SH. Perilunate injuries: diagnosis and treatment. J Am Acad Orthop Surg 1998;6(2):114–120

[6] Muppavarapu RC, Capo JT. Perilunate Dislocations and Fracture Dislocations. Hand Clin 2015;31(3):399–408

[7] Adkison JW, Chapman MW. Treatment of acute lunate and perilunate dislocations. Clin Orthop Relat Res 1982(164):199–207

[8] Apergis E, Maris J, Theodoratos G, Pavlakis D, Antoniou N. Perilunate dislocations and fracture-dislocations. Closed and early open reduction compared in 28 cases. Acta Orthop Scand Suppl 1997;275:55–59

[9] Vitale MA, Seetharaman M, Ruchelsman DE. Perilunate dislocations. J Hand Surg Am 2015;40(2):358–362, quiz 362

[10] Sawardeker PJ, Kindt KE, Baratz ME. Fracture-dislocations of the carpus: perilunate injury. Orthop Clin North Am 2013;44(1):93–106

[11] Budoff JE. Treatment of acute lunate and perilunate dislocations. J Hand Surg Am 2008;33(8):1424–1432

[12] Knoll VD, Allan C, Trumble TE. Trans-scaphoid perilunate fracture dislocations: results of screw fixation of the scaphoid and lunotriquetral repair with a dorsal approach. J Hand Surg Am 2005;30(6):1145–1152

[13] Park MJ, Ahn JH. Arthroscopically assisted reduction and percutaneous fixation of dorsal perilunate dislocations and fracture-dislocations. Arthroscopy 2005;21(9):1153

[14] Herzberg G, Burnier M, Marc A, Merlini L, Izem Y. The role of arthroscopy for treatment of perilunate injuries. J Wrist Surg 2015;4(2):101–109

[15] Kim JP, Lee JS, Park MJ. Arthroscopic reduction and percutaneous fixation of perilunate dislocations and fracture-dislocations. Arthroscopy 2012;28(2):196–203.e2

[16] Jeon IH, Kim HJ, Min WK, Cho HS, Kim PT. Arthroscopically assisted percutaneous fixation for trans-scaphoid perilunate fracture dislocation. J Hand Surg Eur Vol 2010;35(8):664–668

[17] Liu B, Chen SL, Zhu J, Wang ZX, Shen J. Arthroscopically assisted mini-invasive management of perilunate dislocations. J Wrist Surg 2015;4(2):93–100

[18] Oh WT, Choi YR, Kang HJ, Koh IH, Lim KH. Comparative Outcome Analysis of Arthroscopic-Assisted Versus Open Reduction and Fixation of Trans-scaphoid Perilunate Fracture Dislocations. Arthroscopy 2017;33(1):92–100

[19] Weil WM, Slade JF III, Trumble TE. Open and arthroscopic treatment of perilunate injuries. Clin Orthop Relat Res 2006;445(445):120–132

[20] Inoue G, Imaeda T. Management of trans-scaphoid perilunate dislocations. Herbert screw fixation, ligamentous repair and early wrist mobilization. Arch Orthop Trauma Surg 1997;116(6–7): 338–340

[21] Slade JF III, Grauer JN, Mahoney JD. Arthroscopic reduction and percutaneous fixation of scaphoid fractures with a novel dorsal technique. Orthop Clin North Am 2001;32(2):247–261

29 Radiocarpal Pain and Stiffness

Christoph Pezzei, Stefan Quadlbauer

Abstract

Pain and stiffness of the wrist present a difficult problem which has significant implications. Several causes account for loss of range of motion (ROM) and pain following trauma to the distal radius and carpus. Extra-articular ones include heterotypic ossification and changes in joint geometry, and the intra-articular ones include malunion, steps in articular surface, carpal injuries, and instability. The method for treating stiffness and pain of the wrist depends on the needs of the individual patient, age, residual wrist mobility, level of physical activity, functional demands, and radiographic changes. Persistent pain is the main reason for dissatisfaction, so reduction should not be compromised to preserve mobility. Conservative treatment options include nonsteroidal antirheumatic drugs, steroid infiltration, splinting of the wrist, and hand therapy. If conservative intervention shows no improvement of ROM or pain, then several surgical treatment options such as wrist denervation, arthroscopic or open arthrolysis, partial wrist arthrodesis (PWA), total wrist arthrodesis (TWA), or wrist arthroplasty (WA) can be considered.

Keywords: distal radius fractures, pain, stiffness, denervation, wrist arthrolysis, RSL-arthrodesis, wrist arthroplasy, total wrist arthrodesis

29.1 Introduction

Pain and stiffness of the wrist presents a difficult problem which has significant implications. Several causes account for loss of range of motion (ROM) and pain following trauma to the distal radius and carpus. These can be classified into extra-articular and intra-articular. Extra-articular ones include heterotypic ossification and changes in joint geometry, and the intra-articular ones include malunion, steps in articular surface, carpal injuries, and instability.[1] This chapter will focus on stiffness and pain after distal radius fracture (DRF). Carpal injuries and instability will be discussed in other chapters of this book.

DRFs are the most common fractures of the upper extremities with an incidence of approximately 190/100.000 per year.[2,3,4] Over the last decades, the trend has moved away from stabilizing DRF with Kirschner wires (K-wires) or external fixator, toward open reduction and internal fixation using volar angular stable locking plates. Dorsally displaced DRF can also be stabilized from volar aspect, which simultaneously reduces the risk of extensor tendon irritation when compared to dorsal plating.[5,6]

Complication rates following surgically treated DRF are low and well-documented in the literature,[7,8] but stiffness of the wrist is seldom mentioned.[9] Early mobilization of the wrist after DRF leads to better functional results and, as reported in the literature, reduces the risk for restricted ROM.[5] As early as 1814, Colles warned his colleagues about prolonged wrist immobilization after DRF that could lead to potential impairment.[10] Nevertheless, some studies have demonstrated that the recovery period in the first 2 months significantly influence the ultimate functional outcome.[11]

Wrist stiffness and pain after surgically treated DRF is often caused by loss of reduction, screw penetration into the radiocarpal joint, or malunion with an intra-articular step-off. Knirk and Jupiter have shown that a step-off greater than 2 mm in the radiocarpal joint has a higher risk for posttraumatic radiographic degenerative arthritis, leading to pain and functional impairment. Young patients are more prone to develop degenerative arthritis if the DRF heals with malalignment in the radiocarpal joint.[12]

Routine daily activities require a ROM of at least 30 to 50 degrees of extension, 5-degree flexion, 10 degrees of radial deviation, and 15 degrees of ulnar deviation.[13,14] The method for treating stiffness and pain of the wrist depends on the needs of the individual patient. Conservative treatment options include nonsteroidal antirheumatic drugs, steroid infiltration, splinting of the wrist, and hand therapy. If conservative intervention shows no improvement of ROM or pain, then several surgical treatment options such as wrist denervation, arthroscopic or open arthrolysis, partial wrist arthrodesis (PWA), total wrist arthrodesis (TWA), or wrist arthroplasty (WA) can be considered.

29.2 Surgical Techniques

29.2.1 Denervation of the Wrist

Denervation of the wrist is an established procedure for treating chronic pain when conservative treatment fails. An advantage of wrist denervation is pain relief without the risk of stiffness. Should neurectomy prove unsuccessful, then alternative treatments options are still possible.

The concept of total wrist joint denervation (TWJD) was first described by Albrecht Wilhelm in 1966[15] and includes five skin incisions to access all ten terminal nerve branches of the wrist. Complete denervation has been considered to be the most effective method to achieve pain relief, while preserving the highest degree of mobility in the wrist. A disadvantage of this technique is the possible loss of skin sensitivity and protective proprioception. The literature describes many modifications of this procedure, but to date no definitive technique has been established. Although TWJD is very popular, partial wrist joint denervation (PWJD) is still performed more frequently.

PWJD was first described by Berger in 1998[16] in a single-incision technique with complete neurectomy of the anterior interosseous nerve (AIN) and the posterior interosseous nerve (PIN). Studies have shown that a neurectomy of the PIN and AIN may influence the proprioception of the wrist.[17] The PIN sends fibers to the central part of the dorsal wrist and is the primary dorsal innervator. The AIN innervates the volar capsule, periosteum, and ligament insertions as shown by Van de Pol et al.[18]

The PIN and AIN are accessed via a 3 to 4 cm longitudinal dorsal incision between radius and ulnar one finger-breath proximal the ulnar head. The PIN is identified after the dissection between the extensor digitorum communis and extensor indicis proprius overlying the interosseous membrane. After longitudinal incision of the interosseous membrane, the AIN is presented. Neurectomy is performed by resecting 2 cm of each nerve.

Weinstein et al[19] described outcomes after PWJD as did Hofmeister et al.[20] Both studies reported pain relief between 50 and 80% and a reduced DASH score. Of note, 85 to 90% of the patients were satisfied with the result. However, the success rate after 28 to 31 months dropped to 68 to 85%.

The diagnostic value of preoperative diagnostic nerve block remains unclear. Many authors describe and discuss a diagnostic nerve block prior to surgery, but the outcome remains controversial. No strong correlations between diagnostic pain relief and severity of postoperative pain can be proved.[16] Two possibilities could explain the differing results in literature. Either the anesthetic injections failed to block the affected nerve or the interosseus branches were missed during surgery.

29.2.2 Wrist Arthrolysis

Both open and arthroscopic wrist arthrolysis is not very frequently documented in the literature. Surgical intervention is indicated if patients present with persistent, disturbing ROM restriction despite a minimum of at least 6 months conservative treatment. Capsular contracture should be the main criteria for restricted ROM, and other reasons such as radiocarpal malalignment should be excluded. The resulting stiffness in the wrist should also be painless in the restricted ROM.

If pronation and supination are affected, then open or arthroscopic arthrolysis of the distal radial ulnar joint (DRUJ) is preferred. Del Piñal et al[21] reported about arthroscopic arthrolysis of the DRUJ in six patients with a posttraumatic loss of supination of at least 90 degrees. Only the adherences between the volar capsule and the ulnar head were released. At the follow-up after 3 years, mean supination was 76 degrees and the mean improvement in supination was 80 degrees. Kleinman and Graham[22] showed in an anatomical and clinical study

that DRUJ capsulectomy can markedly improve forearm rotation.

Kamal and Ruch et al[23] reported the open volar capsular release after DRF in eleven patients and a mean follow-up of 4.5 months. Wrist extension, flexion, and DASH score improved after surgery, but were lower than the minimal clinical difference. Pain according to the visual analogue scale was not affected as a result of the arthrolysis.

Arthroscopic arthrolysis has the advantage of small skin incisions, which lowers the risk of tissue scarring. Verhellen and Bain[24] performed an anatomical study on two patients with posttraumatic wrist stiffness. They found a mean distance of 6.9 mm from the capsule to the median nerve, 6.7 mm to the ulnar nerve, and 5.2 mm to the radial artery. ROM improved in both patients, in extension as well as flexion. Luchetti et al[25] performed an arthroscopic release of the wrist in 22 patients after DRF and reported an increase of ROM from 84 to 99 degrees in extension/flexion. Osterman et al[26] reviewed 54 patients with an arthroscopic release of the wrist and DRUJ, or both. At a mean follow-up of 62 months, ROM in extension and flexion improved from 35 to 41 degrees, but a loss of wrist motion of 30% was noted over time. Hatorri et al[27] retrospectively analyzed 11 patients with posttraumatic wrist contracture and a mean follow-up of 13 months. They found a mean improved ROM in extension by 9 degrees and flexion of 13 degrees. Mean arc of wrist extension/flexion improved significantly from 76 to 98 degrees.

Arthrolysis of the radiocarpal joint is only applicable under specific criteria. Patients should present with no anatomical malalignment and a painless wrist, which is reduced in extension/flexion. Literature suggests an improved ROM, but simultaneously this gain lessens over time. Nevertheless, this ROM improvement should be critically addressed. Does this minimal clinical difference become a recognizable improvement for the patient?

29.2.3 Partial Wrist Arthrodesis

The principle of PWA fuses the painful arthritic components of the joint and shifts the movement axis to an intact component of the joint. This depends on the damaged area of the articular surface, because malunion or cartilage damage after DRF leads to secondary arthritic changes in the radiocarpal joint. The lunate facet is one of the key areas in DRF that is frequently and precociously involved in arthritic changes. The mediocarpal joint is generally not affected.

Radioscapholunate Arthrodesis

Posttraumatic radiocarpal osteoarthritis with radiolunate and radioscaphoid joint involvement can be treated with radioscapholunate (RSL) arthrodesis. It requires an intact mediocarpal joint. Many studies report successful RSL arthrodesis for degenerative joint disease (DJD) in rheumatoid arthritis, but very few exist after malunited DRF.[28,29] RSL arthrodesis is typically carried out using a dorsal approach with different fixation options.

We prefer the volar approach for RSL arthrodesis after operatively treated DRF as most surgeons are familiar with this technique using it in volar plating, and in addition the extensor tendons remain preserved when hardware is inserted. Existing hardware can also be removed without an additional incision.[30] Distal scaphoidectomy (DSE) in RSL arthrodesis was first reported by Garcia-Elias et al in 2001[31] and 2005[32] and resulted in improved pain relief, better flexion, and radial deviation. They also

showed a union rate of 100% of the RSL arthrodesis carried out with additional DSE.[31,32]

Surgical Technique of Volar Radioscapholunate

The volar RSL incision uses the preexisting incision for both hardware removal and RSL arthrodesis. It is extended distally to the radial side, to sufficiently expose the scaphoid. The hardware is removed and a capsulotomy is performed to examine the carpus and subsequently the radiocarpal articulation (▶ Fig. 29.1d). The complete palmar rim of the radius is planed using a chisel (▶ Fig. 29.1e). The distal quarter of the scaphoid is resected (▶ Fig. 29.1f). This unlocks the

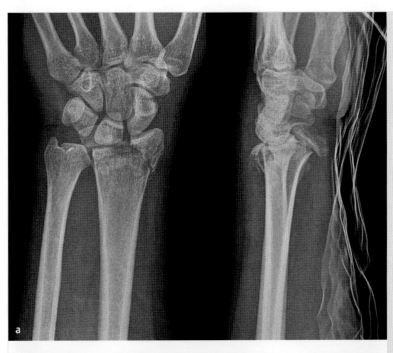

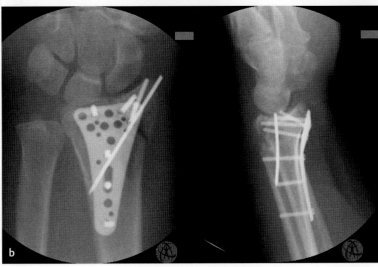

Fig. 29.1 (a) Case example: A 40-year-old man after a fall from 7 m. Multiple fractures in both arms. Preoperative left side view of distal radius fracture (DRF). **(b)** Postoperative view after open reduction and fixation with angle stable plate and additional Kirschner wires (K-wires).

▶ Continued

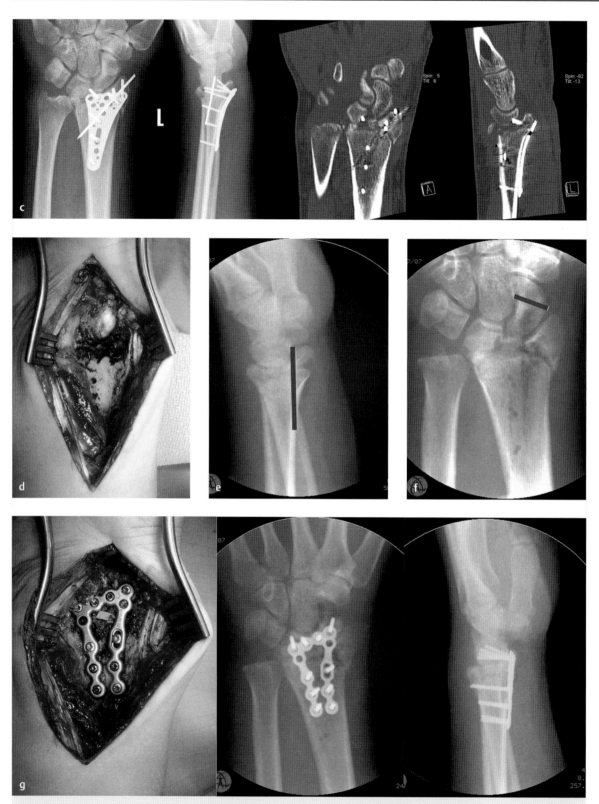

Fig. 29.1 (*Continued*) (c) Loss of reduction and screw penetration into the joint destroying the radiocarpal surface (d) view into the destroyed radiocarpal joint after hardware removal. (e) The complete palmar rim of the radius is planed using a chisel. (f) The distal quarter of the scaphoid is resected to unlock the scaphotrapeziumtrapezoid (STT) joint to improve range of motion and pain relief. (g) Final fixation with a straight polyaxial, 2.5 locking frame plate (APTUS Medartis, Switzerland); 2 screws placed in the lunate and scaphoid, in this case one cortical and one fixed angle screw, each under image intensification and postoperative X-ray control.

(*Continued*)

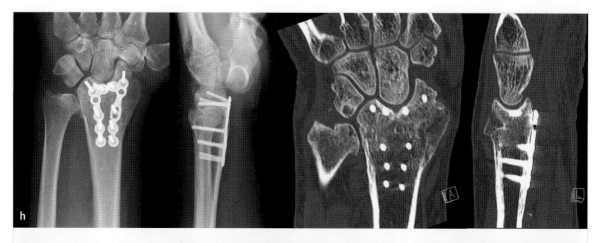

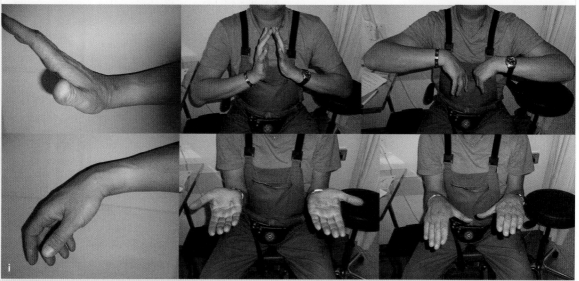

Fig. 29.1 (*Continued*) (**h**) Radiological result after 5 years: complete bony healing, no sign of midcarpal arthritis, exact positioning of the lunate in the lateral view, and ideal screw placement in lunate and scaphoid. (**i**) Functional result after 5 years: visual analogue scale (VAS) is 0.

scaphotrapeziumtrapezoid (STT) joint. Maximal extension of the wrist enhances visualization and exposes the proximal articular surfaces of the scaphoid, lunate, and distal radius. To denude the cartilage surface, we use a rongeur or a burr until cancellous bone is exposed. If the scapholunate ligament is intact and stable, decortication of this area is not necessary. In cases of instability or malalignment between the scaphoid and lunate, the scapholunate area must be denuded and filled with a cancellous bone graft. A K-wire is temporarily inserted to maintain the correct alignment between the scaphoid and lunate. The extracted part of the scaphoid and palmar rim of the radius can be used for the cancellous bone graft. No additional bone harvesting is necessary. The radiocarpal joint is filled with cancellous bone graft. K-wires in the scaphoid and lunate are used as joysticks for correct positioning and then the carpal bones are temporarily fixed to the radius.

For the final fixation, a straight polyaxial, 2.5 locking frame plate (APTUS Medartis, Switzerland) (▶ Fig. 29.1g), is used. The plate must be precisely placed to avoid screw penetration into the midcarpal joint. Fixation to the radius shaft occurs in the long-leg hole using a cortical screw. Two screws are then placed in the lunate and scaphoid under image intensification.

After distal resection of the scaphoid, and in the presence of scapholunate ligament instability, it may be helpful to fix the scaphoid to the plate with an additional cortical screw. The variable angled locking system allows exact screw placement in the carpal bones. Fixation to the shaft is completed using fixed angular stable screws. The K-wires are removed and the cancellous bone graft is compacted into the arthrodesis site.

Postoperative immobilization uses a thermoplastic short-arm orthosis for 5 weeks. After 2 weeks, the orthosis may be removed for hand therapy with active wrist

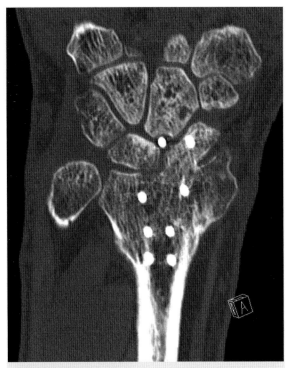

Fig. 29.2 Screw penetration into the midcarpal joint. The plate was placed too far distally.

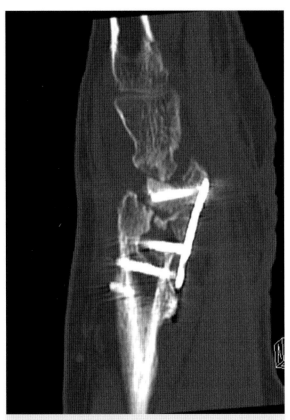

Fig. 29.3 Dorsal intercalated segment instability (DISI) or volar intercalated segment instability (VISI) position of the lunate lead to midcarpal arthritic changes within a short period of time.

and finger motion. Bony fusion of the RSL arthrodesis can be expected approximately 3 months after surgery, after which normal activities may be resumed.

Results of Volar Radioscapholunate

From 2006 to 2014, 14 patients with malunited DRF and DJD limited to the radiocarpal joint underwent volar RSL arthrodesis and DSE. Eleven patients with a mean follow-up of 63 months (range: 30–97 months) were included in the final analysis.

All patients showed union and no midcarpal DJD in the CT scans at the final follow-up. The mean ROM in extension was 53, flexion 42, supination 81, pronation 85, radial deviation 10, and ulnar deviation 25. The ROM in extension, extension/flexion arc, and supination improved significantly after the surgery. Patients achieved a mean of 80% of grip strength compared to the healthy hand.[12]

Pitfalls of Volar Radioscapholunate

It is important that the plate is not placed too distally to avoid screw penetration into the midcarpal joint. The precise use of an image intensifier while inserting the distal screws is essential to avoid this complication (▶ Fig. 29.2).

Dorsal intercalated segment instability or volar intercalated segment instability position of the lunate leads to

secondary arthritic changes in the midcarpal joint associated with pain and may therefore be a precursor for a total wrist fusion (▶ Fig. 29.3).

Tips and Tricks of Volar Radioscapholunate

A plane fixed-angle plate is used to avoid flexor tendon irritation. By means of a chisel, the complete palmar rim of the radius is planed which enables the precise positioning of the plate. The extracted bone is used as the cancellous bone graft (▶ Fig. 29.1e).

The exact placement of the lunate in a neutral position is important to avoid secondary arthritic changes in the midcarpal joint. The K-wire used as a joystick helps to position the lunate correctly (▶ Fig. 29.1h).

Removing the distal pole of the scaphoid unlocks the STT joint and decreases the rate of nonunion.

29.2.4 Wrist Arthroplasty

The first wrist arthroplasty was performed in 1890 by Themistocles Gluck.[33] The implant was made of ivory and used a ball-and-socket design. Total wrist implants have evolved from silicone implants to metacarpal fixation and further to modern designs that maximize bone stock and minimize instability.

Modern implants incorporate porous coating technology for better bone ingrowth. Studies investigated outcomes of modern implants and demonstrated improved pain scores and validated performance measures. The 5-year survival rate was reported up to 97%.[34] As designs are still evolving and new models are emerging, long-term outcomes are still pending.

Patients undergoing wrist arthroplasty with posttraumatic or primary osteoarthritis are often younger and more active than patients with rheumatoid arthritis. Therefore, longevity of the implants and the ability to withstand greater stresses should be considered when performing a wrist arthroplasty in young patients.

Complication rates are still high for total wrist arthroplasty and range from 10 to 21%. Yet, serious complications such as intraoperative fractures at 2% and deep infections at about 1.4% are rare.[34]

The indications for treating young patients with posttraumatic or primary osteoarthritis is still unclear as there is not enough evidence to prove that they will truly benefit, considering their high physical demands.

29.2.5 Total Wrist Arthrodesis

TWA includes fusion of the carpus to the radius witch eliminates wrist motion. It is a well-established procedure to relieve pain in patients with advanced pancarpal degenerative or posttraumatic arthritis.

Mannerfelt and Malmsten[35] were the first to perform internal fixation of TWA in 1971, using a retrograde rush pin from the third metacarpal bone to the distal radius. Rotational stability was ensured by using one or more staples. The technique was improved by some authors and in 1996 Hastings et al[36] were the first to use the Association for Osteosynthesis (AO) /Association compression plate. Their results showed significantly higher union and lower complication rates, when compared to other techniques. The literature documents complications with 29% (19% major and 10% minor complications) and radiocarpal nonunion ranges at about 4.4%.[37]

In a systemic review, Cavaliere and Chung[38] compared TWA with WA and found 100% patient satisfaction, although TWA showed better pain relief, lower complications rates, and less revision rates than WA. Interestingly, only 3 out of 14 studies that dealt with the outcome of ROM in WA determined a return to a functional arc of motion. They concluded that WA should only be recommended until TWA produces superior results.

Including the carpometacarpal (CMC) joint into the fusion mass to obtain rigid fixation remains controversial. Hardware-related complications are well-reported in the literature. Micromotion at the CMC joint leads to hardware failure with screw loosening or breakage. Painful CMC nonunion after spanning plate arthrodesis has been reported to up to 43%.[39] Today's newer plates exclude the metacarpal bone fixation in the wrist arthrodesis thus preventing the metacarpal joint stiffening.

29.3 Conclusion

The etiology and various stages of posttraumatic DJD allow certain therapeutic options, but several factors determine the final procedure. These include age of patient, residual wrist mobility, level of physical activity, functional demands, and radiographic changes.

Complete denervation can be recommended to patients with sufficient residual mobility of the wrist because of the low morbidity rate. Further procedures are still possible, even if wrist denervation should prove unsuccessful.

PWA, such as RSL arthrodesis, is applicable if osteoarthritis is limited to the radiocarpal joint and the mediocarpal joint remains unaffected. Biomechanical studies have shown improved ROM when the distal pole of the scaphoid is resected. Clinical studies have only shown a significantly better ROM in radial deviation, but higher union rates with unlocking the STT joint[40] and pain relief.[32] Surgery after DRF in posttraumatic radiocarpal arthritis, using a palmar approach and additional scaphoidectomy showed a significantly improved ROM in extension, extension/flexion, and supination. Nevertheless, volar locking plating showed union in all treated patients.

Total wrist fusion is usually recommended in young patients who perform heavy manual labor, especially if ROM of the wrist is very restricted and all other reconstructive procedures are inadequate. The complication rates are low compared to wrist arthroplasty.

Only few studies reported a recovery of ROM higher than the functional ROM for wrist arthroplasty. Particularly in young patients the longevity and load bearing of the implants should be considered when planning the intervention. New implants for wrist arthroplasty are emerging on the market, but to date insufficient data are available to make any conclusive statements regarding the longevity of the implants. Even though recent studies show promising results, the long-term experience is pending and requires further research.

References

[1] Bergman J, Bain G. Arthroscopic release of wrist contracture. In: Slutsky DJ, Osterman AL, eds. Fractures and Injuries of the Distal Radius and Carpus. Philadelphia, PA: W.B. Saunders; 2009:501–506

[2] Bonafede M, Espindle D, Bower AG. The direct and indirect costs of long bone fractures in a working age US population. J Med Econ 2013;16(1):169–178

[3] Bässgen K, Westphal T, Haar P, Kundt G, Mittlmeier T, Schober HC. Population-based prospective study on the incidence of osteoporosis-associated fractures in a German population of 200,413 inhabitants. J Public Health (Oxf) 2013;35(2):255–261

[4] Court-Brown CM, Caesar B. Epidemiology of adult fractures: a review. Injury 2006;37(8):691–697

[5] Quadlbauer S, Pezzei C, Jurkowitsch J, et al. Early rehabilitation of distal radius fractures stabilized by volar locking plate: a prospective randomized pilot study. J Wrist Surg 2017;6(2):102–112

[6] Quadlbauer S, Pezzei C, Jurkowitsch J, Keuchel T, Hausner T, Leixnering M. Spontaneous radioscapholunate fusion after septic

arthritis of the wrist: a case report. Arch Orthop Trauma Surg 2017;137(4):579–584

[7] Johnson NA, Cutler L, Dias JJ, Ullah AS, Wildin CJ, Bhowal B. Complications after volar locking plate fixation of distal radius fractures. Injury 2014;45(3):528–533

[8] Figl M, Weninger P, Liska M, Hofbauer M, Leixnering M. Volar fixed-angle plate osteosynthesis of unstable distal radius fractures: 12 months results. Arch Orthop Trauma Surg 2009; 129(5):661–669

[9] Yu YR, Makhni MC, Tabrizi S, Rozental TD, Mundanthanam G, Day CS. Complications of low-profile dorsal versus volar locking plates in the distal radius: a comparative study. J Hand Surg Am 2011;36(7):1135–1141

[10] Colles A. The classic. On the fracture of the carpal extremity of the radius. Abraham Colles, Edinburgh Med. Surg. J., 1814. Clin Orthop Relat Res 1972;83(83):3–5

[11] MacDermid JC, Roth JH, Richards RS. Pain and disability reported in the year following a distal radius fracture: a cohort study. BMC Musculoskelet Disord 2003;4:24

[12] Quadlbauer S, Leixnering M, Jurkowitsch J, Hausner T, Pezzei C. Volar radioscapholunate arthrodesis and distal scaphoidectomy after malunited distal radius fractures. J Hand Surg Am 2017;42(9): 754.e1–754.e8

[13] Brigstocke G, Hearnden A, Holt CA, Whatling G. The functional range of movement of the human wrist. J Hand Surg Eur Vol 2013;38(5):554–556

[14] Palmer AK, Werner FW, Murphy D, Glisson R. Functional wrist motion: a biomechanical study. J Hand Surg Am 1985;10(1):39–46

[15] Wilhelm A. Denervation of the wrist. Tech Hand Up Extrem Surg 2001;5(1):14–30

[16] Berger RA. Partial denervation of the wrist: a new approach. Tech Hand Up Extrem Surg 1998;2(1):25–35

[17] Burke D, Gandevia SC, Macefield G. Responses to passive movement of receptors in joint, skin and muscle of the human hand. J Physiol 1988;402(1):347–361

[18] Van de Pol GJ, Koudstaal MJ, Schuurman AH, Bleys RLAW. Innervation of the wrist joint and surgical perspectives of denervation. J Hand Surg Am 2006;31(1):28–34

[19] Weinstein LP, Berger RA. Analgesic benefit, functional outcome, and patient satisfaction after partial wrist denervation. J Hand Surg Am 2002;27(5):833–839

[20] Hofmeister EP, Moran SL, Shin AY. Anterior and posterior interosseous neurectomy for the treatment of chronic dynamic instability of the wrist. Hand (N Y) 2006;1(2):63–70

[21] Del Piñal F, Moraleda E, Rúas JS, Rodriguez-Vega A, Studer A. Effectiveness of an arthroscopic technique to correct supination losses of 90° or more. J Hand Surg Am 2018;43(7):676.e1–676.e6

[22] Kleinman WB, Graham TJ. The distal radioulnar joint capsule: clinical anatomy and role in posttraumatic limitation of forearm rotation. J Hand Surg Am 1998;23(4):588–599

[23] Kamal RN, Ruch DS. Volar Capsular Release After Distal Radius Fractures. J Hand Surg Am 2017;42(12):1034.e1–1034.e6

[24] Verhellen R, Bain GI. Arthroscopic capsular release for contracture of the wrist: a new technique. Arthroscopy 2000;16(1):106–110

[25] Luchetti R, Atzei A, Fairplay T. Arthroscopic wrist arthrolysis after wrist fracture. Arthroscopy 2007;23(3):255–260

[26] Osterman AL, Culp RW, Osterman MN. Arthroscopic release of wrist contractures. Plast Reconstr Surg 2010;126

[27] Hattori T, Tsunoda K, Watanabe K, Nakao E, Hirata H, Nakamura R. Arthroscopic mobilization for contracture of the wrist. Arthroscopy 2006;22(8):850–854

[28] Sturzenegger M, Büchler U. Radio-scapho-lunate partial wrist arthrodesis following comminuted fractures of the distal radius. Ann Chir Main Memb Super 1991;10(3):207–216

[29] Inoue G, Tamura Y. Radiolunate and radioscapholunate arthrodesis. Arch Orthop Trauma Surg 1992;111(6):333–335

[30] Argintar E, Edwards S. Volar radioscapholunate arthrodesis for malunited distal radius fracture with unsalvageable wrist articular degeneration: case report. J Hand Surg Am 2010;35(7):1089–1092

[31] Garcia-Elías M, Lluch A. Partial excision of scaphoid: is it ever indicated? Hand Clin 2001;17(4):687–695, x

[32] Garcia-Elias M, Lluch A, Ferreres A, Papini-Zorli I, Rahimtoola ZO. Treatment of radiocarpal degenerative osteoarthritis by radioscapholunate arthrodesis and distal scaphoidectomy. J Hand Surg Am 2005;30(1):8–15

[33] Ritt MJ, Stuart PR, Naggar L, Beckenbaugh RD. The early history of arthroplasty of the wrist. From amputation to total wrist implant. J Hand Surg [Br] 1994;19(6):778–782

[34] Halim A, Weiss AC. Total Wrist Arthroplasty. J Hand Surg Am 2017;42(3):198–209

[35] Mannerfelt L, Malmsten M. Arthrodesis of the wrist in rheumatoid arthritis. A technique without external fixation. Scand J Plast Reconstr Surg 1971;5(2):124–130

[36] Hastings H II, Weiss AP, Quenzer D, Wiedeman GP, Hanington KR, Strickland JW. Arthrodesis of the wrist for post-traumatic disorders. J Bone Joint Surg Am 1996;78(6):897–902

[37] Wei DH, Feldon P. Total wrist arthrodesis: indications and clinical outcomes. J Am Acad Orthop Surg 2017;25(1):3–11

[38] Cavaliere CM, Chung KC. A systematic review of total wrist arthroplasty compared with total wrist arthrodesis for rheumatoid arthritis. Plast Reconstr Surg 2008;122(3):813–825

[39] Nagy L, Büchler U. AO-wrist arthrodesis: with and without arthrodesis of the third carpometacarpal joint. J Hand Surg Am 2002;27(6):940–947

[40] Mühldorfer-Fodor M, Ha HP, Hohendorff B, Löw S, Prommersberger KJ, van Schoonhoven J. Results after radioscapholunate arthrodesis with or without resection of the distal scaphoid pole. J Hand Surg Am 2012;37(11):2233–2239

30 Ulnar Pain and Pronosupination Losses

Riccardo Luchetti, Andrea Atzei

Abstract

Posttraumatic painful limitation of pronosupination of the wrist is frequently secondary to wrist sprain or fracture. Persistent rigidity of distal radioulnar joint (DRUJ), due to capsular contracture and/or joint adherences, may be treated by arthroscopic or open release. Particular attention is paid in the description of both the procedures. More complex conditions are related to both distal radius and ulna malunion in which a correction osteotomy is needed; ulna head conflict in which a wafer resection is suggested; ulna subluxation or dislocation in which ulna relocation is mandatory; extensor digiti minimi (EDM) tendon DRUJ interposition in which the tendon should be repositioned; malpositioned screw into the DRUJ in which the screw removing restore the pronosupination. Finally, ulna head and/or sigmoid notch chondropathy or osteochondropathy are situations in which salvage procedures are requested.

Keywords: wrist rigidity, pronosupination loss, pronosupination stiffness, arthroscopic wrist arthrolysis, open wrist arthrolysis, DRUJ rigidity, DRUJ stiffness, DRUJ release, DRUJ arthrolysis

30.1 Introduction

Painful limitations of pronosupination are frequently seen after distal radius fracture (DRF), of both intra- and extra-articular type.[1,2,3,4] Associated fractures of ulna and ulnar styloid may be another cause of limited pronosupination.

Primary goal of any DRF treatment, either conservative or surgical, is to obtain healing of the fracture with good final functional recovery.

However, when treatment requires prolonged immobilization, it may yield to capsule contracture and articular adherences, causing wrist stiffness (►Fig. 30.1 and ►Fig. 30.2).

Frequently, wrist stiffness can be improved by an adequate rehabilitation treatment. However, cases in which the limitation of pronosupination persists after rehabilitation must be treated surgically.[2,5,6,7,8,9]

When pain is also present, it may recognize several causes, mostly, but not exclusively, joint damage, thus it requires a thorough investigation before any treatment.

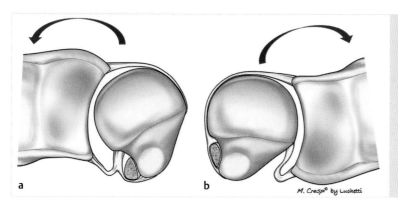

Fig. 30.1 Normal motion of the distal radioulnar joint (DRUJ): **(a)** supination, **(b)** pronation. Note the behavior of the palmar and the dorsal capsule.

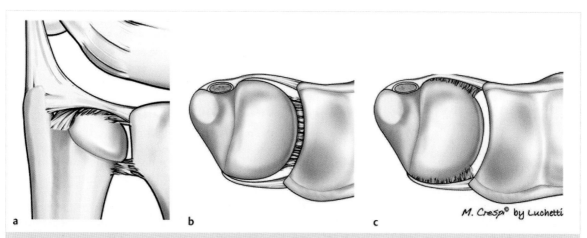

Fig. 30.2 Adherences of the distal radioulnar joint (DRUJ): **(a)** sagittal view of the DRUJ with adherence between the triangular fibrocartilage complex and the ulnar head and between the neck of the ulna and the radius; **(b)** axial view of the DRUJ showing the adherence between the neck of the ulna and the radius; **(c)** axial view showing the adherences between palmar and dorsal capsule and the ulna head.

30.2 Indication

Wrist stiffness is a common finding after either conservative or surgical treatment of DRF and is usually managed by standard physical rehabilitation program.

Surgical arthrolysis is indicated when rehabilitation fails to restore or improve pronosupination. Typical indication is the capsular contracture due to prolonged immobilization for extra-articular or intra-articular DRF that occurs in a congruent distal radioulnar joint (DRUJ).

However, rigidity of the DRUJ may develop even after proper closed fracture reduction and cast immobilization, due to contracture of the volar and dorsal capsule (▶Fig. 30.2).

When pain is present, a more accurate evaluation of the wrist condition before surgery is suggested as to investigate presence of associated damage of cartilage or ligaments, especially of the triangular fibrocartilage complex (TFCC).

Concomitant joint or ligament damage should not be treated at the same time of arthrolysis because of different rehabilitation protocols.

If DRUJ stiffness is associated with a loss of DRUJ congruence, due to a damage of either the articular surface of the ulna head or the sigmoid notch, it is not good candidate for arthrolysis. In the latter cases, arthrolysis should be performed after joint reconstruction.

30.3 Diagnostic Imaging

Diagnostic imaging is essential to understand the causes of rigidity. Appropriate investigation may include various assessments from simple radiography to magnetic resonance imaging (MRI).

30.3.1 Radiography

Radiographic images of the injury are fundamental to define original fracture line and its possible orientation toward the DRUJ and its consequent involvement. Radiographic comparison with the healthy wrist should be performed in order to consider the following parameters: (1) shape and inclination of the DRUJ; (2) ulna variation; (3) posttraumatic changes of both the ulna head and the sigmoid notch; (4) position of the ulna relative to the radius in the lateral view.

30.3.2 CT Scan

The computed tomography (CT) scan allows to obtain further details on the anatomical profile of the radius and the ulna and on their relationships. Seldom, it must be performed bilaterally, for comparison. CT scan may also be performed in neutral position, maximum supination and pronation, in order to confirm the degree of pronosupination loss and mostly to reveal any bone conflicts, subluxations or dislocations of DRUJ.

30.3.3 Magnetic Resonance Imaging

MRI is useful for the evaluation of the ligament lesions and degree of bone and cartilage involvement. It is particularly indicated in case of persistent posttraumatic pain: as it may show areas of bone marrow edema or osteochondral damage of the ulna head, the ulnar styloid and/or the carpal bones, or residual signs of both the distal radius and ulnar head fractures. However, MRI accuracy in the assessment of chondral lesion is rather low. Also, it does not show any capsular contractures or if there are articular adhesions that may cause DRUJ stiffness.

30.3.4 Arthrography, ArthroCT, and ArthroMRI

Arthrography[10] is an examination that is no longer performed except in association with CT scan and MRI. The value of this test in wrist stiffness is to confirm the adhesive capsulitis and arthrofibrosis, as only a little amount of contrast medium can be introduced into the joint. In normal subjects, the wrist may be injected with 2 to 3 cc of liquid. When the joint is affected by arthrofibrosis or adhesive capsulitis, injection is rather difficult and the volume of liquid is drastically reduced to less than 1 cc, which is also frequently dispersed into the surrounding soft tissues. Noticeably, arthroCT and arthroMRI have less significance and clarity to show associated osteoarticular disorders as compared to patients without arthrofibrosis or adhesive capsulitis.

30.4 Surgical Options

Surgical arthrolysis of pronosupination loss consists of releasing capsular contracture and intra-articular adherences of the DRUJ: it can be performed either by an open approach[4,11,12] or by arthroscopic procedure.[2,5,6,13,14,15]

30.4.1 Open Arthrolysis

Appropriate forearm positioning is the key. Vertical position is recommended in order to allow unrestricted control of forearm rotation. Use of a simple traction tower, as from wrist or shoulder arthroscopy, may be beneficial.[7]

The DRUJ is approached through a dorsal access (▶Fig. 30.3). The dorsal capsule is reached through the fifth dorsal compartment. Incision of the capsule starts at the level of the ulnar neck up to just proximal to the dorsal DRUJ ligament, taking care to preserve it. A freer periosteal elevator is introduced through this approach and the adherences at the level of the neck are released. The maneuver is continued just proximal to the ulnar head, permitting the resection of fibrotic bands between the ulna head and the TFCC (▶Fig. 30.4). The release is continued dorsally up to the extensor carpi ulnaris (ECU) tendon sheath to separate the capsule from the ulna head (▶Fig. 30.4). Gentle forearm rotation is performed to stretch

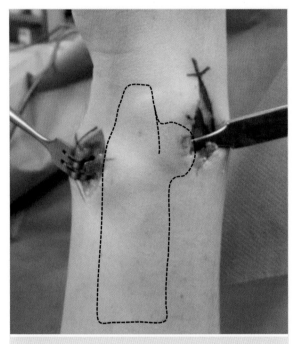

Fig. 30.3 Open arthrolysis of the distal radioulnar joint (DRUJ) using a dorsal and palmar skin incision: the periosteal elevator pass forms dorsal to palmar through the DRUJ. Ulna is designed on the skin to show the relationship between the periosteal elevator and the ulna head.

remaining adherences and evaluate the amount of motion obtained.

Sharp resection may be repeated as necessary, until complete pronation is reached. If supination is still limited, a second step of surgery is performed. From the same dorsal access, the periosteal elevator is driven under the ulnar neck more palmarly (▶Fig. 30.4) to detach the anterior capsule from the ulnar head. Some lateral sliding maneuvers around the shape of the ulnar head will improve supination (▶Fig. 30.5a–d).

Actually, this is a blind maneuver performed with the tip of the elevator. It frequently detaches part of the capsule from the radius, producing the same effect as the actual release of the capsular adherences.

The detachment of the palmar capsule produces an improvement in supination, and the detachment of the posterior capsule improves the pronation.

When the supination loss persists after capsular release, the attention should be addressed to an ischemic retraction of the pronator quadratus muscle.[12] Then, a 3-cm ulnar skin incision is made at the level of the ulnar neck (▶Fig. 30.6), the pronator quadratus muscle insertion is identified and the muscle fibers are detached from the ulna (preserving the deep insertion on the radial border of the ulna). Thus, a further improvement of the supination should be obtained without provoking DRUJ instability.

30.4.2 Arthroscopic Arthrolysis

Standard vertical position with elbow counter-traction of about 3 kg is used for proper joint distraction. Finger traps are applied to the index and middle finger to permit a more physiologic joint alignment. Arthroscopy is performed dry in all cases,[16,17] flushing the joint with saline to remove debris, if necessary.[16,17,18,19]

Arthroscopy always starts from the radiocarpal joint through the 3–4 and 6R portals.[7] Often, the radiocarpal space shows some capsular contracture, therefore radiocarpal arthrolysis is performed as needed.

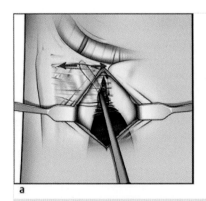
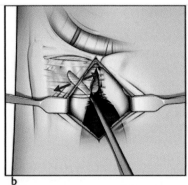
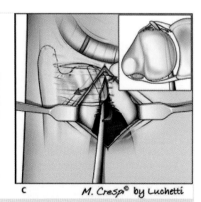

a   b   c   M. Cresp® by Luchetti

Fig. 30.4 Technique of the adherences resection by open arthrolysis using the periosteal elevator. **(a)** resection of the adherences between the triangular fibrocartilage complex (TFCC) and the ulna head; **(b)** resection of the adherences between the dorsal capsule and the ulna head; **(c)** resection of the palmar adherences between the ulna head and the palmar capsule. Note the resection of the dorsal capsule preserving the dorsal branch of the TFCC.

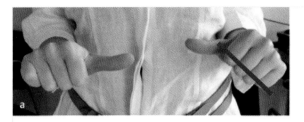
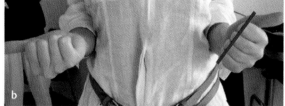
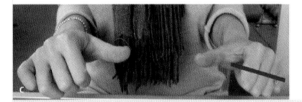
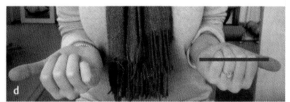

Fig. 30.5 Pronation **(a)** and supination **(b)** loss in patient with distal radius fracture treated with volar plate. Pronation **(c)** and supination **(d)** recovered after volar plate removing and open arthrolysis.

Depending on the integrity of the TFCC, arthroscopic treatment may be performed in three different modalities which are as follows:

1. When the central disc of the TFCC is intact, DRUJ arthrolysis is required by DRUJ arthroscopy (▶ Fig. 30.7). Arthroscopy of the fibrotic DRUJ is even more difficult than in standard cases, as the joint space is almost completely occupied by adherences and synovial tissue, and joint visualization is very poor. Therefore, after the DRUJ portal is placed and proper intra-articular location is confirmed with scope, a periosteal elevator is introduced into the DRUJ portal to create some working space by resecting the adherences between the TFCC and the ulna head with a gentle blind maneuver.[7] Then the scope is introduced again in the DRUJ portal and both the ulna head and the proximal part of the TFCC are explored (▶ Fig. 30.8a, b). In addition, a proximal DRUJ portal may be created at the level of the ulnar neck to introduce a periosteal elevator and resect any adherences within the sigmoid notch (▶ Fig. 30.9b). A volar DRUJ portal may be created using an in-out technique, a periosteal elevator is introduced to release the anterior capsule (▶ Fig. 30.9a). Then the scope may be shifted to detach the lateral capsule from the ulna head up to the ECU tendon sheath and complete the arthrolysis. Often, the scope can only see the tip of the periosteal elevator as some other blind maneuvers are required (▶ Fig. 30.9). Particularly when the periosteal elevator is driven proximally to achieve a complete release, attention must be given to protect the ulnar neurovascular structures palmarly (▶ Fig. 30.9c) and the ECU tendon dorsally. The patient undergoes immediate and prolonged rehabilitation.

2. As an alternative option, still in case of intact TFCC, DRUJ arthrolysis may be performed with the scope in the radiocarpal joint.[20] The freer elevator, positioned in the 6U or 4–5 portal, is introduced into the DRUJ through a small opening in the central disc close to the volar and the dorsal branches of the DRU ligament. Moving the periosteal elevator around the ulnar head, although in a blind fashion, allows detachment or stretching of the volar and the dorsal capsule thus restoring motion of the DRUJ (▶ Fig. 30.10a–f). Sometimes, the central disc can be resected intentionally to facilitate the procedure.

3. When the central disc of the TFCC is lacerated, the arthroscopic approach becomes much easier. Sometimes, the central disc can be resected intentionally to facilitate the procedure. Although a dorsal DRUJ portal may be useful to work under the TFCC and in the volar and dorsal capsular recesses, the whole procedure can be completed with the scope in the 3–4 portal (or rarely in the 6U portal). The adherences between the volar and the dorsal capsule and the ulna head are resected with the periosteal elevator introduced into the 6U and/or 6R portal (▶ Fig. 30.11).

Management of associated joint damages is more complex. Decision-making depends on the location and extension of the chondropathy. In case of minimal joint damage limited to the periphery of the ulnar head or the edge of the sigmoid notch, DRUJ arthrolysis is still indicated. On the other hand, gross chondral damage should be treated with secondary reconstruction or salvage procedures, and it requires explicit and informed consent by the patient (see Chapter 30.8).

30.5 Results

Two groups of patients were considered. The first group was treated by open DRUJ arthrolysis. All of them underwent DRUJ dorsal and volar release as previously

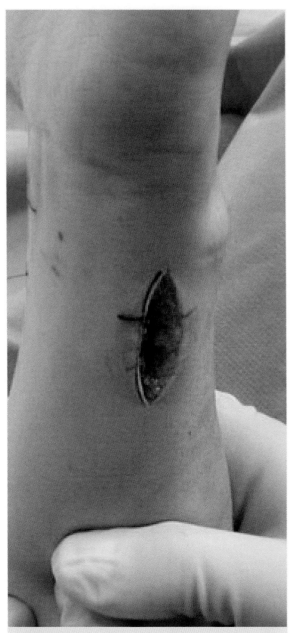

Fig. 30.6 Palmar approach to the pronator quadratus muscle release.

dislocation, ulna head fracture isolated or associated with DRF.

Preoperative pain was always present, mostly under load. No activity was possible for the patients, specifically for those tasks requiring full supination.

In both groups, diagnostic X-ray imaging was performed to assess the damage of the wrist in which the distal radius was frequently affected by fractures healing or malunion or, very rarely, nothing because it was a simple wrist sprain treated by cast immobilization.

MRI showed involvement of several ligaments and especially TFCC that resulted damage almost constantly. However, even when an obvious foveal detachment of the TFCC was evident as MRI showed a foveal detachment of the TFCC, capsular contracture prevented clinical maneuvers to demonstrate DRUJ instability. CT scan was done in a few cases to assess: (1) ulnar head position relative to distal radius; (2) ulnar styloid nonunion; (3) fracture healing; and (4) the malunion of the distal radius.

Arthroscopy of the ulnocarpal compartment showed: (1) fibrotic bands in the ulnocarpal joint between the ulnar border of the radius and the lunotriquetral ligament or lunate bone depending on the type of original damage; (2) osteochondral lesions and articular step-offs were seen on the articular surface of the radius and carpal bones. The latter correlated with residual pain after surgery, giving reason of the worst results in these cases. A hypertrophic dorsal border of the distal radius was resected to improve wrist extension in two cases.

All cases in group 1 were evaluated at 1 to 3 months. No complications were documented. One case failed for obvious joint degeneration due to pre-existing arthritis and was lost at follow-up. Mean improvement of the pronosupination ranged from 112 to 145 degrees. Few cases had improvement in the supination from 0 to 80 degrees. Only one case reached complete supination.

All cases in group 2 were re-evaluated clinically at a mean follow-up of 32 months (range 2–140 months). No complications were documented. One case failed due to wrong indications; one patient expired.

In all the 19 cases, pain was significantly diminished or completely absent and both wrist range of motion (ROM) and grip strength were improved at follow-up.

30.6 Contraindications

DRUJ arthrolysis is not indicated in presence of obvious arthritic joint changes. Combined osteochondritis of the ulna head of the sigmoid notch do not benefit from the arthrolysis (▶ Fig. 30.12). Distal radius malunion that involves the sigmoid notch should be treated by correction osteotomy. Dorsal subluxation of the ulna head must be reduced first, then there should be an adequate period of rehabilitation before arthrolysis. Theoretically, DRUJ reduction and arthrolysis might be performed

described. In the cases where the distal radius volar plate needed removal, the volar approach to the DRUJ was the same as for the plate removal. The volar capsule of the DRUJ was released after plate removal.

The second group was treated by arthroscopic DRUJ arthrolysis. Most of the patients were affected by rigidity of both radiocarpal joint and DRUJ. Overall, the most common scenario was represented by the combined loss of supination and flexion. When isolated DRUJ rigidity was present, supination loss was the most frequent limitation. Causes of rigidity were cast immobilization for DRF, TFCC open and arthroscopic repair of DRUJ

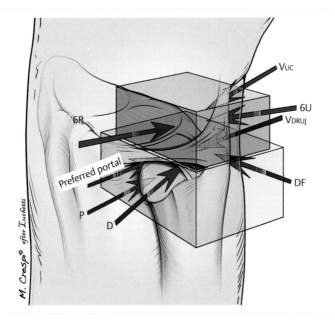

Fig. 30.7 Box theory for arthroscopic approach to the ulnocarpal joint (*red box*) and distal radioulnar joint (DRUJ) (*blue box*). Portals of the ulnocarpal joint (*red arrows*) and DRUJ portals (*blue arrows*).

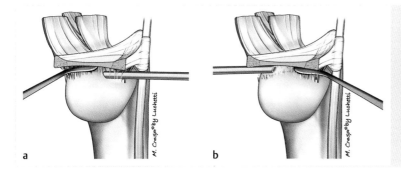

Fig. 30.8 Arthroscopic adherences resection of the distal radioulnar joint. **(a)** Resection of the adherences between the ulna head and triangular fibrocartilage complex (TFCC): scope in dorsal portal and periosteal elevator in the palmar portal; **(b)** scope in palmar portal and dissector in the dorsal portal. Attention should be payed not to damage the foveal insertion of the TFCC.

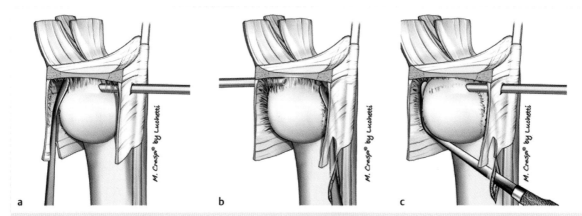

Fig. 30.9 Drawings showing the adherences resection around the ulna head. **(a)** Resection of the palmar adherences between the ulna head and the palmar capsule using the scope in dorsal distal radioulnar joint (DRUJ) and periosteal elevator through a palmar access (palmar DRUJ portal); **(b)** resection of the dorsal adherences between the ulna head and dorsal capsule using the scope in palmar DRUJ portal and periosteal elevator in dorsal DRUJ portal; **(c)** alternative palmar adherences resection through a dorsal portal using a more curved periosteal elevator and scope in dorsal DRUJ portal.

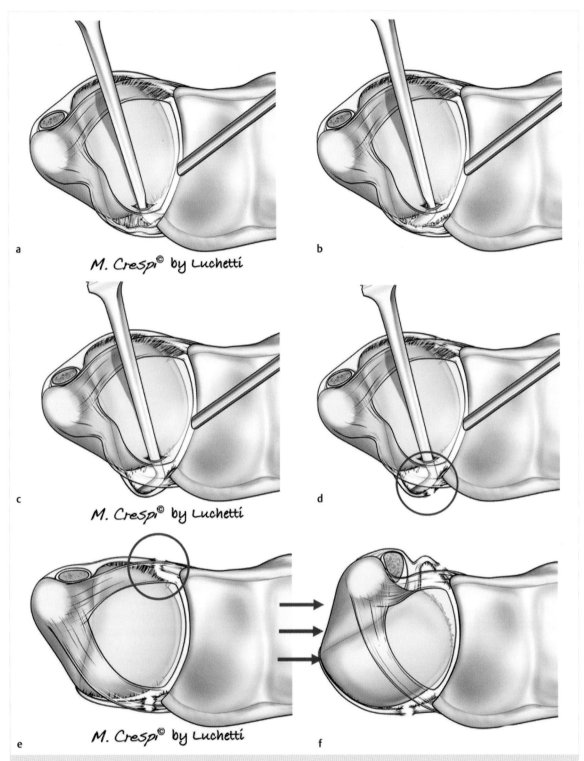

a *M. Crespi© by Luchetti*

b

c *M. Crespi© by Luchetti*

d

e *M. Crespi© by Luchetti*

f

Fig. 30.10 Drawing showing resection of the distal radioulnar joint (DRUJ) adherences maintaining the scope and elevator in the radiocarpal and ulnocarpal joints (according to del Piñal[20]). Scope in 3–4 portal and periosteal elevator in 6R portal. Periosteal is introduced into the anterior part of the DRUJ through a mini incision close to the palmar branch of the triangular fibrocartilage complex. The adherences are resected with gentle maneuvers of motion of periosteal tip **(a, b)** detaching the capsule from the ulna head. Pull maneuver **(c)** of the capsular by periosteal tip determines rupture of the capsule **(d)** close to the border of the radius palmar medial border (*red circle*). Same maneuver is carried out for the palmar capsule **(e, f)** with capsule adherence resection and capsular tear close to the radius dorsal medial border (*blue circle*).

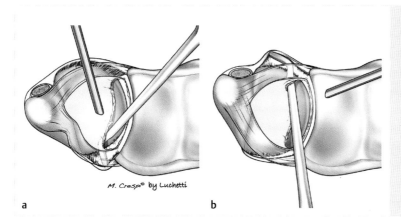

Fig. 30.11 Drawing showing dorsal **(a)** and palmar **(b)** capsular adherences resection through a central triangular fibrocartilage complex pre-existing lesion.

a   b

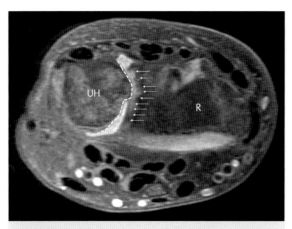

Fig. 30.12 Magnetic resonance axial imaging of ulnar head (*white dotted line*) and sigmoid notch (*white arrows*) posttraumatic deformity causing painful loss of pronosupination. R, radius; UH, ulnar head.

Table 30.1 Preferred technique according to the pathological condition

Pathology	First choice	Second choice
Isolated DRUJ rigidity	Arthroscopic arthrolysis	Open arthrolysis
Complex DRUJ rigidity		
• Distal radius volar plate to be removed	Open arthrolysis	
• Distal radius volar plate not to be removed	Arthroscopic arthrolysis	Open arthrolysis
• Distal radius malunion to be corrected	Open arthrolysis	Arthroscopic arthrolysis
• Ulna dorsal subluxation	Relocation with open arthrolysis	

Abbreviation: DRUJ, distal radioulnar joint.
Note: The abovementioned suggestions are valid for expert arthroscopists. Novice arthroscopists are recommended to consider the open technique.

simultaneously, but immobilization required after joint reduction is very likely to cause a recurrence of capsular contracture and/or adherences formation and consequent recurrence of injury.

Associated peripheral tear of the TFCC is another contraindication to arthrolysis. TFCC repair should be performed after arthrolysis, but it requires postoperative immobilization and thus it may cause recurrence of rigidity.

In summary, any associated surgery that does not allow immediate postoperative mobilization is a real contraindication for the arthrolysis.

Tips and Tricks

To obtain a correct indication and treatment, some suggestions are presented in the ▶ Table 30.1 and ▶ Table 30.2.

30.7 Conclusion

Recent improvements in the arthroscopic field have made it possible to treat wrist stiffness, including DRUJ, in a much less aggressive manner than the open technique, with improved functional results by reducing soft-tissue damage and joint exposure. Recently, the minimal surgical approaches used by open technique in this anatomical area have achieved results similar to the arthroscopic technique. Therefore, the minimal invasive open technique is closing the gap between arthroscopy. Moreover, in case of removal of the distal radius volar plates, the volar part of the DRUJ can be reached through the same surgical access to the radius, thus reducing the need for additional incisions.

The arthroscopic approach to the stiff DRUJ requires considerable experience as this joint is already difficult to manage in anatomically normal situations. Beyond specific instruments such as the 1.9-mm arthroscope, which are extremely delicate, the periosteal elevator is the element with which it is possible to perform the arthrolysis of this joint. In straight or curved shape, it is inserted in the appropriate access and with gentle maneuvers it is possible to detach the adhesions and the fibrotic bands, and resect the volar and dorsal capsule contracture and the TFCC from the head of the ulna

Table 30.2 Open and arthroscopic surgical technique: step by step procedures

- **Open DRUJ Arthrolysis:** Dorsal approach first:

  – Release of adherences between ulna neck and radius using a small periosteal elevator.

  – Release adherences between TFCC and ulna head.

  – Detach dorsal capsule increasing the pronation (protect the ECU tendon).

  – Release the volar capsule producing a sufficient supination of the DRUJ. Insufficient supination: volar approach by in-out technique.

  – Release the volar capsule paying attention not to damage the neurovascular bundle.

  – Release the pronator quadratus muscle if needed.

- **Arthroscopic DRUJ Arthrolysis**

  – 3–4 portal scope, 6R portal instruments.

  – If TFCC is intact, two choice are available: continue with radiocarpal arthroscopy passing through the TFCC (two small holes close to the volar and dorsal branches of the TFCC)[20] or proceed with DRUJ arthroscopy. The second procedure considers DRUJ arthroscopy with the scope in dorsal portal, instrument in volar portal.[7] Release the adherences between TFCC and ulna head first, then release the volar capsule with periosteal elevator from the volar side. The procedure is inverted with scope in volar portal and instrument in dorsal portal: with the periosteal elevator the dorsal capsule is detached. At the end the pronosupination is tested.

  – If TFCC has a central lesion, the scope is introduced in 3–4 portal and instrument in 6R: through the TFCC central lesion the elevator is pushed in the volar side under the volar branch of the TFCC detaching the volar capsule; using the volar portal between the volar ulnocarpal ligaments, the periosteal elevator will be introduced under the dorsal branch of the TFCC detaching the dorsal capsule with gentle maneuver of supination and pronation (the scope should be turned 90° back). At the end, the pronosupination is tested.

Abbreviations: DRUJ, distal radioulnar joint; ECU, extensor carpi ulnaris; TFCC, triangular fibrocartilage complex.

obtaining a valid improvement of the motility of the DRUJ. Various authors have demonstrated this technique to solve the rigidity of DRUJ. Pederzini et al[2] showed that the intraoperative improvement of the DRUJ ROM was maintained postoperatively. On the contrary, radiocarpal arthrolysis has different outcome: the intraoperative radiocarpal joint ROM showed a decrease in the immediate postoperative period and recovered only after adequate rehabilitation. Other authors have published their experience, but only few of them reported their experience on DRUJ arthrolysis.[7] Recently, del Piñal et al[20] described outstanding results with arthroscopic DRUJ arthrolysis using a rib periosteal elevator introduced through a normal TFCC central part from the ulnocarpal joint (▶ Fig. 30.10a–f). Four cases of this series had concomitant major interventions as arthroscopic assisted distal radius corrective osteotomies and associated ulnar styloid resection. Nevertheless, all patients recovered complete supination.

Unfortunately, often capsular contracture or adhesions are not the only cause for DRUJ rigidity. Pronosupination loss may be related, in fact, to several different causes, such as: (1) osteochondrosis; (2) obvious DRUJ arthritis; (3) distal radius or ulnar head malunion; (4) chronic unreducible dorsal dislocation of the ulnar head, even with a locked extensor digiti minimi (EDM) tendon; (5) distal radius volar plate malposition with intra-articular DRUJ screw; (6) ulnar plate malposition for ulna fracture; (7) sequela of joint infection. All these require specific treatment (▶ Table 30.3), more than simple arthrolysis, as shown in Chapter 30.8.

Table 30.3 Posttraumatic DRUJ rigidity and treatment options

Causes	Treatment option
Capsular contracture	Arthrolysis
Distal radius malunion	Correction osteotomy
Ulnar head malunion	Correction osteotomy
Cartilage damage (sigmoid notch, ulnar head)	Arthroplasty
Articular step-off (sigmoid notch, ulnar head)	Correction osteotomy
Dislocation and subluxation (ulnar head)	Relocation
Head and sigmoid notch damaged by K-wires	Arthrolysis/arthroplasty
Tendon interposition (EDM)	Tendon relocation
Articular infection	Debridement

Abbreviations: DRUJ, distal radioulnar joint; EDM, extensor digiti minimi; K-wire, Kirschner wire.

30.8 Types of Painful DRUJ Rigidity

30.8.1 Dislocation or Dorsal Subluxation and Positive Ulna Variation Secondary to Distal Radius Malunion

Block of the pronosupination is determined by a volar dislocation of the ulna head (▶ Fig. 30.13a–j).

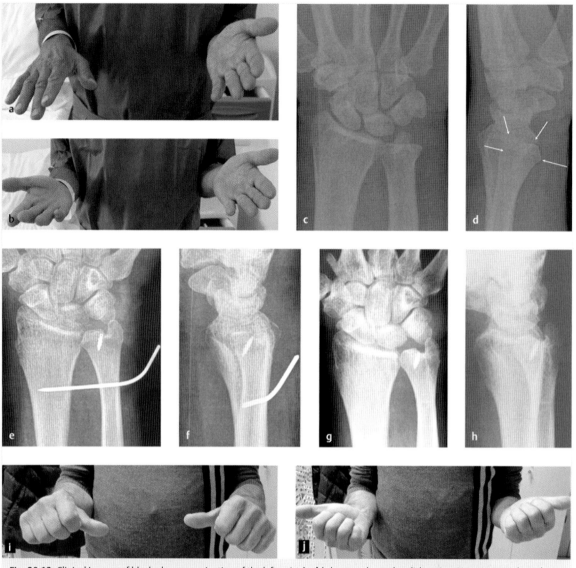

Fig. 30.13 Clinical images of blocked pronosupination of the left wrist **(a, b)** due to palmar ulna dislocation. X-ray images show the ulna dislocation **(c, d)**, the reduction of the dislocation with triangular fibrocartilage complex foveal reattachment with anchor screw and temporary fixation with radioulnar (Kirschner wire) K-wire **(e, f)**, follow-up result after K-wire removing maintaining the correct position of the ulna head **(g, h)**; and final clinical result with recovery of pronosupination **(i, j)**.

Loss of pronosupination due to positive ulnar variance following extra-articular DRF might be due to a shortening malunion of the radius. Ulnar head cannot remain in its anatomical position frequently dorsally dislocated. Associated TFCC tear could be present and all the lesions have to be treated contemporary (▶Fig. 30.14a–l).

Sometimes radiological images show ulnar head impaction against the carpal bones (lunate and triquetrum). Basically, the most appropriate surgical treatment for this condition is the distal radius corrective osteotomy. However, if the ulnar plus variance is around 3 mm, an acceptable alternative is the wafer resection of the ulna head that can be performed by open or arthroscopic technique. As it allows immediate rehabilitation, DRUJ

arthrolysis may also be associated with the wafer resection (▶Fig. 30.15). Positive ulnar shaft shortening is indicated for ulnar variance greater than 3 mm.

In intra-articular distal radius malunion due to dislocation of the medial part fragment of the radius, particular attention must be paid in the correction plan for both the sigmoid notch and the lunate facet (▶Fig. 30.16a–j). The osteotomy planning must be very precise: the arthroscopic assistance will give great advantages due to the increased accuracy of performing the intra-articular osteotomy, at the same time preserving the ligamentous structures.[21] If a stable fixation of the osteotomy is achieved, time of immobilization can be shortened and rehabilitation can start very early.

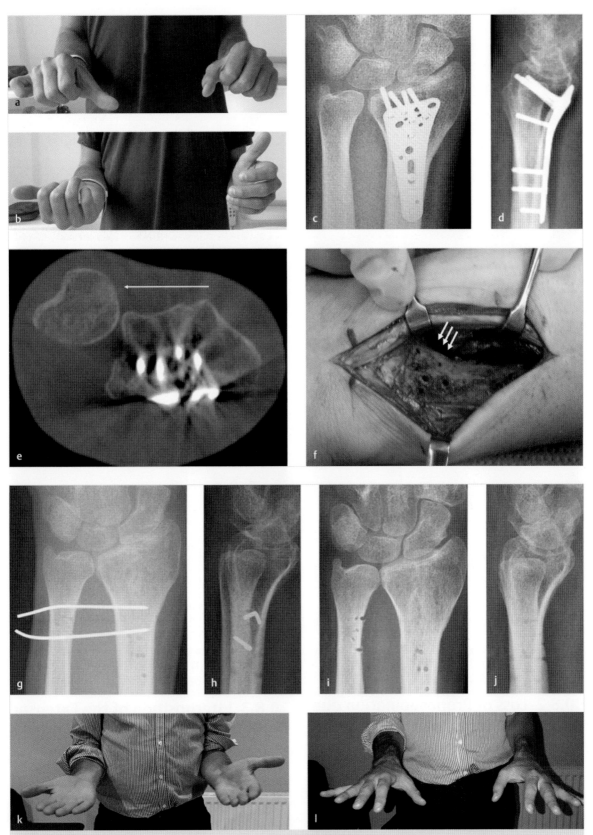

Fig. 30.14 Clinical images of supination loss of the left wrist (a, b) 3 months after distal radius fractures treated with volar plate (c, d). CT scan axial images showing the dorsal subluxation (*white arrow*) of the ulna head (e). Intraoperative images (f) of volar plate removing and palmar distal radioulnar joint (DRUJ) adherences and capsule resection (*white arrows*). X-ray images of temporary radioulna fixation with two Kirschner wires (K-wires) after reduction of the subluxation (g, h) and DRUJ position maintained after K-wires removing (i, j). Clinical final result with recovery of the pronosupination (k, l).

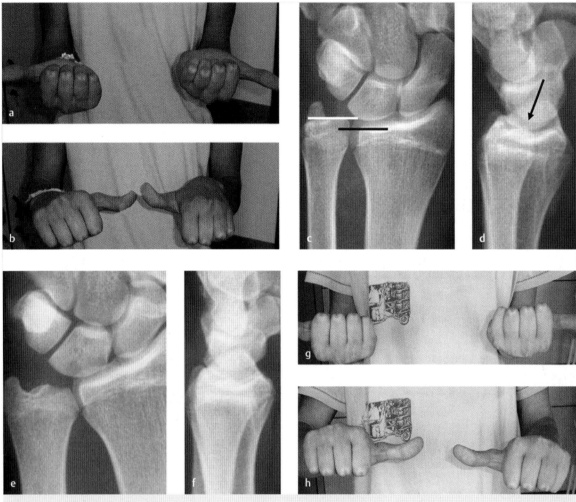

Fig. 30.15 Ulna impaction syndrome due to positive ulna variance of the left wrist. **(a, b)** Clinical wrist motion: note the reduction of pronation of the left wrist. **(c, d)** X-ray images of positive ulna variance (*black* and *white lines* in the anteroposterior view and *black arrow* in the lateral view). **(e, f)** X-ray images showing the wafer resection of the ulna head. **(g, h)** Complete recovery of the pronation and supination at follow-up.

Even in this condition, associated ligament injuries can be found. Ligament injuries can be treated at the same time or secondarily. Treatment requires an immobilization period which is in contrast with the postoperative protocol of arthrolysis.

30.8.2 Loss of Pronosupination due to Screws Interposed into the DRUJ

This is a condition in constant increasing due to volar plate fixation for DRF.

The most distal and medial screw is malpositioned into the DRUJ (▶Fig. 30.17a) and surgeon failed to recognize the incorrect position of the screw during the intraoperative fluoroscopy. The simple maneuver of intraoperative

pronosupination should be helpful in hearing noise due to the contact of the screw with the ulnar head.

CT scan is mandatory (▶Fig. 30.17b) and the screw removing allows to obtain the complete pronosupination with painless wrist.

30.8.3 Interposition of the Extensor Digiti Minimi

Rarely, a strong limitation or block of the DRUJ motion might be due to the interposition of the EDM into the DRUJ (▶Fig. 30.18). The cause of this situation is the fracture of the distal radius associated with dorsal dislocation of the ulna head which collects the tendon in the DRUJ.

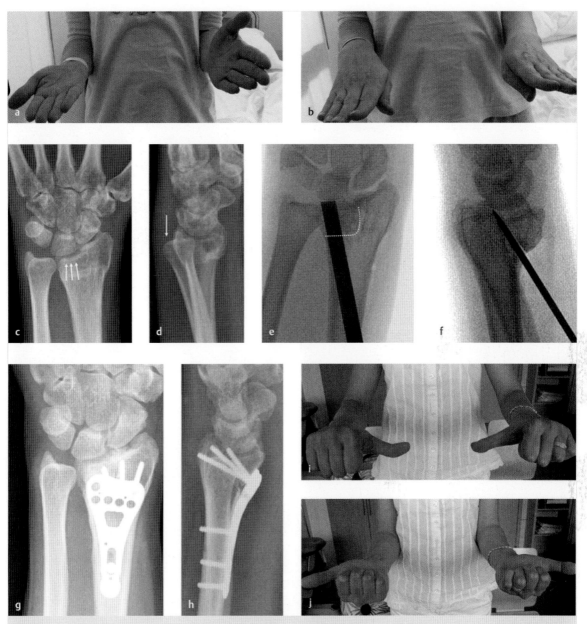

Fig. 30.16 Clinical images of supination loss of left wrist **(a, b)** due to distal radius malunion (**c**; *white arrows*) and dorsal subluxation of ulna head (**d**; *white arrow*). X-rays images **(e, f)** of intra-articular correction osteotomy (*dotted line*) and volar plating. **(g)** with relocation of the ulna head **(h)**. Clinical result at follow-up with complete recovery of supination **(i, j).**

Tendon entrapment determines decrease in motility of the fifth finger and sometime a radiological DRUJ diastasis may be evident. Ultrasound and MRI are helpful. The surgeon can help the radiologist addressing the diagnosis on this cause. Wrist arthroscopy is not very useful in these cases and the risk of erroneous interpretation is high.

The surgical procedure provides a posterior approach through fifth dorsal extensor compartment and the EDM into the DRUJ is found. After its relocation, the TFCC is repaired and the dorsal joint capsule is closed.

30.8.4 Ulna Malunion

The fractures of the ulna can be of the head, neck, and diaphysis or may be associated.

All of them can be a cause of reduction in the pronosupination and rise in ulnar pain. Unfortunately, even a correct treatment can incur a painful rigidity of the DRUJ as described in the previous paragraph, obviously if the initial treatment has led to a correct skeletal consolidation the stiffness can be solved with rehabilitation or DRUJ arthrolysis.

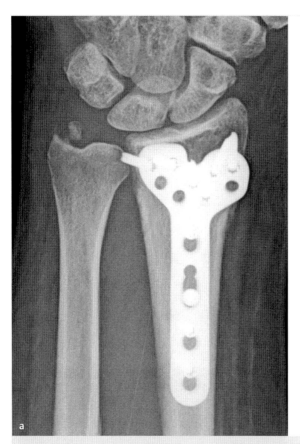

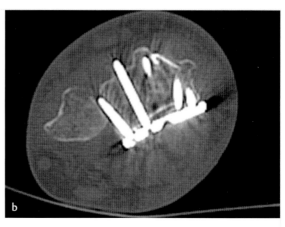

Fig. 30.17 (a) X-ray image of distal radius fracture with volar plate in which the medial screw is into the distal radioulnar joint (DRUJ). (b) CT scan axial image showing the medial screw into the DRUJ.

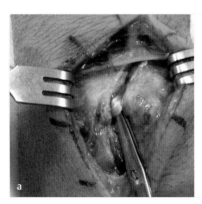

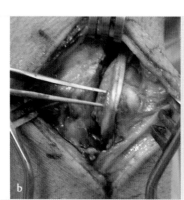

Fig. 30.18 Intraoperative images of extensor digiti minimi (EDM) tendon into the distal radioulnar joint (DRUJ) (a, b), a typical cause of pronosupination loss.

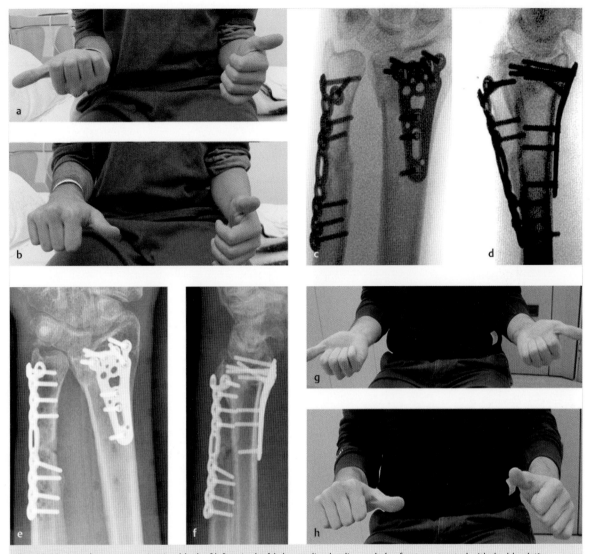

Fig. 30.19 Complete pronosupination block of left wrist **(a, b)** due to distal radius and ulna fractures treated with double plating **(c, d)**. Note the uncorrected reduction and fixation of the ulna. X-ray images. **(e, f)** showing the correction of the malposition of the ulna and fixation with new plate obtaining a relocation of the ulna. Clinical result of supination and pronation recovery **(g, h)**.

If there is a malunion of the ulna, which causes a marked reduction in the motility of the DRUJ, the treatment should be addressed to the bone structure by corrective osteotomy (▶ Fig. 30.19a–h).

Much more difficult is the diagnosis of an ulna malunion due to diaphysis fracture. Comparative X-rays and comparative CT scan in supination, pronation, and neutral position are required. Specific treatment is the corrective osteotomy of the ulna (derotation + plate fixation).

Distal ulna malunion is much easier to diagnose, but corrective osteotomy still remains the treatment of choice.

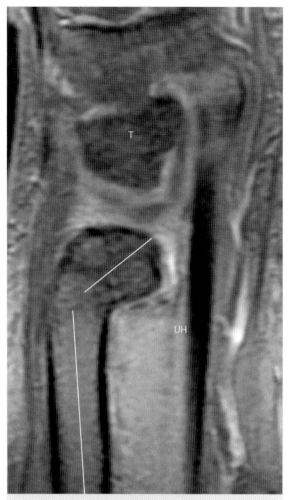

Fig. 30.20 Magnetic resonance image of ulna head with flexion deformity. T, triquetrum; UH, ulnar head.

The situation is more problematic when the head of the ulna is involved (▶ Fig. 30.20). Stiffness is not always correctable and the problem may not be resolved due to joint damage.

References

[1] Altissimi M, Rinonapoli E. Le rigidità del polso e della mano. Inquadramento clinico, valutazione diagnostica e indicazioni terapeutiche. Giornale Italiano di Ortopedia e Traumatologia, LXXX Congresso 1995;21:187–192 (suppl)

[2] Pederzini L, Luchetti R, Montagna G, Alfarano M, Soragni O. Trattamento artroscopico delle rigidità di polso. Rivista "il Ginocchio". 1991;XI-XII:1–13

[3] Hanson EC, Wood VE, Thiel AE, Maloney MD, Sauser DD. Adhesive capsulitis of the wrist. Diagnosis and treatment. Clin Orthop Relat Res 1988(234):51–55

[4] Kleinman WB, Graham TJ. The distal radioulnar joint capsule: clinical anatomy and role in posttraumatic limitation of forearm rotation. J Hand Surg Am 1998;23(4):588–599

[5] Osterman AL, Culp RW, Bednar JM. The arthroscopic release of wrist contractures. Scientific Paper Session A1. Presented at the American Society of Hand Surgery Annual Meeting, Boston, MA, 2000

[6] Verhellen R, Bain GI. Arthroscopic capsular release for contracture of the wrist: a new technique. Arthroscopy 2000;16(1):106–110

[7] Luchetti R. The role of arthroscopy in post-traumatic stiffness. In: del Piñal F et al, eds. Arthroscopic Management of Distal Radius Fractures. Berlin, Springer. 2010:151–173

[8] Kleinman WB. DRUJ contracture release. Tech Hand Up Extrem Surg 1999;3(1):13–22

[9] Luchetti R, Atzei A, Fairplay T. Arthroscopic wrist arthrolysis after wrist fracture. Arthroscopy 2007;23(3):255–260

[10] Maloney MD, Sauser DD, Hanson EC, Wood VE, Thiel AE. Adhesive capsulitis of the wrist: arthrographic diagnosis. Radiology 1988;167(1):187–190

[11] af Ekenstam FW. Capsulotomy of the distal radio ulnar joint. Scand J Plast Reconstr Surg Hand Surg 1988;22(2):169–171

[12] Garcia-Elias M. Management of lost pronosupination. In: Slutsky DJ, ed. Principles and Practice of Wrist Surgery. Philadelphia, PA: WB Saunders; 2010:507–514

[13] Bain GI, Verhellen R, Pederzini L. Procedure artroscopiche capsulari del polso. In: Pederzini L, ed. Artroscopia di polso. Milan: Springer-Verlag Italia; 1999:123–128

[14] Luchetti R, Atzei A, Mustapha B. Arthroscopic wrist arthrolysis. Atlas Hand Clin 2001;6:371–387

[15] Luchetti R, Atzei A. Artrolisi artroscopica nelle rigidità posttraumatiche. In: Luchetti R, Atzei A, eds. Artroscopia di polso. Fidenza: Mattioli 1885 Editore, 2001:67–71

[16] Atzei A, Luchetti R, Sgarbossa A, Carità E, Llusà M. [Set-up, portals and normal exploration in wrist arthroscopy] Chir Main 2006;25(Suppl 1):S131–S144

[17] del Piñal F, García-Bernal FJ, Pisani D, Regalado J, Ayala H, Studer A. Dry arthroscopy of the wrist: surgical technique. J Hand Surg Am 2007;32(1):119–123

[18] Luchetti R, Bain G, Morse L, McGuire D. Arthroscopic arthrolysis. In: Randelli et al, eds. Arthroscopy. Berlin, Heidelberg: Springer-Verlag; 2016:935–951

[19] McGuire DT, Luchetti R, Atzei A, Bain GI. Arthroscopic arthrolysis. In: Geissler WB, ed. Wrist and Elbow Arthroscopy. New York: Springer Science Business Media. 2015:165–175

[20] Del Piñal F, Moraleda E, Rúas JS, Rodriguez-Vega A, Studer A. Effectiveness of an arthroscopic technique to correct supination losses of 90° or more. J Hand Surg Am 2018;43(7):676.e1–676.e6

[21] Luchetti R. Arthroscopic ulnar head resection and Sauvé-Kapandji. In: del Piñal F, et al, eds. Arthroscopic Management of Ulnar Pain. Berlin, Springer; 2012:315–334

31 Chronic Distal Radioulnar Joint Instability

Michael C. K. Mak, Pak-Cheong Ho

Abstract

Chronic distal radioulnar joint instability is caused by disruption of its stabilizers of which the triangular fibrocartilage complex (TFCC) has a key role, and it is the aim of this chapter to illustrate a minimally invasive method to reconstruct the TFCC anatomically by means of an arthroscopic-assisted approach. Any causative skeletal malalignment must be identified and corrected before TFCC reconstruction is considered. The current concept of anatomical reconstruction, first proposed by Adams, aims to restore the volar and dorsal radioulnar ligaments and their radial and foveal insertions with uniform tension. An arthroscopic-assisted method of reconstruction was developed and the technique was illustrated. Open capsulotomies are avoided and scarring is minimized, and accurate placement of the foveal insertion is possible by arthroscopic visualization. Outcomes in 28 consecutive cases performed over a period of 17 years in our center were favorable and showed a potential advantage in preserving the range of motion.

Keywords: TFCC reconstruction, TFCC tear, DRUJ instability, TFCC reconstruction, wrist arthroscopy, arthroscopic technique

31.1 Introduction

31.1.1 Distal Radioulnar Joint Anatomy and Its Stabilizers

Distal radioulnar joint (DRUJ) straddles between the forearm and the wrist joint. Being the distal articulation of the forearm, its related structures are also important parts of the wrist. Its stability is conferred by its bony configuration and soft tissue stabilizers, of which there are static and dynamic components. The bony articulation consists of a semicylindrical ulnar seat with a mean radius of curvature of 8 mm[1] and a shallower concave sigmoid notch with a radius of 15 mm (▶ Fig. 31.1). The centers of the subtended arcs of these curvatures do not meet and thus the intrinsic congruence of the DRUJ is nonconcentric, which also limits the articulation contact area. DRUJ rotation results in a combined roll and slide motion of the radius with respect to a fixed ulna, where supination brings the volar rim of the radius closer in contact with the ulna and pronation the dorsal rim. There is no single isometric point of rotation but rather a centrode of rotation located near the center of the ulnar head.[2] This configuration accounts for 20% of the stability in a volar–dorsal direction.[3] Thus, DRUJ stability heavily relies on soft tissue stabilizers, which include capsular, ligamentous, and musculotendinous components. The DRUJ capsule, triangular fibrocartilage complex (TFCC), and interosseous membrane (IOM) provide static stability, while the pronator quadratus and extensor carpi ulnaris (ECU) provide dynamic stability. The TFCC was found to be the most important stabilizer, with the volar radioulnar ligament providing almost 50% of the constraint in preventing dorsal subluxation of the ulnar head in relation to the radius in all positions.[3] Division of the TFCC alone results in DRUJ dislocation in all positions even with intact DRUJ capsule and pronator quadratus.[4] The IOM and in particular its distal portion, the distal oblique bundle (DOB), assume a significant stabilizing role if the TFCC is injured.[5] However, in the presence of an intact TFCC, sectioning of the distal IOM resulted in minimal change in stability.[6] Given its key role in stabilization, restoring normal TFCC integrity is most important in the surgical treatment of DRUJ instability.

The TFCC is a blend of ligamentous, fibrous, and fibrocartilaginous components that function to stabilize the DRUJ and bear force in the ulnocarpal joint while allowing smooth motion. It consists of the articular disc, meniscus homolog, volar and dorsal radioulnar ligaments, subsheath of the ECU, ulnar capsule, and ulnolunate and ulnotriquetral ligaments. Of these, the volar and dorsal radioulnar ligaments are the most important stabilizing structures.[1,6-8] It is now known that different parts of these two ligaments have different stabilizing roles as the forearm rotates. The foveal insertion is contributed by deep fibers of the radioulnar ligaments and the more ulnar and distal styloid insertion is contributed by superficial fibers. Superficial dorsal and deep volar fibers of the radioulnar ligaments tighten and provide stability in pronation, whereas superficial volar and deep dorsal ligaments stabilize in supination.[1,9] The foveal insertion is recognized as the more important,[10] acting as the anchor of a hammock-like structure.[11]

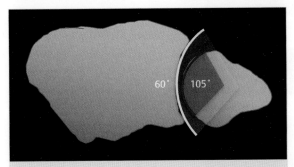

Fig. 31.1 The shallower sigmoid notch has mean radius of curvature of 15 mm while that of the ulnar head is 8 mm. The centers of the two curvatures do not meet.

31.2 Indications

As a sequela of distal radius fractures, chronic DRUJ instability may cause persistent pain, weakness of grip or rotation, or clunking after resolution of the acute injury.

Studies showed that 43 to 78% of distal radius fractures are associated with TFCC injuries detected by arthroscopy[12,13] and 10 to 19% of distal radius fractures are associated with DRUJ instability.[14,15] On physical examination, there may be the prominence of the ulnar head, with a positive piano key sign indicating overt instability.[16] Local tenderness is an important sign to localize the specific lesion present. The sites that have to be covered include the dorsal TFCC, foveal region,[17] the soft spot between the ulnar head, triquetrum, flexor carpi ulnaris (FCU), and ECU tendons, the DRUJ dorsal capsule, lunate, triquetrum, lunotriquetral ligament, and the volar TFCC. Passive pronosupination of the forearm may elicit pain. DRUJ ballottement test in neutral, supination, and pronation is performed, with up to 5 mm of dorsovolar translation of the DRUJ present in the normal wrist. Any translation in maximal pronosupination should be regarded as abnormal. Furthermore, in full pronation, pain and instability elicited by the dorsal push of the ulnar head relative to the radius indicate tear of the deep palmar radioulnar ligament; whereas in full supination, positive signs on the volar push of the ulnar head indicate tear of the deep dorsal radioulnar ligament. The ulnocarpal ligament stress test is performed with the forearm in neutral rotation and the wrist in radial deviation, in which the ulnar head is balloted as in the DRUJ ballottement test. Abnormal increase in translation indicates ulnocarpal ligament tear. There may be pain on resisted supination and pronation, which is alleviated by a volar push on the dorsal ulnar head. In addition to plain radiographs, computed tomography may be useful in the analysis of skeletal malalignment, in particular, sigmoid notch configuration. Magnetic resonance arthrography is useful in diagnosing TFCC tears and other ligament injuries, and with wrist traction applied, can accurately detect 98% of TFCC tears.[18]

31.2.1 Correction of Skeletal Deformity

Post-traumatic DRUJ instability results from malunion, leading to bony malalignment or incompetence of soft tissue stabilizers or both (▶Fig. 31.2).

Skeletal malalignment affecting the DRUJ include intra-articular malunion and incongruity of the sigmoid notch and ulnar head, displaced basilar ulnar styloid fracture, shortening of the radius, dorsal tilting, and coronal shift.

Although a positive correlation between ulnar styloid process fractures and TFCC tears was reported in some studies,[12,19] a recent meta-analysis found no correlation between ulnar styloid fracture and subsequent DRUJ instability or symptoms.[20] Therefore, an ulnar styloid nonunion itself may not be the prime culprit of DRUJ instability; rather, distal radius malunion is a more important factor. An intra-articular malunion that results in flattening of the sigmoid notch may lead to instability despite intact radioulnar ligaments, for which a sigmoid notch osteotomy can be performed to increase its concavity.[21] Extra-articular malalignment in each of the three planes, past a certain extent, causes DRUJ instability. Dorsal tilt of more than 10° was shown in a biomechanical study to cause DRUJ diastasis, changes in the IOM, and limitation of pronosupination.[22] A 2-mm radial translation of the distal radius, in the presence of an ulnar styloid fracture, is associated with an increased dorsal volar DRUJ displacement due to the loss of tension of the DOB.[23] Finally, shortening of the distal radius was found to be correlated with DRUJ subluxation and limitation of pronation due to stretching and incompetence of the TFCC.[24] A three-dimensional realignment is thus necessary if deformity correction is to be undertaken.

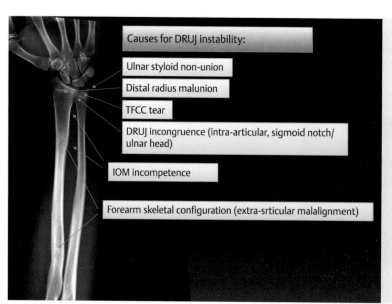

Causes for DRUJ instability:

Ulnar styloid non-union

Distal radius malunion

TFCC tear

DRUJ incongruence (intra-articular, sigmoid notch/ulnar head)

IOM incompetence

Forearm skeletal configuration (extra-srticular malalignment)

Fig. 31.2 Causes of distal radioulnar joint (DRUJ) instability.

31.2.2 Triangular Fibrocartilage Complex Reconstruction

If there is no significant bony malalignment or if instability is not completely restored after corrective osteotomy, restoring a functional TFCC is the key to regaining stability.

Arthroscopy is the gold standard in the assessment of the TFCC and to provide information on the extent of injury, reparability, and cartilage condition. TFCC reconstruction with tendon graft is indicated in irreparable TFCC with symptomatic DRUJ instability, which may happen with a neglected chronic injury, a massive tear with tension on apposition, or suboptimal healing after conservative treatment or surgical repair. In these situations, the remaining TFCC substance may be too thinned and friable for robust healing.

With the current understanding of the functional anatomy of the TFCC, anatomical reconstruction of the volar and dorsal radioulnar ligaments, first described by Adams,[25] is now widely adopted.[26,27] This method aims to restore normal DRUJ kinematics by using a single tendon graft with uniform tension, which is passed through the edges of the sigmoid notch and through the ulna at the foveal insertion site (▶Fig. 31.3, ▶Fig. 31.6a). Based on this method of anatomical reconstruction, since 2000, we have developed and utilized an arthroscopic-assisted technique.[28,29] In this minimally invasive technique, open capsulotomy and capsular dissection were not necessary, minimizing soft tissue scarring, fibrosis, and stiffness and allowing earlier rehabilitation. Under arthroscopic control, the fovea is clearly located, allowing accurate placement of the graft at the isometric point. Contraindications include significant symptomatic DRUJ arthritis and forearm rotational instability due to insufficiency of the IOM. A diagnostic arthroscopy could be performed before or at the same time as the definitive reconstruction to establish reparability of the TFCC.

31.3 Surgical Technique

31.3.1 Setup and Instruments

The patient is positioned supine with longitudinal wrist traction of 10 to 15 lb. A tourniquet is applied over the arm. Instruments employed include:

- A 1.9-mm or 2.7-mm arthroscope.
- Motorized full-radius shaver (2.0/2.9 mm) and radiofrequency probe.
- Powered instruments, including cannulated drills.
- The 2-mm arthroscopic graspers and suction punch.
- Fluoroscopic image intensifier.

Step 1: Wrist Arthroscopy and Triangular Fibrocartilage Complex Central Opening Preparation

The assessment of the radiocarpal joint with standard 3/4 viewing and 4/5 working portals is done to look for any associated chondral or ligamentous injuries. The integrity of the TFCC is assessed by probing of the volar and dorsal periphery, the trampoline test, and the hook test. TFCC reconstruction is indicated when the foveal detachment is beyond repair. As direct access to the foveal insertion is essential for passage of the graft, a central TFCC perforation is required. If the central part of the TFCC is intact, a central perforation is created with an arthroscopic knife or radiofrequency ablation. Any pre-existing central perforation is enlarged to 5 to 6 mm (▶Fig. 31.4), the ulnar head is exposed, and the edge is smoothened to ensure easy passage of the graft.

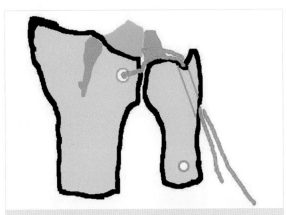

Fig. 31.3 Anatomical reconstruction of volar and dorsal radioulnar ligaments and their insertions into the fovea.

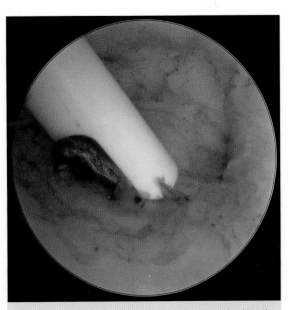

Fig. 31.4 Enlarging a triangular fibrocartilage complex (TFCC) central perforation with radiofrequency ablation.

Step 2: Harvesting of Tendon Graft

A 2-cm volar longitudinal incision is made midway between palmaris longus (PL) tendon and radial border of FCU tendon at the level of the proximal wrist crease (▶Fig. 31.5b). The PL tendon is harvested in full length with a tendon harvesting stripper.

The flexor tendons and median nerve are retracted radially, and the FCU, ulnar nerve, and artery are retracted ulnarly to expose the distal radius. The distal border of the pronator quadratus marks the approximate level of the radial tunnel.

Step 3: Radial Tunnel Preparation with Passage of Tendon Graft

A 2-cm dorsal longitudinal incision is extended proximally from the 4/5 portal (▶Fig. 31.5a). A window is made in the extensor retinaculum over the fourth extensor compartment. The extensor tendons were retracted to the radial side to expose the edge of the sigmoid notch. A 1.1-mm guide pin is inserted on the dorsal surface of distal radius radial to the sigmoid notch, 5 mm proximal to the articular surface of lunate fossa, and 5 mm radial to the sigmoid fossa with a volar tilt of 10 to 15° parallel to the surface of the lunate fossa (▶Fig. 31.6b). Tendons and neurovascular structures on the volar side are gently retracted by an assistant, while the guide pin is advanced with direct visualization of the tip (▶Fig. 31.7). After guide pin position is confirmed by fluoroscopy, the tunnel is enlarged to 2.2 to 2.5 mm, depending on the caliber of the tendon graft using cannulated drill bits and soft tissue protection by drill sleeves at both entry and exit sites.

Step 4: Ulnar Tunnel Preparation

A 3-cm longitudinal incision was made over the subcutaneous border of ulna from 1 cm proximal to the tip of ulnar styloid (▶Fig. 31.5c). A 1.1-mm guide pin is inserted from 1.5 to 2 cm proximal to the tip of ulnar styloid at an acute angle targeting at the fovea of the ulnar head (▶Fig. 31.6c), parallel to the ulna in the sagittal plane. This can be facilitated by placing the thumb on the ulnar styloid as a reference to gauge position. It is necessary to ensure, under direct arthroscopic view, that the guide pin exits at the center of the fovea, which is now the isometric point of insertion (▶Fig. 31.8). Cannulated drills are passed over the guide pin in a stepwise manner up to 2.9 or 3.2 mm, depending on the caliber of the graft. The tip of the guide pin is clamped with a hemostat passing through the 4/5 portal to avoid iatrogenic damage of articular cartilage.

Step 5: Passing of the Volar Limb of Tendon Graft into Joint and Exteriorization through Ulnar Tunnel

A 2-mm arthroscopic grasper is inserted through the bone tunnel in the radius from dorsal to volar, grasping the tendon graft and passing it through the tunnel from volar to dorsal (▶Fig. 31.6d). A volar capsular window at the interval between the ulnolunate and short radiolunate ligaments is created bluntly using the trocar of a 2.7-mm scope introduced from the 4/5 portal (▶Fig. 31.9). Through this window, the volar limb of the tendon graft is pulled into the joint by a 2-mm arthroscopic grasper introduced from the 4/5 portal (▶Fig. 31.6e, ▶Fig. 31.10). This tendon graft is then grasped and pulled through the ulnar tunnel to the exterior by a grasper introduced through the ulnar tunnel exiting the fovea (▶Fig. 31.6f).

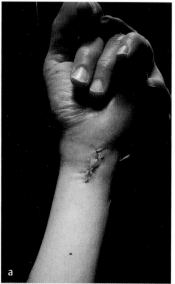
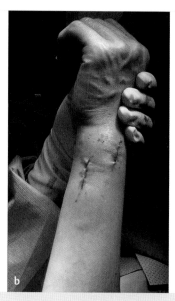
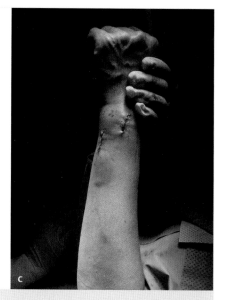

Fig. 31.5 (a–c) Volar and dorsal incisions.

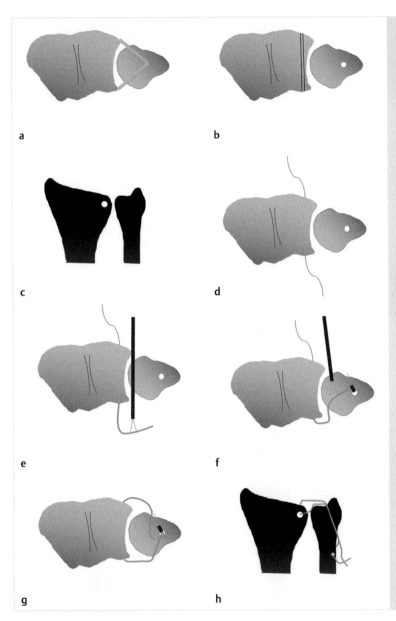

Fig. 31.6 (a) Anatomical reconstruction of volar and dorsal radioulnar ligaments and their insertions into the fovea. **(b)** A bone tunnel is created in the ulnar aspect of the distal radial subarticular bone. **(c)** A second bone tunnel is created in the ulna from 1.5 to 2 cm proximal to the ulnar styloid to the fovea, with arthroscopic confirmation. **(d)** Tendon graft (blue) is passed into the bone tunnel from volar to dorsal by a grasper. **(e)** A grasper is introduced into the 4/5 portal and passed through a capsular window between the short radiolunate and ulnolunate ligaments to the exterior. **(f)** The volar limb of the tendon graft is retrieved into the joint, and with a second grasper, passed through the ulnar tunnel and to the exterior. **(g)** The dorsal limb of the tendon graft is pushed into the joint through the 4/5 portal and passed into the ulnar tunnel. **(h)** A third transverse bone tunnel is made 1 cm proximal to the oblique tunnel in the ulna. Through this tunnel, one limb of the graft is passed and tied with the other limb.

Step 6: Passing of the Dorsal Limb of Tendon Graft into Joint and Exteriorization through Ulnar Tunnel

The dorsal limb of the tendon graft is braided with suture at its end. It is then grasped and pushed into the joint through the 4/5 portal with an artery forceps or grasper deep to the extensor tendons. It is then pulled through the ulnar bone tunnel in the same way as the volar limb, the tendon end being pulled outside using a grasper inserted through the ulnar tunnel (▶Fig. 31.6g, ▶Fig. 31.11).

Step 7: Tensioning and Tying around Ulnar Neck

The tendon graft should have a smooth course and uniform tension throughout. The stabilization effect is checked by manually tightening both limbs of the graft and balloting the DRUJ. Another transverse bone tunnel is made about 1 cm proximal to the oblique tunnel at the distal ulna using a 2.5-mm drill bit, one limb of the graft is passed through and then tied with the other limb in a shoelace manner (▶Fig. 31.6h, ▶Fig. 31.12), in maximal tension in neutral forearm rotation. The tendon knot is locked using Ethibond suture. The wounds were then closed in layers.

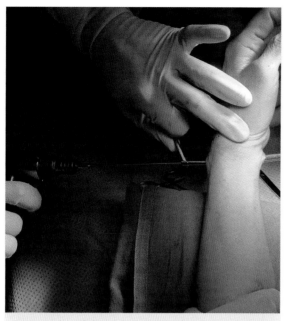

Fig. 31.7 The radial tunnel is created under direct visualization on the volar and dorsal sides while tendons and neurovascular structures are protected.

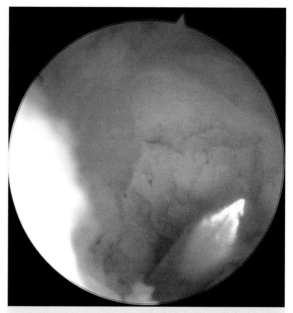

Fig. 31.8 The correct placement of the foveal guide pin is ensured under arthroscopic view.

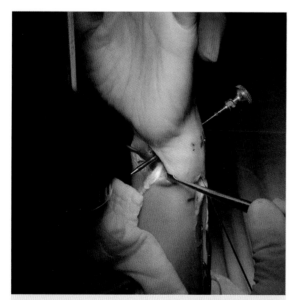

Fig. 31.9 A volar capsular window at the interval between the ulnolunate and short radiolunate ligaments is created bluntly using the trocar of a 2.7-mm scope introduced from the 4/5 portal.

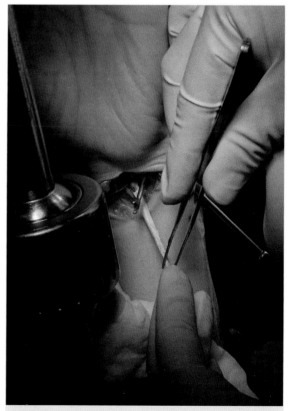

Fig. 31.10 The volar limb of the tendon graft is pulled into the joint by a 2-mm arthroscopic grasper introduced from the 4/5 portal.

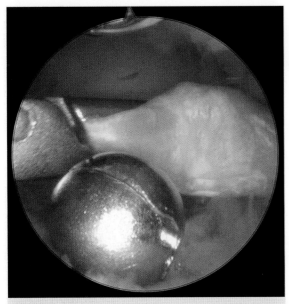

Fig. 31.11 Both limbs of the tendon graft are pulled through the ulnar bone tunnel by graspers, one after the other.

31.4 Rehabilitation

A long-arm cast is applied to immobilize the forearm in neutral rotation for 3 weeks. An elbow hinged brace is then given for 3 weeks to allow elbow flexion and extension while blocking forearm rotation. Alternatively, a sugar tong splint can be given with similar effect. Once the cast is removed, supervised midrange active and passive forearm rotation exercise and free wrist flexion and extension exercise out of splint are started. By the seventh week after operation, mobilization exercise with no range limitation and strengthening exercise are started and no immobilization is required in the daytime. A below-elbow wrist splint is worn at rest for 3 more weeks and then only at night for another 3 weeks.

31.5 Outcomes and Complications

A total of 28 patients received arthroscopic-assisted TFCC reconstruction for 28 wrists in our center between 2000 and 2016 (▶Table 31.1). There were 15 males and 13 females with an average age of 35 years at operation (ranging from 17 to 58). The average follow-up duration was 62 months (range: 3–138). A history of injury was present for all patients resulting in persistent ulnar wrist pain and weakness. Cases with previous skeletal deformity or malunion, DRUJ arthrosis, and ulna impaction syndrome were excluded. There were 16 subjects who previously received surgery on their affected wrists (5 had arthroscopic debridement, 1 had open and 9 had

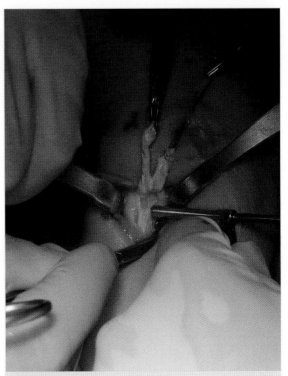

Fig. 31.12 A transverse bone tunnel is made 1 cm proximal to the oblique tunnel at the distal ulna using a 2.5-mm drill bit. One limb of the graft is passed through and then tied with the other limb in a shoelace manner.

arthroscopic TFCC repair, and 1 had ulnar styloid fixation with capsular repair), 2 patients with history of polyarticular gouty arthritis, and 2 patients with rheumatoid arthritis and systemic lupus erythematosus, respectively, at quiescent stage. Thirteen patients were injured at work.

Postoperatively, mean grip power increased from 58.6 to 71.6% of the contralateral nonaffected hand at the final assessment (▶Table 31.2), the mean pronosupination range improved from 84.6% of the normal side to 91.2% at the final postoperative assessment compared with the preoperative range of motion, and flexion–extension range improved from 77.1 to 83.71% (▶Fig. 31.13). The mean Mayo wrist score was 58 preoperatively and was 79 at the final assessment, with a 36% increase. The scores were excellent or good in 19 patients. The mean visual analog scale pain score decreased from 5.9 ± 1.5 preoperatively to 3 ± 2.5 postoperatively. Of five patients who were not able to return to work, four had causes unrelated to the wrist, which were back pain, disabling gouty arthritis, depression, and stroke with hemiplegia, respectively. The radiographic assessment revealed no widening, subluxation, or arthrosis of the DRUJ on follow-up. Bony erosion over distal ulna was noted in one patient, likely related to the friction with the tendon knot. There was no progressive enlargement of the tunnels.

Table 31.1 Patient demographics

Patient no. and initials	Sex	Age	Injury side D: dominant	Symptom duration (mo)	Previous surgery	Arthroscopic findings	Outcome	Complications
1. SWW	F	47	L	11	Arthroscopic TFCC repair	Massive dorsal tear	Unemployed	Nil
2. LYK	F	23	L (D)	22	Arthroscopic debridement	TFCC radial tear	RTW	Nil
3. YOF	M	42	L	17	Arthroscopic TFCC repair	TFCC volar central tear	RTW	Nil
4. YPK	M	34	L (D)	9	Ulnar styloid fixation + soft tissue reconstruction	Ulnar styloid nonunion	RTW	Nil
5. LPC	M	28	R (D)	21	Arthroscopic TFCC repair	Massive central tear	RTW	Nil
6. TKW	M	49	R (D)	24	Arthroscopic debridement	Massive tear with urate crystal and SNAC 2	Unemployed	Nil
7. SPK	M	23	L	12	No	Large foveal tear	RTW	Nil
8. YYM	M	17	R (D)	13	No	Massive dorsal tear	RTW	Nil
9. WFM	F	45	L	10	No	Massive central tear and villonodular synovitis	RTW	Nil
10. TLT	F	20	R (D)	8	No	Large foveal tear	RTW	Nil
11. WKY	F	22	R (D)	28	Arthroscopic debridement	Large foveal tear	RTW	Nil
12. FMY	F	41	L	23	Open TFCC repair	Massive central tear	RTW	Nil
13. CWC	M	28	R (D)	18	Arthroscopic TFCC repair	Large foveal tear	Unemployed	Dystonia
14. TYL	F	45	L	4	No	Radial tear	RTW	Graft rupture at 18 mo
15. WLK	F	36	L	14	No	Massive dorsal tear	RTW	Graft rupture at 14 mo
16. TLT	M	20	R (D)	132	No	Complete foveal tear, and dorsal TFCC synovitis and scar	RTW	Nil
17. WKY	F	22	R (D)	28	Arthroscopic synovectomy	Complete foveal tear	RTW	Nil
18. FMY	F	41	L	23	Arthroscopic foveal repair	Complete foveal tear	RTW	Graft rupture at 8 mo
19. FCF	F	52	R (D)	20	Diagnostic arthroscopy	Massive central to dorsal tear	RTW	Nil
20. LHY	M	20	R (D)	60	No	Central and complete foveal tear	RTW	Nil
21. NCP	M	32	R (D)	61	Arthroscopy and triquetral-hamate ligament thermal shrinkage for midcarpal instability and arthroscopic TFCC repair	Massive central to dorsal tear	RTW	Ulnar nerve entrapment by graft and neurolysis performed at 2 wk
22. LSH	M	19	R	7	Arthroscopic foveal repair	Complete foveal tear	RTW	Graft loosening at 4 wk (external to bone tunnel)
23. WYW	M	58	R (D)	38	Arthroscopic debridement of TFCC central tear and ulnar shortening osteotomy	Healed central tear with lax TFCC	RTW	Nil

Table 31.1 Patient demographics (*Continued*)

Patient no. and initials	Sex	Age	Injury side D: dominant	Symptom duration (mo)	Previous surgery	Arthroscopic findings	Outcome	Complications
24. WPH	F	48	L	19	Arthroscopic debridement of TFCC central tear	Massive central tear with dorsal fibrosis	Unemployed	Graft rupture at 12 mo
25. CCP	M	48	L	30	Arthroscopic foveal repair	Complete foveal tear	Unemployed	Nil
26. LKW	M	31	R (D)	27	Arthroscopic foveal repair	Complete foveal tear	RTW	Nil
27. CHM	F	36	L	156	No	Complete foveal tear	Housewife	Nil
28. YC	M	51	R (D)	21	Diagnostic arthroscopy	Complete foveal tear and massive central tear	RTW	Nil

Abbreviations: RTW, returned to work; SNAC, scaphoid nonunion advance collapse; TFCC, triangular fibrocartilage complex.
Source: Reprinted from Mak MCK, Ho PC. Arthroscopic-Assisted Triangular Fibrocartilage Complex Reconstruction. Hand Clin 2017;33(4):625–637, Copyright 2017, with permission from Elsevier.

Table 31.2 Summary of outcomes

	Preoperation		Latest follow-up	
	Average and SD	Range	Average and SD	Range
Pronation	67.9 ± 22	6–94	76.3 ± 9.7	55–90
Supination	74.5 ± 25.8	0–95	81.5 ± 17.8	40–115
Pronation (%)	82.8 ± 26.4	10–124	92.3 ± 12	68.7–114.3
Supination (%)	85.1 ± 27.1	0–105	95.1 ± 34.6	40–242.8
Pronation + supination (%)	84.7 ± 21.8	10–114	91.1 ± 16	52.7–126
Extension + flexion (%)	77.1 ± 25.4	7–126.3	83.7 ± 28	42–131.6
Radial + ulnar deviation (%)	71.4 ± 25.2	18–132.5	83.5 ± 21.9	50–119
Grip strength (%)	58.6 ± 29.1	6.6–114	71.6 ± 26.2	16.7–106
Mayo wrist score	57.6 ± 15	15–90	79.3 ± 13.1	25–100
VAS pain score	5.9 ± 1.5	2–9	3 ± 2.5	0–7

Abbreviations: SD, standard deviation; VAS, visual analog scale.
Source: Reprinted from Mak MCK, Ho PC. Arthroscopic-Assisted Triangular Fibrocartilage Complex Reconstruction. Hand Clin 2017;33(4):625–637, Copyright 2017, with permission from Elsevier.

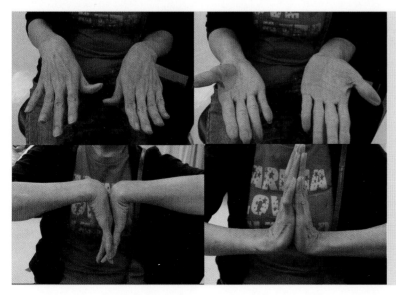

Fig. 31.13 Postoperative motion of one patient.

No fracture or tendon injury occurred intraoperatively. There was one case of broken Kirschner wire, which was removed from the joint. Ulnar nerve entrapment by the tendon graft occurred in one case, resulting in transient partial ulnar nerve palsy. Revision of the tendon graft and ulnar nerve release was performed, with full nerve recovery subsequently. Two other patients developed transient neurapraxia of the ulnar nerve due to nerve retraction during operation. Both had complete recovery within a few weeks. Three patients complained of discomfort due to scar hypersensitivity and graft knot irritation. No paresthesia was noted over the territory of dorsal cutaneous branch of the ulnar nerve.

There were four cases of graft rupture, which presented at 10, 12, 14, and 18 months. Two of these occurred from new injuries of their wrists after the operation, and two occurred without reinjury. Arthroscopic debridement of the torn tendon graft edges was performed in these four cases. Revision tendon grafting was performed in two cases. One patient had the resolution of symptoms, while the other patient continued to be symptomatic. In one patient, loosening of the graft external to the ulnar bone tunnel occurred at 4 weeks postoperatively and revision with graft retightening was performed. Subsequent recovery was smooth and he became a league handball player.

Adams and Berger reported their outcome of open TFCC reconstruction in 2002.[25] Pain relief was achieved in 12 out of 14 patients and there were 2 recurrences. The postoperative grip strength reached 85% of the opposite hand and the range of pronation and supination was 90 and 87% compared to the preoperative range. Our results with a less invasive technique were at least comparable with the established open reconstruction, with a potential advantage in restoring range of motion. In our series, there was 12 and 9% increase in pronation and supination range, respectively, compared with preoperative values. This could be attributed to the less invasive nature of the technique and not having the need for a dorsal DRUJ capsular flap. As a result, the motion is started earlier in our rehabilitation protocol beginning at the fourth week, while in Adams series, immobilization was required for 6 weeks. An extensive capsulotomy could also result in fibrosis with reduced range of motion.

31.6 Conclusion

Reconstruction of the TFCC with autologous tendon graft is indicated in chronic DRUJ instability with irreparable TFCC tears. The procedure, described by Adams and Berger, reconstructs the volar and dorsal radioulnar ligaments, the main stabilizers of the DRUJ, and their anatomical foveal insertion, to restore native DRUJ kinematics. Based on this reconstruction design, an arthroscopic-assisted technique is a less invasive alternative, which offers several advantages. Arthroscopy offers a clear visualization of the TFCC tear for an accurate assessment of its reparability. Capsulotomies at the DRUJ and radiocarpal joints are no longer necessary for placement of the tendon graft inside the joint. The ulnar bone tunnel can be created with precision at the isometric foveal insertion point under a direct and magnified view. Our results show that arthroscopic anatomical TFCC reconstruction is a safe and effective alternative to the original open technique with comparable results and complication rates, and may achieve better range of motion through preservation of soft tissue and capsular integrity and earlier rehabilitation.

Tips and Tricks

- The central portion of the remaining TFCC is debrided to allow clear visualization of the foveal attachment.
- Smooth gliding of the tendon graft along its course ensures uniform tension throughout.
- Bone tunnels are created in a stepwise manner by cannulated drill bits, while neurovascular structures and tendons on the dorsal and volar sides are carefully protected.
- To avoid blowout, bone tunnels are placed at least 5 mm from the edges of the ulnar and distal edges of the distal radius.
- The graft is tied in tension with the forearm in neutral rotation.

References

[1] af Ekenstam F, Hagert CG. Anatomical studies on the geometry and stability of the distal radio ulnar joint. Scand J Plast Reconstr Surg 1985;19(1):17–25

[2] King GJ, McMurtry RY, Rubenstein JD, Gertzbein SD. Kinematics of the distal radioulnar joint. J Hand Surg Am 1986;11(6):798–804

[3] Stuart PR, Berger RA, Linscheid RL, An KN. The dorsopalmar stability of the distal radioulnar joint. J Hand Surg Am 2000;25(4):689–699

[4] Palmer AK, Werner FW. The triangular fibrocartilage complex of the wrist—anatomy and function. J Hand Surg Am 1981;6(2):153–162

[5] Moritomo H. The distal oblique bundle of the distal interosseous membrane of the forearm. J Wrist Surg 2013;2(1):93–94

[6] Ward LD, Ambrose CG, Masson MV, Levaro F. The role of the distal radioulnar ligaments, interosseous membrane, and joint capsule in distal radioulnar joint stability. J Hand Surg Am 2000;25(2):341–351

[7] Ishii S, Palmer AK, Werner FW, Short WH, Fortino MD. An anatomic study of the ligamentous structure of the triangular fibrocartilage complex. J Hand Surg Am 1998;23(6):977–985

[8] Schuind F, An KN, Berglund L, et al. The distal radioulnar ligaments: a biomechanical study. J Hand Surg Am 1991;16(6):1106–1114

[9] Xu J, Tang JB. In vivo changes in lengths of the ligaments stabilizing the distal radioulnar joint. J Hand Surg Am 2009;34(1):40–45

[10] Haugstvedt JR, Berger RA, Nakamura T, Neale P, Berglund L, An KN. Relative contributions of the ulnar attachments of the triangular fibrocartilage complex to the dynamic stability of the distal radioulnar joint. J Hand Surg Am 2006;31(3):445–451

[11] Nakamura T, Yabe Y. Histological anatomy of the triangular fibrocartilage complex of the human wrist. Ann Anat 2000;182(6):567–572

[12] Lindau T, Arner M, Hagberg L. Intraarticular lesions in distal fractures of the radius in young adults. A descriptive arthroscopic study in 50 patients. J Hand Surg [Br] 1997;22(5):638–643

[13] Geissler WB, Freeland AE, Savoie FH, McIntyre LW, Whipple TL. Intracarpal soft-tissue lesions associated with an intra-articular fracture of the distal end of the radius. J Bone Joint Surg Am 1996;78(3):357–365

[14] Geissler WB, Fernandez DL, Lamey DM. Distal radioulnar joint injuries associated with fractures of the distal radius. Clin Orthop Relat Res 1996;(327):135–146

[15] Kazemian GH, Bakhshi H, Lilley M, et al. DRUJ instability after distal radius fracture: a comparison between cases with and without ulnar styloid fracture. Int J Surg 2011;9(8):648–651

[16] Morrissy RT, Nalebuff EA. Dislocation of the distal radioulnar joint: anatomy and clues to prompt diagnosis. Clin Orthop Relat Res 1979;(144):154–158

[17] Tay SC, Tomita K, Berger RA. The "ulnar fovea sign" for defining ulnar wrist pain: an analysis of sensitivity and specificity. J Hand Surg Am 2007;32(4):438–444

[18] Lee RK, Griffith JF, Ng AW, Nung RC, Yeung DK. Wrist Traction During MR Arthrography Improves Detection of Triangular Fibrocartilage Complex and Intrinsic Ligament Tears and Visibility of Articular Cartilage. AJR Am J Roentgenol 2016;206(1):155–161

[19] Geissler WB. Arthroscopically assisted reduction of intra-articular fractures of the distal radius. Hand Clin 1995;11(1):19–29

[20] Mulders MAM, Fuhri Snethlage LJ, de Muinck Keizer RO, Goslings JC, Schep NWL. Functional outcomes of distal radius fractures with and without ulnar styloid fractures: a meta-analysis. J Hand Surg Eur Vol 2018;43(2):150–157

[21] Thomas J, Large R, Tham SK. Sigmoid notch osteotomy for posttraumatic dorsal dislocation of the distal radioulnar joint: A case report. J Hand Surg Am 2006;31(10):1601–1604

[22] Kihara H, Palmer AK, Werner FW, Short WH, Fortino MD. The effect of dorsally angulated distal radius fractures on distal radioulnar joint congruency and forearm rotation. J Hand Surg Am 1996;21(1):40–47

[23] Dy CJ, Jang E, Taylor SA, Meyers KN, Wolfe SW. The impact of coronal alignment on distal radioulnar joint stability following distal radius fracture. J Hand Surg Am 2014;39(7):1264–1272

[24] Omori S, Moritomo H, Murase T, et al. Changes in length of the radioulnar ligament and distal oblique bundle after Colles' fracture. J Plast Surg Hand Surg 2013;47(5):409–414

[25] Adams BD, Berger RA. An anatomic reconstruction of the distal radioulnar ligaments for posttraumatic distal radioulnar joint instability. J Hand Surg Am 2002;27(2):243–251

[26] Shih JT, Lee HM. Functional results post-triangular fibrocartilage complex reconstruction with extensor carpi ulnaris with or without ulnar shortening in chronic distal radioulnar joint instability. Hand Surg 2005;10(2–3):169–176

[27] Teoh LC, Yam AK. Anatomic reconstruction of the distal radioulnar ligaments: long-term results. J Hand Surg [Br] 2005;30(2):185–193

[28] Tse WL, Lau SW, Wong WY, et al. Arthroscopic reconstruction of triangular fibrocartilage complex (TFCC) with tendon graft for chronic DRUJ instability. Injury 2013;44(3):386–390

[29] Mak MCK, Ho PC. Arthroscopic-Assisted Triangular Fibrocartilage Complex Reconstruction. Hand Clin 2017;33(4):625–637

Index

Note: Page numbers set in **bold** or *italic* indicate headings or figures, respectively.